PRACTICAL PERIODONTAL DIAGNOSIS AND TREATMENT PLANNING

PRACTICAL PERIODONTAL DIAGNOSIS AND TREATMENT PLANNING

Serge Dibart, DMD
Professor and Director of Post-Graduate Program of Periodontology and Oral Biology
Boston University School of Dental Medicine

Thomas Dietrich, MD, DMD, M.P.H.
Professor and Head of Oral Surgery
The School of Dentistry, University of Birmingham

WILEY-BLACKWELL

A John Wiley & Sons, Ltd., Publication

Edition first published 2010
© 2010 Blackwell Publishing

Blackwell Publishing was acquired by John Wiley & Sons in February 2007. Blackwell's publishing program has been merged with Wiley's global Scientific, Technical, and Medical business to form Wiley-Blackwell.

Editorial Office
2121 State Avenue, Ames, Iowa 50014-8300, USA

For details of our global editorial offices, for customer services, and for information about how to apply for permission to reuse the copyright material in this book, please see our website at www.wiley.com/wiley-blackwell.

Library of Congress Cataloging-in-Publication Data

Practical periodontal diagnosis and treatment planning / [edited by] Serge Dibart, Thomas Dietrich.
    p. ; cm.
   Includes bibliographical references and index.
   ISBN-13: 978-0-8138-1184-0 (alk. paper)
   ISBN-10: 0-8138-1184-8 (alk. paper)
   1. Periodontal disease. I. Dibart, Serge. II. Dietrich, Thomas, 1969-
   [DNLM: 1. Periodontal Diseases–diagnosis.
2. Periodontal Diseases–therapy. 3. Evidence-Based Dentistry–methods. 4. Patient Care Planning.
WU 240 P895 2010]
   RK361.P734 2010
   617.6′32–dc22

                              2009023103

A catalog record for this book is available from the U.S. Library of Congress.

Set in 9.5 on 12 pt Helvetica Light by SNP Best-set Typesetter Ltd., Hong Kong
Printed in Singapore

Disclaimer

The contents of this work are intended to further general scientific research, understanding, and discussion only and are not intended and should not be relied upon as recommending or promoting a specific method, diagnosis, or treatment by practitioners for any particular patient. The publisher and the author make no representations or warranties with respect to the accuracy or completeness of the contents of this work and specifically disclaim all warranties, including without limitation any implied warranties of fitness for a particular purpose. In view of ongoing research, equipment modifications, changes in governmental regulations, and the constant flow of information relating to the use of medicines, equipment, and devices, the reader is urged to review and evaluate the information provided in the package insert or instructions for each medicine, equipment, or device for, among other things, any changes in the instructions or indication of usage and for added warnings and precautions. Readers should consult with a specialist where appropriate. The fact that an organization or Website is referred to in this work as a citation and/or a potential source of further information does not mean that the author or the publisher endorses the information the organization or Website may provide or recommendations it may make. Further, readers should be aware that Internet Websites listed in this work may have changed or disappeared between when this work was written and when it is read. No warranty may be created or extended by any promotional statements for this work. Neither the publisher nor the author shall be liable for any damages arising herefrom.

1   2010

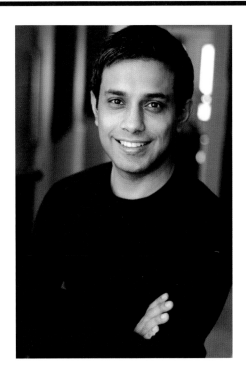

IN MEMORY OF DR. SHEILESH DAVE
September 3, 1967–March 7, 2009

Dr. Sheilesh Dave's dental career began after he graduated from the Faculty of Dentistry, University of Alberta, in 1992. He practiced in Calgary, Alberta, for 10 years, and then took his ambitions to Boston University, where he attended the Faculty of Periodontics, graduating from BU's periodontal program in 2004. For him periodontology was a specialty that provided the right mix of manual skill and intellectual prowess. He proved to be an excellent, studied surgeon and enjoyed the academic underpinnings of our profession. He was an outstanding student, well respected by his fellow graduates and the faculty and staff at Boston University. Following his graduation, Sheilesh returned to his roots, and set up a thriving practice in Calgary.

Always challenging himself, never content with the status quo was the key to his success. In his sadly short career Sheilesh earned a reputation among his colleagues for his honed skills as a periodontist, for always pursuing the academic side of periodontics, always trying to be on the cutting edge of his work, and for being a kind, warm, funny person. Apart from his career, Sheilesh was an accomplished pianist, having studied seriously both classical and jazz; he could be heard playing with a jazz combo on Tuesday evenings. He was finally on the cusp of enjoying the fruits of his labor, enjoying his family and life, when a tragic accident suddenly took him from us.

Sheilesh's premature departure leaves behind his loving parents and his lovely wife and their two children, a son and a daughter. He also leaves behind his sister and her husband and their two children.

He will be remembered for his kind, gentle, generous, loving, spirited soul, and for being a most authentic and special person. He walks among the daffodils now.

Contents

Contributor List

Geoffrey John Bateman, BDS, MFDS, MRD, MMedEd, FDS (Rest Dent)
Consultant in Restorative Dentistry
The School of Dentistry
University of Birmingham
St. Chad's Queensway
Birmingham
B4 6NN
United Kingdom
geoffrey.bateman@sbpct.nhs.uk

Melanie Campese, DMD, MS
Department of Periodontology and Oral Biology
Boston University School of Dental Medicine
100 East Newton Street
Boston, MA 02118
melcampese@hotmail.com

Sheilesh Dave, DDS, MSD,CAGS, deceased
Practice limited to Periodontology and Implant Dentistry
1333 8th Street SW
Calgary, Alberta
Canada T2R 1M6

Serge Dibart, DMD
Professor of Periodontology and Oral Biology
Director, Post-Graduate Program and 2nd Floor Specialty Clinics
Boston University School of Dental Medicine
100 East Newton Street
Boston, MA 02118
Tel: (617) 638-4762
sdibart@bu.edu

Thomas Dietrich, MD, DMD, M.P.H.
Professor and Head of Oral Surgery
The School of Dentistry
University of Birmingham
St. Chad's Queensway
Birmingham
B4 6NN
United Kingdom
Tel: +44-121-237-2825
Fax: +44-121-237-2825
t.dietrich@bham.ac.uk

Paul S. Farsai, DMD, MPH, FACD
Associate Professor, Director of Evidence-based Dentistry and Behavioral Sciences
Department of General Dentistry
Boston University School of Dental Medicine
72 East Concord Street—Robinson Room 334
Boston, MA 02118-2526
Tel: (617) 414-1146
Fax: (617) 414-1061
pfarsai@bu.edu

Joseph P. Fiorellini, DMD, DMSc
Professor and Chair, Department of Periodontics
University of Pennsylvania School of Dental Medicine
Robert Schattner Center, Evans Building
240 S. 40th Street
Philadelphia, PA 19104-6030
Tel: (215) 898-3268
Fax: (215) 573-3939
jpf@dental.upenn.edu

Adnan Ishgi, BDS
Senior Resident, Doctor of Science in Dentistry degree candidate in Prosthodontics, Division of Postdoctoral Prosthodontics Department of Restorative Sciences and Biomaterials
Boston University School of Dental Medicine
100 East Newton Street
Boston, MA 02118
ishgi@bu.edu

Raman Kohli, DDS, MSc, FRCD(c)
Practice limited to Periodontology and Implant Dentistry
3155 Harvester Rd., Suite 401
Burlington, Ontario
Canada L7N 3V2
Tel: (905) 681-3240
rkperio@gmail.com

Luca Landi, MD, DDS
Practice limited to Periodontology and Implant Dentistry
Via della Balduina 114
00136 Roma
Italy
Tel/Fax: +39.0635403508
lulandi@fastwebnet.it
studio.ric@tin.it

Cataldo W. Leone, DMD, DMSc
Professor of Periodontology and Oral Biology
Associate Dean for Academic Affairs
Diplomate, American Board of Periodontology
Boston University Goldman School of Dental Medicine
100 East Newton Street
Boston, MA 02118
Tel: (617) 638-5241
cleone@bu.edu

Yves Macia, DDS, MS (anthropology)
Practice limited to Periodontology and Implant Dentistry
13, Boulevard Lord Duveen
13008 Marseille, France
yvesmacia@free.fr

Steven M. Morgano, DMD
Professor and Director, Division of Postdoctoral
Prosthodontics Department of Restorative Sciences and
Biomaterials
Boston University School of Dental Medicine
100 East Newton Street
Boston, MA 02118
Tel: (617) 638-5429
smorgano@bu.edu

Christoph A. Ramseier, MAS, DMD
Periodontist SSO, EFP
Assistant Professor
Department of Periodontology
School of Dental Medicine
University of Berne
Freiburgstrasse 7
3012 Bern
Switzerland
Tel: +41 31 632-2589/2540 (direct)
Fax +41 31 632-4915
christoph.ramseier@zmk.unibe.ch

Carlos Eduardo Sabrosa, DDS, MSD, DScD
Associate Professor
Department of Operative Dentistry
Universidad do Estado do Rio de Janeiro
Pavilhão Paulo de Carvalho, Anexo Mário Franco Barrozo
Av. 28 de Setembro, 157—2° andar
Vila Isabel—Rio de Janeiro—RJ
Brazil CEP 20551-030
Tel: (21) 2587-6313
Fax: (21) 25876861

Dimitra Sakellari, DDS, PhD
Assistant Professor
Department of Preventive Dentistry, Periodontology, and
Implant Dentistry
Aristotle University of Thessaloniki Dental School
212 A. Vas. Olgas Avenue
Thessaloniki, Greece 55133
Tel: + 30 2310 281900,403839
Fax: + 30 2310 281901
dimisak@med.auth.gr

Mehmet Ilhan Uzel, DMD, DSc
Clinical Associate Professor, Department of Periodontics
Director, International Program in Periodontics and
Implant Dentistry
University of Pennsylvania School of Dental Medicine
Robert Schattner Center, Evans Building
240 S. 40th Street
Philadelphia, PA 19104-6030
ilhanuzel@comcast.net

Thomas Van Dyke, DDS, PhD
Professor, Department of Periodontology and Oral Biology
Director, Clinical Research Center
Boston University School of Dental Medicine
100 East Newton Street
Boston, MA 02118
Tel: (617) 638-4758
tvandyke@bu.edu

Clemens Walter, DMD
Department of Periodontology, Endodontology, and
Cariology
School of Dentistry
University of Basel
Hebelstrasse 3
CH-4056 Basel
Switzerland
clemens.walter@unibas.ch

PRACTICAL PERIODONTAL DIAGNOSIS AND TREATMENT PLANNING

Chapter 1 The Necessity of an Evidence-based Approach to Diagnosis and Treatment

Today, the concept of evidence-based health care surrounding our clinical practice of dentistry is discussed more than ever. However, many times this term has been used to define anything *but* "evidence-based dentistry" (EBD).

The term "evidence-based" has evolved through certain iterations through the years. It was first used in 1992 when a paper was published by a clinical epidemiology group at McMaster University in Canada (Evidence Based Medicine working group 1992). Their article described their challenge to adopt an "evidence-based practice" (EBP) approach since it "de-emphasizes intuition, unsystematic clinical experience and pathophysiological rationale as sufficient grounds for clinical decision making." The paper was written with the clear intent of placing a greater emphasis on a systematic appraisal of the evidence.

The first use of the term "evidence-based" in the UK was in a 1996 *British Medical Journal* article by David Sackett et al. and was defined as the "… conscientious, explicit and judicious use of current best evidence in making decisions about the care of individual patients. …"

The term "current best evidence" is the operative word here because it implies that our best available evidence should by definition change as we progress through more research findings, to the point that what was true as the best available evidence even as recently as ten years ago in dentistry in some respects is not even true today. Many examples come to mind, such as the new adhesive systems, a newer generation of composites, more non-surgical periodontal therapy, more procedure-specific use of biomaterials due to better-applied research results, and so on.

The American Dental Association (ADA) has defined the concept of EBD as:

> "An approach to oral health care that requires the judicious integration of systematic assessments of clinically relevant scientific evidence, relating to the patient's oral and medical condition and history, with the dentist's clinical expertise and the patient's treatment needs and preferences."

EBD has five components. This premise is simply based on the notion that to perform a scientific search for the current best evidence, one must be able to interpret the clinical scenario, translate it into searchable terminology, and then find the best evidence by critically assessing the quality and the appropriateness of the published evidence to address the identified clinical scenario. The five components are:

1. **Translate a clinical problem into a question.** For example: A new patient who is pregnant comes to see you with a chief complaint that she wants a second opinion on her need for periodontal surgery. She has heard periodontal disease may cause low-birth-weight babies and asks, "Do I really need surgery or could I just have dental cleanings (scalings) to prevent a low-birth-weight baby?" An easy method to translate a clinical scenario into a searchable format is by using the PICO structure. PICO is an acronym for **P**roblem, **I**ntervention (or Index, i.e., a category or condition), **C**omparison, and **O**utcome. So, by using PICO, one would devise the following structured format for the example described above:

   How would I describe the dental **P**roblem or population?

   "In *pregnant patients* …"

   Which main **I**ntervention or index am I considering?

   "With *periodontal disease* …"

   What is the main **C**omparison or alternative?

   "Compared to *pregnant people (patients) without periodontal disease* …"

   What is the **O**utcome to be studied?

   "Is there a greater risk of *low-birth-weight babies*?"

2. **Effectively search for the best evidence.** For this component, one must determine which databases to search and then use the appropriate databases and search filters to find the best evidence. The most common database is Medline (accessible via many free Internet portals such as www.pubmed.gov); however, there are many highly specialized databases such as Psychlit for behavioral research, Cancerlit for cancer literature, and NHSEED for economic evaluation research (UK) (see Chapter 4). As a source of high-level study designs, the Cochrane Oral Health Group (OHG), which originated in New England in 1994 and moved to Manchester (UK) in 1996, now has a registry of 83 reviews, 53 protocols, and 26 titles in dentistry (Clarkson et al. 2003). OHG specifically reviews a particular type of study design, randomized controlled trials (RCT), which are suitable study designs

for treatment-based clinical decisions. Summaries of the reviews are listed on the OHG website (http://www.ohg.cochrane.org/).

The term "filter" refers to the strategy for condensing thousands of articles into a more refined or limited set of relevant data. Filtration could be based on "human" topics, "English" language articles, a certain period of time (certain decade of research and beyond), and so on (many more filtration strategies are available). For the above-mentioned example, a search of the best evidence yielded the following number of articles (at the time of print):

- 97,702 articles that include the word "pregnant"

- 60,671 articles that include the words "periodontal disease"

- 243 articles that include the words "pregnant" and "no periodontal disease"

- 30,539 articles that include the words "low-birth-weight": Clearly, reading more than 180,000 articles to address our clinical scenario is neither indicated nor necessary. By using just "human" subjects and "English" language as our limits for our filtration strategy, we came up with 186 articles that describe the association (or lack thereof) between periodontal disease in pregnant patients and low-birth-weight babies. A further review of the articles and additional filtration (specificity and sensitivity) yielded 21 articles that describe the potential link between pregnant patients with periodontal disease and the risk for pre-term and low-birth-weight babies.

3. **Critically appraise the evidence.** One must critically read and evaluate the basis of the articles at hand (all 21 of the articles). This means that for this component level, one must assess at some foundational level the quality of the research methodology, the study design, the statistical analyses, and the conclusions that are published in each research article. It should be noted that the mere fact that an article is published (in a reputable journal or otherwise) does *not* mean that the study design, the research methods, the statistical analyses, or the conclusions were/are appropriate. Certain clinical or patient-centered questions can be best answered and more scientifically based if they are investigated through specific research designs or methods. For example, randomized control trials are suitable and indicated for the majority of therapeutic interventions, whereas cohort studies are suitable in design to answer questions on prognosis. Critical appraisal skills are evaluative skills that are taught and developed over time with appropriate supervision from knowledgeable and skilled individuals.

For our example, there are 21 studies that show some level of association between low-birth-weight and periodontal disease. The discrepancies come from the use of methods used in conducting the research, the appropriateness of the statistical analyses in interpreting the data, the various study designs compared in the studies, the process by which the data were collected, the criteria used for inclusion or exclusion of risk factors, or the lack of such parameters, and so on.

4. **Apply appraisal results to clinical practice.** At this time, if one critically appraises and assesses the quality of the research findings for our above-mentioned clinical scenario, the evidence is mounting and suggests a new risk factor—periodontal disease. Pregnant women who have periodontal disease may be seven times more likely to have a baby that is born too early and too small.

More research is certainly needed to confirm how periodontal disease may affect pregnancy outcomes. It appears that periodontal disease triggers increased levels of biological fluids that induce labor. Furthermore, data suggest that women whose periodontal condition worsens during pregnancy have an even higher risk of having a premature baby.

Therefore, by using the most current published clinical evidence available, clinicians in private practice can make the judicious recommendation to their patients that periodontal disease may in fact be a significant risk for a pre-term, low-birth-weight baby.

I ask you, the reader, a rhetorical question now: Is this in fact what we are currently telling our patients? If not, then why? More importantly, what is the level of appropriate scientific evidence that supports these communications or recommendations with our patients? Certainly, then, an understanding of the levels of evidence in scientific research becomes necessary for any clinician to judiciously take the research recommendations and translate them to his clinical practice (see Chapter 4).

5. **Evaluate application step and outcomes.** As with any treatment modality, good science and good patient care must be evaluated once it is rendered. Some therapy or treatment (or preventive care) can be assessed shortly after it has been rendered, and for other occasions, the evaluation of the applied care must be assessed within a much wider time span. Nevertheless, evaluation of outcomes is a necessary component of responsible and appropriate evidence-based healthcare.

From a study design standpoint, identifying whether periodontal disease actually causes pre-term, low-birth-weight babies is very difficult to measure with the presence of other variables.

Ethical issues also arise in a clinical trial if periodontal treatment is withheld for an indefinite period from half of the subjects, so technically this question cannot be measured well.

Regardless of whether this association is proven or not, dentists have nothing to lose by encouraging their patients to take care of their teeth.

PROBLEMS WITH INTRODUCING EBD

Amount of Evidence

There are currently about 500 journals related to dentistry and not all are relevant to all areas of dental practice, nor can a busy practitioner read any more than a small handful of articles routinely.

Quality of Evidence

Because enhancing career prospects in academia is partially tied to the number of publications one authors, much of the ever-increasing volume of evidence produced is not necessarily to increase the knowledge base, which in essence compromises quality. In addition, a number of publications that are widely read are not subject to peer review, and even when peer review exists, there is always the unfortunate reality of publication bias (defined as the tendency by both researchers and editors to publish positive reviews or results).

Dissemination of Evidence

History has shown that even in the presence of good evidence, the application phase of EBD can take many years to become the norm or standard in practice. Unless good methods of dissemination are available, good evidence can go to waste.

Practice Based on Authority Rather Than on Evidence

Common practice in professional development and continuing education demonstrates that the dental school model, which uses techniques or therapies based on views of authority rather than evidence, may lead to the wrong or outdated treatment being performed.

ADVANTAGES OF EBD

What Constitutes Evidence?

Personal clinical examination, including specific findings from history and results from tests, constitutes evidence. Research evidence is a manifestation of a much larger scale of interventions and, therefore, becomes a stronger tool for clinical decision making because it extends beyond individual experience. This should not, however, replace individual experience but rather anchor our clinical experience from years of prac-

tice. Sound reproducible research outcomes should enable clinicians to recognize gaps and uncertainties in their knowledge rather than wait for the next patient to expose our inadequacies. This implies a marriage between the research process and the clinical application of that process, hence the need for a continuous process of reading, learning, and applying a dynamic field of information.

What is Good Evidence?

The RCT study design is the gold standard for evidence for treatment-related questions. An even better level of evidence is a systematic review or a meta-analysis of a series of RCTs. However, this is only true for the clinical question regarding therapeutics. For other clinical questions, a study design hierarchy exists to determine the levels of evidence (see Chapter 4). This means that in the EBD process, no evidence is considered to be bad evidence; there are just levels of applicable good, better, and best evidence.

Finding and Making Sense of Evidence

After finding the evidence, one needs to make sense of it. This appraisal should be critical; after all, no research design is perfect and the health status of a person is at stake. The Critical Appraisal Skills Program (CASP) at Oxford University has developed a worksheet that can be used while reading and interpreting published articles to make sense of the evidence (http://www.phru.nhs.uk/Pages/PHD/CASP.htm). The aim of the critical appraisal is to systematically consider the validity, results, and relevance to our own clinical practice.

EBD improves the effective use of research evidence in clinical practice. If used judiciously, it favors the early uptake of new and better treatments or results in the early rejection of ineffective treatments.

It uses resources more effectively. For example, a systematic review of materials may lead to the earlier adoption of the most effective ones and the subsequent reduction in replacement levels, thereby saving resources.

EBD relies on evidence rather than authority for clinical decision making. Regular reviewing of currently available literature should develop us as practitioners so we attain the skills to evaluate evidence for ourselves based on our own experiences rather than have someone interpret the data for us.

To use this approach, we need to develop new interpretive skills for identifying clinical problems, searching literature by using conventional and electronic means, and critical appraisal. In the same spirit, this book encompasses practical evidence-based developments in diagnosis and treatment planning for a periodontal patient.

REFERENCES

Clarkson J, Harrison JE, Ismail AI, Needleman I, and Worthington H. 2003. Evidence based dentistry for effective practice. Dunitz Martin Publishers. pp 97–99.

EBM Working Group. 1992. Evidence based medicine. JAMA. 268:2420–2425.

Sackett DL, Rosenberg WM, Gray JA, Haynes RB, and Richardson WS. 1996. Evidence based medicine: what it is and what it isn't. BMJ. 312(7023):71–72.

Chapter 2 Classification of Periodontal Diseases and Conditions

From October 30 to November 2, 1999, the American Academy of Periodontology assembled an International Workshop for a Classification of Periodontal Diseases and Conditions, which resulted in a new classification (Armitage, 1999). The periodontal diseases discussed here reflect the new classification system.

I. GINGIVAL DISEASES

These diseases are classified according to the patient's symptoms, medical and dental history, and clinical examination. This evaluation consists of describing the physical aspect of lesions and their distribution, spread, and duration, as well as their radiological aspects and microbiological profiles if required.

A. Dental plaque-induced gingival diseases

Whether they are associated with hormonal imbalances, mediations, systemic disorders, or malnutrition, these gingival diseases have the following characteristics in common (Mariotti, 1999):

— The signs and symptoms are confined to the gingiva.

— Plaque is the main etiological factor which will initiate or exacerbate the gingival lesions.

— Inflammation of the gingival tissues will produce changes in color (transition to a red/bluish-red hue), shape (enlarged gingival contours due to edema or fibrosis), texture, bleeding upon stimulation, and elevated sulcular temperature (Figure 2.1).

— There is no alveolar bone loss and pocket depth; clinical attachment levels around teeth are stable.

— This is a reversible condition which resolves upon removal of the etiological factors.

— Possible role as a precursor to attachment loss around teeth.

Gingivitis primarily induced by dental plaque includes the following disease subdivisions:

1. Gingivitis associated with dental plaque only: Signs and symptoms typical of gingivitis can be observed at all ages of dentate populations and this disease has been considered to be the most common form of periodontal disease (Page, 1985). The disease can be observed in a child as young as five years of age, progress with a peak during puberty, and remain present throughout life at various extents. Plaque is present at the gingival margin and a positive correlation exists between gingivitis and plaque accumulation.

There is no pathognomonic flora associated with gingivitis, although the dental plaque in gingivitis differs from that present in gingival health (Ranney, 1993). Note that gingivitis may also occur on a reduced periodontium (decreased amount of alveolar bone height and connective tissue support around teeth) which was previously surgically treated for a periodontitis. This situation is encountered when there is a recurrence of inflammation of the marginal gingiva on a periodontium with previous attachment loss but without any evidence of progressive attachment loss (no indication of active disease) (Mariotti, 1999).

a. Without local contributing factors

b. With local contributing factors (see VIII A, below):

— Artefacta gingivitis (automutilation)

2. Gingival diseases modified by systemic factors:

a. Associated with the endocrine system

This type of gingivitis is caused by a combination of plaque and steroid hormones. The composition of dental plaque remains non-specific (non-related to the microbiological analysis).

1) Puberty-associated gingivitis: A rise in gingival inflammation and gingival volume is noted during puberty in both sexes without necessarily seeing a rise in the quantity of plaque (Sutcliffe, 1972). The incidence of the severity of gingivitis in adolescence is not only related to the rise in steroid hormones but is also influenced by a variety of factors such as dental caries, mouth breathing, teeth crowding, and tooth eruption (Stamm, 1986). These changes are reversible after puberty. More specifically, hyperplastic gingivitis often seen during the adolescence period can be associated with:

— Orthodontic treatment: Note that fibrotic tissue tends to recur if surgical removal is attempted during orthodontic treatment.

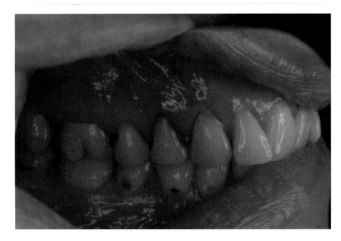

Figure 2.1. Localized gingivitis, characterized by bleeding upon probing. There is no attachment loss.

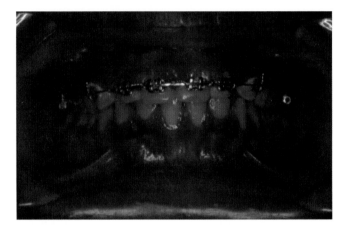

Figure 2.2. Maxillary generalized moderate gingivitis following the placement of braces. Notice the difference with the mandibular arch, which does not have braces.

It is recommended to wait until orthodontic appliances are removed before surgically removing excess tissue (Figure 2.2).

— Mouth breathing: Mouth breathing, which often accompanies Angle's classification 2 division 1 malocclusion, is considered to be an exacerbating factor to gingivitis (Lindhe, 2003). Gingival hyperplasia tends to affect mostly the anterior superior region and is also prone to recurrence if surgical removal is performed without any correction of the actual mouth breathing through orthodontic treatment or cessation of habit.

2) Menstrual-cycle-associated gingivitis: The most common sign is a minor gingival inflammation during ovulation; gingival exudate has been shown to increase at least 20% in 75%

of women (Hugoson, 1971). This situation is reversible after ovulation.

Note: Hormonal gingivitis or post-menopausal gingivitis can be seen in women taking hormone replacement therapy. Signs and symptoms may involve atrophic, thin, erythematous gingival tissues and patient complaints of gingival sensitivity to spicy foods and acidic beverages. Palliative treatment is suggested.

3) Pregnancy-associated:

a) Gingivitis: A combination of pregnancy hormones and dental plaque may increase the severity of gingivitis in women sensitive to local irritants. In addition to the typical gingivitis signs, severe inflammation can develop in the presence of relatively low amounts of dental plaque (Hugoson, 1971). It will usually affect pregnant women in their second or third trimester, and is reversible after child delivery.

b) Pyogenic granuloma: This refers to a mass of hyperplastic gingival tissue principally found in the interdental maxillary regions (Figure 2.3). It is not a tumor but an exaggerated inflammatory response to irritation resulting in a solitary poliploid capillary hemangioma which can easily bleed upon mild provocation (Sills et al. 1996). Pregnancy-associated pyogenic granuloma presents clinically as a painless protuberant exophytic mass attached by a sessile or pedunculated base from the gingival margin. It has been reported to occur

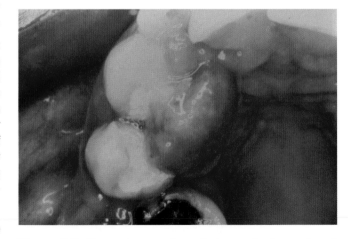

Figure 2.3. Pyogenic granuloma between teeth number 4 and 5. Reprinted with permission from Chapple and Hamburger, 2006.

in 0.5% to 5% of pregnancies and can develop as early as the first trimester (Mariotti, 1999). It usually regresses or completely disappears following parturition. If needed, surgical excision can be performed post-partum. The treatment for pregnancy-associated gingivitis and pyogenic granuloma during pregnancy is an impeccable control of the etiological factors (scaling, prophylaxis, and chlorhexidine rinses).

4) Diabetes-mellitus-associated gingivitis: Diabetes mellitus is a complex disease with varying degrees of systemic and oral complications involving abnormalities in insulin production, fat, proteins, and sugar metabolism, and resulting in an impaired vascular and immune system as well as an inadequate inflammatory response. Diabetes mellitus is categorized as Type 1 and Type 2. Type 1 develops due to impaired production of insulin and Type 2 is caused by deficient utilization of insulin. There is evidence to suggest that uncontrolled Type 1 diabetes in children is associated with exaggerated response of the gingival tissues to dental plaque (Lindhe, 2003). It is a reversible condition once the diabetes is under control and the dental plaque is removed.

b. Associated with blood dyscrasias

1) Leukemia-associated gingivitis: Leukemia is a progressive malignant hematological disease characterized by the development of abnormal leukocytes and leukocytes precursors in the blood and bone marrow. Leukemia is classified according to disease progression (acute or chronic), cell types involved (myeloid or lymphoid), and cell numbers in blood (leukemic or aleukemic). The oral manifestations are acute, consisting of cervical adenopathies, petechia, gingival enlargements, and mucous ulcers. Dental plaque can exacerbate the gingival inflammatory changes which include swelling, redness/blueness, sponginess, and glazed appearance of the gingiva which is infiltrated with leukemic cells (Lindhe, 2003). Persistent and unexplained gingival bleeding may indicate an underlying thrombocytopenia associated with the leukemic condition. Lesions are often found in the acute monocytic type, and consist of a modified gingival volume and bleeding of gingiva upon touch. Symptoms

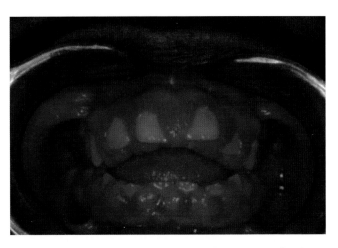

Figure 2.4. Gingival diseases modified by medications. cyclosporine-A-induced gingival enlargement in a 16-year-old after heart transplant.

lessen when antiseptic mouthwashes are used and plaque volume is reduced.

2) Other

3. Gingival diseases modified by medications:

a. Drug-influenced gingival diseases

1) Drug induced gingival enlargement: Three commonly used classes of medications create these lesions:

— Anti-convulsant drug used for treatment of epilepsy: Dilantin (Phenytoin sodium), 50% incidence

— Immunosuppressant drug used to avoid host rejection of grafted tissues: Cyclosporin A, 25% to 30% incidence (Over time, this drug is tapered and the gingival enlargements become easier to control.) (Figure 2.4)

— Calcium channels blocking agents used as hypertensive drugs: Nifedipine, Verapamil, Diltiazem, 15% to 20% incidence

Individuals taking these medications may develop gingival enlargements leading to pseudopockets. Characteristics of drug-influenced gingival enlargement include (Mariotti, 1999):

— Predilection of anterior gingiva; starts interproximally and expands

— Higher prevalence in children

— Onset within the first three months of taking the drug

— Enlargement of the gingival contours appears

- Stippling is present in the gingiva

- Pronounced inflammatory response in relation to the plaque volume

- Not associated with attachment loss but can be found in periodonitums with and without bone loss

  Treatment consists of control of etiological factors followed by full mouth gingivectomy. Gingivectomy (full mouth or local) may need to be performed annually. If possible, the drugs can also be changed or dosages adjusted to improve the oral condition.

2) Drug influenced gingivitis:

a) Oral contraceptives: Studies have shown that women taking oral contraceptive drugs have a higher incidence of gingival enlargement in comparison to women who do not take the medications (Kaufman, 1969). Pronounced inflammation (change in gingival contour, color, exudate) is seen and is reversible upon removal of medications (Figure 2.5).

b) Other

4. Gingival diseases modified by malnutrition:

a. Ascorbic acid deficiency gingivitis: Nutritional deficiencies such as ascorbic acid (vitamin C deficiency) can significantly exacerbate the response of the gingiva to plaque bacteria (Mariotti, 1999). The clinical description of severe vitamin C deficiency or scurvy consists of bulbous, spongy, hemorrhagic, swollen, and erythematous gingival lesions (Charbeneau et al., 1983). This condition is unusually seen in areas of adequate food supply but can potentially affect infants of low socioeconomic families, institutionalized elderly individuals, and alcoholics.

b. Other

B. Non-dental-plaque-induced gingival lesions

Although these gingival lesions are not produced by plaque and do not disappear when plaque is removed, it should be noted that the severity of the clinical manifestation can often be related to the presence of bacterial plaque.

1. Gingival lesions of specific bacterial origin:

   These types of gingivitis and stomatitis can be found in immunocompromised and immunocompetent individuals. They occur when the microorganisms surpass innate host resistance. Clinical signs may range from painful, edematous ulcerations to asymptomatic cancres, mucosal patches, or atypical non-ulcerated inflamed gingiva. Lesions elsewhere on the body may also be present. Gingival lesions may occur due to infections with *Neisseria gonorrhea*, *Treponema pallidum*, streptococci, or other organisms.

   a. *Neisseria-gonorrhea*-associated lesions: Gonorrhea is a sexually transmitted disease which can affect the oropharyngeal region in approximately 20% of infected individuals (Neville, 2002). Diffuse erythema, small erosive pustules, and edema can be seen in this region as well as on tonsils and uvula. Gingivitis and stomatitis, as well as a sore throat and a cervical or submandibular lymphadenopathy may also be present.

   b. *Treponema-pallidum*-associated lesions: Syphilis is a chronic infection produced by *Treponema pallidum*. The primary modes of transmission are sexual contact or mother to fetus. The infection undergoes a characteristic evolution that classically proceeds through three stages: In primary syphilis, an asymptomatic contagious chancre appears three to four weeks post contact at the site of inoculation. When affecting the oral cavity, it can affect the lips, gingiva, tonsils, tongue, and palate. It leaves a scar and heals spontaneously. In secondary syphilis, whitish mucous patches as well as maculopalular cutaneous rashes are often present and are still contagious at this point. In tertiary syphilis, a noncontagious granulomatous inflammation (gumma) reaction appears which can often cause necrosis

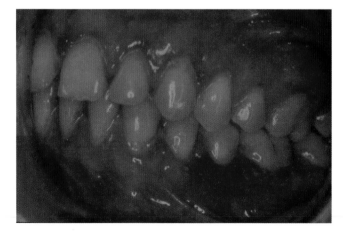

Figure 2.5. Oral-contraceptive-induced gingivitis in a female patient. Notice the "red patch" in the lower left quadrant. Photo courtesy of Iain Chapple.

and perforation of the tongue or palate. Serious systemic conditions are involved (Neville, 2002).

c. Streptococcal-species-associated lesions: An upper respiratory tract infection usually causes fever and accompanies a diffuse gingivitis, tonsillitis, pharyngitis and ulceration of the oral mucosa. One of the most common species involved is the group A, β-hemolytic streptococci (Neville, 2002).

d. Other

2. Gingival diseases of viral origin: Several viral infections are known to cause gingivitis. Most of them enter the body during childhood and may give rise to the disease followed by periods of latency.

a. herpesvirus infection

1) Primary herpetic gingigostomatitis: Herpes simplex virus type 1 (and occasionally type 2) is responsible for causing the primary infection which involves painful severe gingivitis with ulcerations (on keratinized and non-keratinized tissues) and edema followed by stomatitis. High fever and malaise is generally present. Vesicles on lips can produce a crusty lips appearance after rupturing (Miller, 1992) (Figure 2.6).

Palliative treatment only is required. The infection lasts approximately 10 days. During this period, the patient must be well hydrated with liquids and topical application of anesthetic agents is also indicated. Chlorhexidine and an antibiotic may be needed to prevent a super-infection. In the adult infection, antiviral drugs such as Zovirax, #70, 200 mg, 1 tab qid, for 2 weeks can be prescribed.

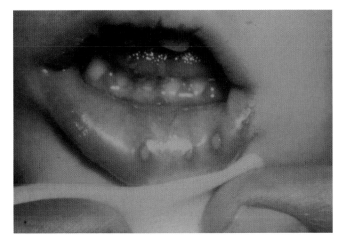

Figure 2.6. Primary herpetic gingivostomatitis in a child. Notice the characteristic lesions on the lower lip. Photo courtesy of Iain Chapple.

2) Recurrent oral herpes: Reactivation of the virus resulting in recurrent infections occurs in 20% to 40% of individuals with the primary infection (Greenberg, 1996). These lesions (vesicles which become ulcers) usually only affect the keratinized tissues and are usually present unilaterally or locally. The treatment, if any, can consist of topical antiviral ointment or tablets.

3) Varicella-zoster infection: Varicella-zoster virus causes varicella (chickenpox) as the primary self-limiting infection. The virus then remains latent and can be reactivated resulting in the herpes zoster infection. This painful unilateral infection is often seen in older individuals and is accompanied by cutaneous lesions of the affected nervous territory (Miller, 1996).

b. Other: Such as herpangina, caused by the Coxsackie virus species.

3. Gingival diseases of fungal origin: The most frequent oral fungal infections consist of candidosis and histoplasmosis.

a. Candida-species infections: *C. albicans* is one of the most frequent candida species affecting the oral cavity. It is considered an opportunistic infection occurring when the host resistance is diminished. Most subtypes of candidosis can be treated with anti-fungal medications (Ketoconazole 200 mg, 1 tab/day, 10 days, or Fluconazole 100 mg, 1 tab/day, 14 days).

1) Generalized gingival candidosis include:

— Acute types:

* Pseudomembranous candidosis: This type of infection produces soft white patches disseminated throughout the oral mucosa. These patches can be removed with an instrument leaving behind an erythematous mucosal surface.

* Atrophic or erythematous candidosis: This type of infection produces red lesions spreading all over the oral mucosa. They are associated with severe pain and discomfort.

— Chronic types:

* Hyperplasic candidosis: Typically, the lesion is longstanding and presents itself as a thick white patch which cannot be rubbed off (leukoplakia correlation).

* Mucocutaneous: This type of candidosis mostly affects the skin, scalp, and nails; much more rarely it affects the gingiva.

— Prosthetic stomatitis (types 1,2,3)

b. Linear gingival erythema: This disease was initially termed "HIV-related gingivitis." It mostly affects immunocompromised individuals or HIV patients. The unusual pattern of inflammation appears as a distinctive linear band of erythema which involves 2 to 3 mm of marginal gingival (Neville, 2002). Redness can be circumscribed or diffused and can spread until it passes the mucogingival junction. It is often generalized in the oral cavity, but can be localized to just a few teeth. The main characteristic is that it does not respond to conventional treatment (SRP and plaque control).

Note: the HIV patient is also more prone to:

— Hyperplasic candidosis

— Pseudomembranous candidosis

— Cheilitis

— Ulcerative necrotizing gingivitis, ulcerative necrotizing periodontitis

— Hairy leukoplakia

— Kaposi's sarcoma

c. Histoplasmosis: Histoplasmosis is a granulomatous disease caused by *Histoplasma capsulatum* and represents one of the most frequent systemic mycoses in the United States. The frequently seen subclinical development of infection usually includes either a pulmonary chronic histoplasmosis (30% have oral manifestations) or a disseminated form found primarily in HIV patients (60% have oral manifestations). Oral findings can consist of painful granulomatous ulcerations (Holmstrup, 1999).

d. Other

4. Gingival lesions of genetic origin:

a. Hereditary gingival fibromatosis: This gingival hyperplasia (ginvival overgrowth) is an uncommon condition of genetic origin. Of idiopathic etiology, this condition develops irrespective of effective plaque removal. Hereditary gingival fibromatosis can be an isolated condition or part of a syndrome or systemic condition (Gorlin et al., 1990) (Figure 2.7).

b. Other

5. Gingival manifestations of systemic conditions:

a. Mucocutaneous disorders: Many dermatologic diseases present with gingival manifestations in the form of desquamative, ulcerative, or erythematous gingival lesions. The most relevant ones are presented in the following below:

1) Lichen planus: Lichen planus is one of the most common dermatological diseases affecting the

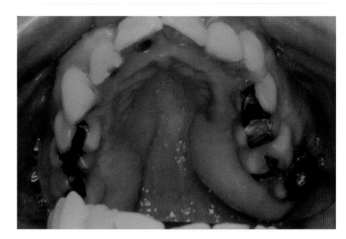

Figure 2.7. gingival fibromatosis. Reprinted with permission from Chapple and Hamburger, 2006.

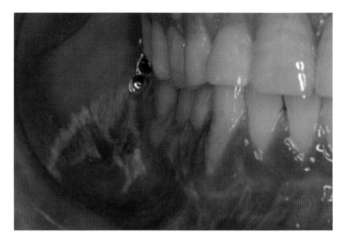

Figure 2.8. Lichen-planus-associated gingivitis. Notice the white striation—a characteristic reticular pattern.

oral cavity. Of autoimmune etiology, it can be classified according to the following subtypes: reticular, atrophic, plaque, erosive, and bullous. The characteristic clinical appearance resembles desquamative chronic gingivitis with the presence of white papules and white striations which often form a reticular pattern, also known as the Wickam striae (Thorn et al., 1988) (Figure 2.8).

2) Pemphigoid: Pemphigoid is a group of disorders in which autoantibodies are directed toward components of the basement membrane, resulting in the detachment of the epithelium from the connective tissue. This may occur on the skin (bullous pemphigoid) and mucous membranes. When only mucous membranes are involved, it is termed benign mucous membrane pemphigoid. The main manifestation is desquamative lesions of the gingiva, presenting intensely ery-

thematous lesions. This type of benign epithelial lesion arises from underneath the basement membrane, producing a desquamation more resistant to detachment during the clinical examination.

3) Pemphigus vulgaris: Pemphigus is a group of autoimmune diseases characterized by the formation of intraepithelial bulla in skin and mucous membranes. One of the most common and serious subtypes of this disease is pemphigus vulgaris. Clinically, it presents as painful desquamative lesions of the gingiva, as erosions or ulcerations which are remains of ruptured bullae (Sciubba, 1996). As a diagnostic tool, the histological analysis can reveal that the bullae contain non-adhering free epithelial cells (Tzank cells). It also will respond positively to the Nicholski test. This disease can be fatal if left untreated.

4) Erythema multiforme: Erythema multiforme is an acute vesiculobullous disease affecting mucous membranes and skin. This inflammatory reaction produces bullae which rupture and leave extensive ulcers covered by yellowish fibrinous exudates, sometimes described as pseudomembranes, on the gingival tissues. Another characteristic oral lesion is the typically swollen lips with crust formation of the vermillion border. "Target lesions," which can be described as a central bulla surrounded by an erythematous halo, can be found on the skin of the hands and feet (Lozada-Nur et al., 1989). The pathogenesis of this disease remains obscure, but an autoimmune reaction is suspected as the main underlying etiological factor. Two main forms of the disease have been described, minor form (limited affection) and major form (Stevens-Johnson syndrome).

5) Lupus erythematosus: Lupus erythematosus represents a group of autoimmune connective tissue disorders in which antibodies are directed toward the individual's cellular components. Two major forms exist: the discoid form (chronic type) and the systemic form. The typical lesions that can be seen on the gingiva appear as small, white dots of central atrophy surrounded by irradiating fine white striae with a periphery of telangiectasia. The characteristic "butterfly" skin lesions are photosensitive, scaly, erythematous macules located on the bridge of the nose and cheeks (Schiodt, 1984).

6) Drug induced

7) Other

b. Allergic reactions: Oral mucosa presents a large concentration of allergens which can stimulate oral allergic reactions of two types: Type I (immediate reaction mediated by IgE) and type IV (retarded contact allergy mediated by T lymphocyte).

1) Dental restorative materials: A Type IV allergic reaction can occur 12 to 48 hours after the oral mucosa has contacted a dental material:

a) Mercury

b) Nickel

c) Acrylic

d) Other

2) Reactions are attributable to:

a) Toothpastes (hypersensitivity reactions to additives and preservatives)

b) Mouthwashes

c) Chewing gum additives

d) Foods and additives (type I or IV reactions)

3) Other: Note that these allergy-associated lesions can appear as reddish to white ulcerations that will disappear when the antigen is removed.

6. Traumatic lesions (factitious, iatrogenic, accidental):

a. Chemical injury or toxic reaction: Toxic gingival reaction can be caused by chemical injury of the mucosa as seen in surface etching of the tissue by toxic products. For example, chlorhexidine can cause desquamation of mucosa; paraformaldehyde can give rise to inflammation and tissue necrosis. Other reactions can be attributed to aspirin, cocaine, or toothpaste rubbed on the gingival tissues (Figure 2.9).

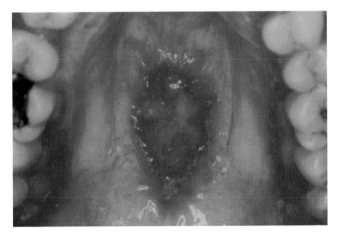

Figure 2.9. Aspirin-induced chemical injuries to the palate and gingiva. This is characteristic of patients sucking on and keeping the aspirin tablets in their mouths instead of swallowing them. Photo courtesy of Iain Chapple.

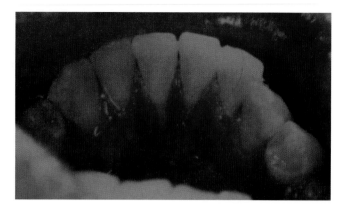

Figure 2.10. Lingual gingival recessions on teeth number 24 and 25 due to chronic trauma from repeated contact with metallic barbell (tongue piercing).

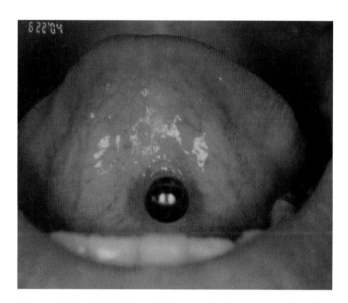

Figure 2.11. Metallic barbell inserted after tongue piercing.

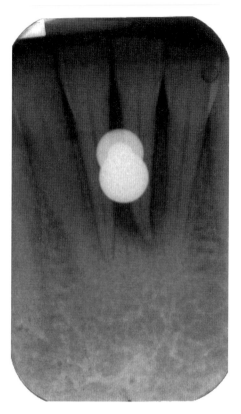

Figure 2.12. Radiograph of teeth number 24 and 25. Notice the extensive bone loss and periodontal ligament (PDL) enlargement following chronic exposure to the deleterious effects of tongue piercing.

II. CHRONIC PERIODONTITIS (DISCARDED OLD TERMINOLOGY: ADULT PERIODONTITIS)

Chronic periodontitis is defined as an infectious disease resulting in inflammation within the supporting tissues of the teeth, progressive attachment loss, and alveolar bone loss (Armitage, 1999). Characterized by pocket formation and gingival recessions, it is recognized as the most frequently occurring form of periodontitis (approximately 80% of all periodontitis cases). It can be present at all ages (adult, child, and adolescent) but is most prevalent in adults (Figure 2.13).

The amount of tissulary destruction is proportional to the quantity of local etiological factors. Subgingival calculus is a frequent finding and variable microbial patterns have been associated with the disease. This disease is often associated with local predisposing factors (dental anatomy or iatrogenous factors) as well as multiple systemic diseases (diabetes mellitus and HIV) and disorders in which the host defense mechanisms play an important role in its pathogenesis. Slow to moderate rates of progression are seen and are usually associated with good prognoses and responses after treat-

    b. Physical or mechanical trauma: Gingival recessions or artefacta gingivitis can be the result of physical traumatic events or bad oral habits (Figures 2.10, 2.11, and 2.12).

    c. Thermal trauma: Minor burns on the oral mucosa can frequently produce painful, vesicle-like lesions of the gingival tissues and palatal and labial mucosa.

7. Foreign body reactions: These may include oral abrasions, cuts, and amalgam tattoos. It is important to verify if the patient has any oral habit such as biting on a stick.

8. Not otherwise specified.

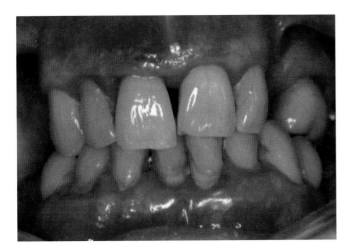

Figure 2.13. Chronic periodontitis in a 45-year-old patient. Notice the obvious etiology (plaque) and related findings (inflammation, suppuration, abscesses, attachment loss …).

ment. The adequate therapy involves the removal of etiological factors by scaling and root planing and reevaluation for periodontal surgery and/or maintenance.

Chronic periodontitis can be further classified according to its extent and severity:

— Classified according to its extent:

  * Localized: 30% or fewer tooth sites are affected.

  * Generalized: More than 30% of tooth sites are affected.

— Classified according to the severity of the clinical attachment loss (CAL):

  * 1 to 2 mm = slight

  * 3 to 4 mm = moderate

  * 5 mm and up = severe

— Classified according to the severity of the probing depths (PD):

  * 3 to 5 mm = mild

  * 5 to 7 mm = moderate

  * 7 mm and up = severe

III. AGGRESSIVE PERIODONTITIS (DISCARDED OLD TERMINOLOGY: EARLY ONSET PERIODONTITIS)

Aggressive periodontitis is a specific type of periodontitis with clearly identifiable clinical and laboratory findings. The definitive diagnosis may be based on clinical, radiographic, and historical data. Primary diagnostic features include:

— Except for the presence of periodontitis, these individuals are otherwise clinically healthy

— Attachment loss and bone destruction is rapid

— Familial (genetic) aggregation. Secondary features that are generally, but not universally present are:

— Amounts of microbial deposits are inconsistent with the severity of the periodontal destruction

— Elevated proportions of *Actinobacillus Actinomycetemcomitans* and, in some populations, *porphyromonas gingivalis*

— Abnormal phagocytary cells and hyper-responding macrophages (elevated levels of PGE2 and IL-1B)

— Progression of attachment bone loss can be self-arresting

Aggressive periodontitis can be further classified in two separate forms:

A. Localized (discarded old terminology: localized juvenile periodontitis):

— Begins at puberty, at around 10 to 12 years of age

— Affects mostly individuals with black-colored skin; males and females are equally affected

— Can often be characterized by small quantities of bacterial plaque in relation to bone destruction, showing limited signs of inflammation (Figure 2.14)

— High immune response (increased immunoglobulin production) to infectious agents

— Higher proportions of *Actinobacillus Actinomycetemcomitans*, serotype b (leukotoxin producing)

— Localized bone loss on first molars and incisors with interproximal attachment loss on at least two permanent teeth, one of which is a first molar, and involving no more than two teeth other than first molars and incisors (Figures 2.15 and 2.16)

  The adequate treatment is to combine systemic antibiotics (Doxicyclin, 200 mg the first day and 100 mg/day for 10 days, or Tetracyclin, 250 mg, qid for 10 days) with scaling and root planing, followed by periodontal surgery if needed, and/or maintenance (Figures 2.17, 2.18, 2.19, and 2.20).

B. Generalized (discarded old terminology: rapidly progressive periodontitis or generalized juvenile periodontitis):

— Usually affects individuals under the age of 30, but not always

— Poor serum antibody response to infecting agents

— Episodic nature of attachment loss

— Generally high levels of inflammation are associated with high levels of bacterial plaque (Figure 2.21).

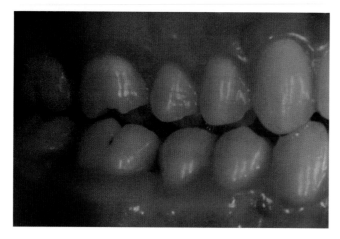

Figure 2.14. Localized aggressive periodontitis in a 15-year-old. Notice the lack of obvious etiology (plaque).

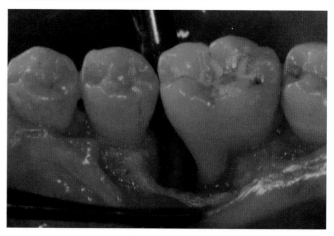

Figure 2.15. Typical bone loss associated with localized aggressive periodontitis and affecting the permanent first molars.

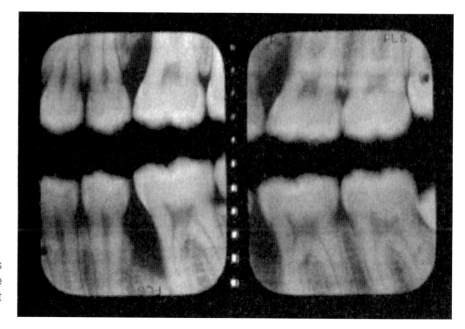

Figure 2.16. Bite wing radiographs showing the typical pattern of bone loss affecting the first permanent molars.

— A more complex microbiota can be found

— May or may not follow the localized form of aggressive periodontitis

— Interproximal attachment loss generally affects at least three permanent teeth other than the first molars/incisors (Figure 2.22).

Secondary descriptive risk factors that can modify the course of all types of periodontitis may include cigarette smoking, emotional stress, drugs, etc. Once again, the treatment may consist of combining systemic antibiotic (Amoxicillin 250 mg and Metronidazole 250 mg, tid for 10 days) and local antiseptic therapy with scaling/root planing and periodontal surgery and/or maintenance if needed.

Note: Refractory periodontitis does not constitute a separate class of disease but can simply additionally qualify a chronic or aggressive periodontitis of refractory by looking at the clinical results. Systemic antibiotic treatment can be considered in the following cases in which more specific microorganisms can be isolated via microbial testing of the subgingival plaque:

— *Porphyromonas gingivalis* and *Prevotella intermedia*: Metronidazole 500 mg tid for seven to 10 days

— *Peptostreptococcus micros*: Clindamycin 300 mg qid for seven days or Augmentin 500 mg tid for 10 days

— *Pseudomonas aeruginosa* or staphylococcus: Ciprofloxacin 500 mg bid for seven days

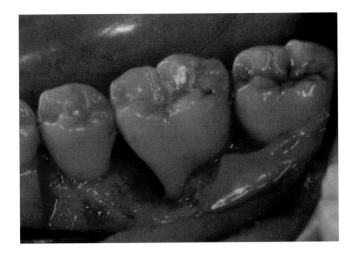

Figure 2.17. One year post therapy (associated with Tetracycline intake); notice partial fill of bony defect.

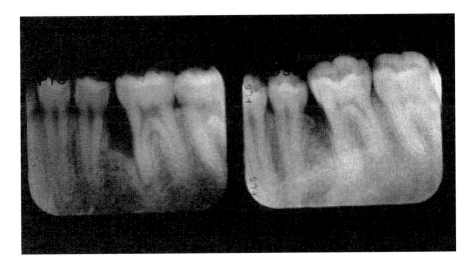

Figure 2.18. Periapical radiographs, before and after treatment at one-year interval.

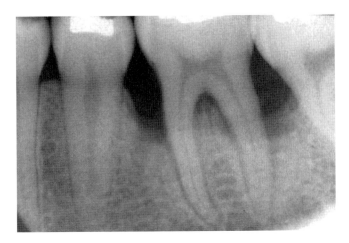

Figure 2.19. Periapical radiograph before treatment in conjunction with antibiotherapy.

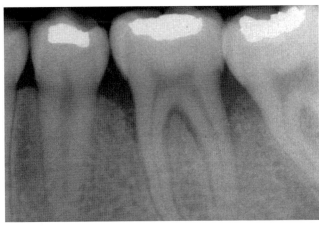

Figure 2.20. Periapical radiograph one year after treatment; notice again the healing of the osseous defect.

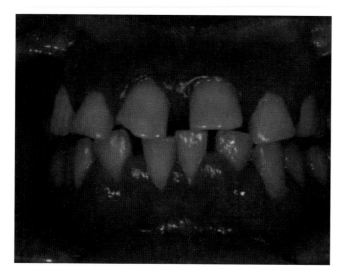

Figure 2.21. Generalized aggressive periodontitis in an 18-year-old patient. Notice the abundance of plaque, unlike that which is found in the localized form.

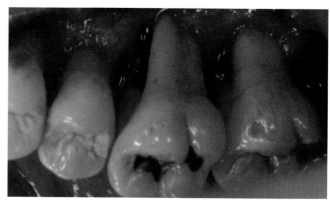

Figure 2.22. Same patient during periodontal surgery; notice the amount and severity of alveolar bone loss.

IV. PERIODONTITIS AS A MANIFESTATION OF SYSTEMIC DISEASES

Bacterial plaque is the original etiologic factor for periodontal disease, but what determines the actual presence or progression of the disease is the immune response of the host. Systemic factors can affect all forms of periodontal diseases by modifying the host's immune and defense mechanisms. Periodontitis forms classified under this category include:

A. Associated with hematological disorders: The blood cells have a vital role in supplying oxygen and assuring hemostasis and protecting of the periodontal tissues. Systemic hematological disorders can have profound effects on the periodontium by denying any of these essential functions. Polymorphonuclear leukocytes (PMN cells) are crucial in the defense of the periodontium. They have protective functions by integrating the following activities: chemotaxis, phagocytosis, and killing/neutralizing the ingested organisms or substances. Individuals with either quantitative (neutropenia or agranulocytosis) or qualitative (chemotactic or phagocytic) PMN deficiencies exhibit severe destruction of the periodontium. The quantitative deficiencies generally affect the periodontium of all teeth, whereas the qualitative ones are associated with the destruction of the periodontium of certain teeth only (Lindhe, 2003).

1. Acquired neutropenia: Neutropenia refers to a decrease in the number of the circulating neutrophils below 1,500/mm3 in an adult, which is also associated with an increased susceptibility to infections (Neville, 2002). Different forms of neutropenia (malignant, chronic, benign, cyclic, and slowly progressing neutropenia) produce variable effects on the periodontium. Generally, oral lesions consist of chronic gingival ulcers which characteristically lack an erythematous periphery and leave a scar once healed.

Cyclic neutropenia is a specific idiopathic disorder (an autosomal dominant pattern of inheritance has been described in a few cases) characterized by regular periodic reductions in the neutrophil population of the affected patient. The underlying cause seems to be related to a defect in the hematopoietic stem cells in the marrow. Beginning in early childhood, the signs and symptoms of cyclic neutropenia last for three to six days and occur in rather uniformly spaced episodes, which usually have a 21-day cycle (Neville, 2002). Patients typically present with fever, anorexia, cervical lymphadenopathy, malaise, pharyngitis, oral mucosal ulcerations, and severe periodontal bone loss with marked gingival recessions and tooth mobility. This alveolar bone loss of both primary and permanent dentitions becomes more accentuated at every recurring episode, leading to the loss of primary teeth at five years of age instead of 11.

2. Leukemias: Leukemias produce excessive numbers of leukocytes in the blood and tissues and also cause a greatly depleted bone marrow function with associated anemia, thrombocytopenia, neutropenia, and reduced range of immune cells. Periodontal bone loss is a consequence of neutrophil functional alterations and deficiencies.

3. Other

B. Associated with genetic disease:

1. Familial cyclic neutropenia

2. Down syndrome

3. Leukocyte adhesion deficiency syndrome (LADS)

4. Papillon Lefevre syndrome

5. Chediak-Higashi syndrome

6. Histiocytosis syndrome

7. Glycogen storage disease

8. Infantile generalized agranulocytosis

9. Cohen syndrome

10. Ehlers-Danlos syndrome

11. Hypophosphatasia

12. Other

V. NECROTIZING PERIODONTAL DISEASE

Necrotizing periodontal diseases have a unique presentation and development with the manifestation of necrotic lesions occurring concomitantly with the immune system depression.

A. Necrotizing ulcerative gingivitis (NUG): This disease is a type of periodontal disease in which the necrosis is limited to the gingival tissues. It has been known for many centuries and has other names such as Vincent's angina, fusospirochetes gingivitis, and trench mouth disease. NUG is an infectious, non-contagious disease, which can undergo dramatic resolution of signs and symptoms once the microbial plaque is eliminated. The following clinical characteristics must be present for diagnosis:

1) Spontaneous bleeding

2) Severe pain

3) Necrosis of gingival papilla (interdental necrosis) leaving crater NUG may also present (Figure 2.23):

4) Formation of white pseudomembranes on gingiva

5) Fever, malaise, lymphadenopathy

6) Increase in salivary flow, submandibular gland enlargement

7) Presence of metallic taste in mouth and oral malodor

Note: Necrosis is limited to the gingival tissues and does not extend to the alveolar bone or outside the periodontium. When the alveolar bone is affected, it is called a necrotic/ulcerative stomatitis or periodontitis.

The epidemiologic and etiologic factors related to NUG are as follows (Rowland, 1999):

— Adolescents and young adults which present poor oral hygiene and a low immunitary defense system are most often affected because of emotional stress, malnutrition, viral infections, smoking, lack of sleep, or concomitant systemic disease (AIDS), or after taking immunosuppressant medications (Figure 2.24).

— *Prevotella intermedia* and spirochetes are characteristic of the microbial flora isolated in these lesions.

B. Necrotizing ulcerative periodontitis (NUP):

Although less frequent then NUG, NUP presents severe erythema of the marginal gingiva and alveolar mucosa accompanied by extensive interproximal tissuary necrosis covered with white pseudomembranes. Spontaneous bleeding and severe loss of attachment around teeth result in the formation of craters interproximally, affecting both hard and soft tissues. Pain, oral malodor, fever, malaise, and lymphadenopathy remain present. NUP can occur after an NUG or in areas in which there already is a chronic periodontitis.

Note: In patients with AIDS, severe bone destruction can produce loss of teeth within three to six months and present bony sequestrum if the disease is not treated. Also, this condition may recur if left untreated.

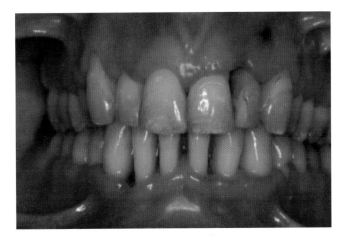

Figure 2.23. Post necrotizing ulcerative gingivitis/periodontitis oral condition. Notice the typical gingival architecture and the "punched out" papillae.

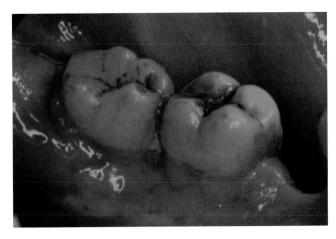

Figure 2.24. Acute necrotizing ulcerative periodontitis in an HIV-positive patient. Notice the denuded mandibular bone. Photo courtesy of Iain Chapple.

A combination of antibiotic therapy (Metronidazole 250 mg, 2 tabs stat, 1 tab qid for seven to 10 days, or Amoxicillin 500 mg, 1 tab tid for seven days), mechanical debridement (scaling and root planing with hand instruments), and antiseptic mouth rinses (chlorhexidine and peroxide) is the treatment of choice for both NUG and NUP (Rowland, 1999).

VI. PERIODONTAL ABSCESS

The classification of periodontal abscesses is primarily based on the location of the infective lesion, which can be defined as a cavity filled with a collection of pus, formed by disintegrated tissue. Abscesses of the periodontium can show various combinations of the following clinical features:

— Pain and sensitivity to touch

— Color change

— Swelling

— Purulence and sinus tract formation

— Pulsative pain, lasting

— Tooth is sensitive to percussion

— Teeth mobility and extrusion

— Fever, lymphadenopathy, and possible radiolucency of the affected alveolar bone

The lesions can be classified as short-lasting (acute: quickly developing) or long-lasting (chronic: developing slowly). They can be further divided into the following three classes:

A. Gingival abscess: Localized purulent infection involving the marginal gingival or the papilla. Generally quickly developing, it becomes fluctuant after 24 to 48 hours and leads to the formation of a purulent orifice. Pulpal hypersensitivity may occasionally be found. No periodontal pockets or alveolar bone loss surround these lesions, although a pseudopocket (gingival pocket) may be present. These lesions are usually rare and are often caused by a foreign body.

Treatment consists of eliminating local etiological factors (see treatment for periodontal abscess).

B. Periodontal abscess: A periodontal abscess is a localized infection within the tissues adjacent to a periodontal pocket that may lead to the destruction of the periodontal ligament and the alveolar bone. These lesions are commonly found in patients suffering from moderate to severe periodontitis. They are precipitated by a change in the subgingival flora, a decrease of host resistance, or both. The tooth is usually vital (Figure 2.25).

The following factors may be associated with periodontal abscesses:

1) Occlusion of the orifice of a periodontal pocket caused by the introduction of food or foreign body or by the incomplete removal of calculus deposits

2) Furcation involvement of periodontal infection

3) Systemic antibiotic therapy given to patients who are untreated for their periodontitis. This situation may lead to a supra-infection by opportunistic microorganisms resulting in a periodontal abscess

4) Diabetic patients have a tendency to develop purulent infections because of their decreased host immune response and their vascular abnormalities

5) Other predisposing factors (enamel pearls, lateral endodontic perforations, etc.) should be evaluated

The appropriate therapy consists of alleviating the pain by either establishing drainage by incision or by local debridement with surgical flap reflected if needed. An antibiotic can be prescribed and the lesion should be reevaluated after the acute phase has passed to detect any underlying periodontal condition.

C. Pericoronaritis (pericoronal abscess): A pericoronal abscess is a localized purulent infection within the tissues surrounding the crown of a partially erupted or difficultly erupting tooth. These abscesses are often seen adjacent to a mandibular third molar. Not only are these teeth difficult to access for proper hygiene, they frequently have difficulty erupting due to their malposition or lack of space. In addition, the already compromised area is often traumatized by occlusion of the opposing antagonist teeth. The recommended immediate treatment is to prescribe a systemic antibiotic and perform a local debridement if possible. Extraction of the tooth (and possibly the antagonist tooth as well) is recommended in the subsequent weeks.

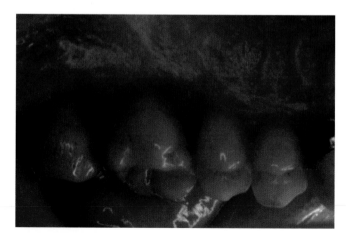

Figure 2.25. Periodontal abscess palatal of tooth number 15. The tooth is vital.

VII. PERIODONTITIS ASSOCIATED WITH ENDODONTIC LESION

A. Combined periodontal and endodontic lesions: Lesions of the periodontal ligament and adjacent alveolar bone may originate from infections of the periodontium or tissue of the dental pulp. A pulpal infection may cause a tissue-destructive process that proceeds from the apical region of a tooth to the marginal gingiva. The term retrograde periodontitis is often used to differentiate this type of lesion from a marginal periodontitis in which the infection spreads from the gingival margin toward the root apex. Another term, pulpodontic-periodontic syndrome, is also used to describe this type of combined lesion in which a tooth suffers from a pulpal/endodontic lesion and periodontitis at the same time (Figure 2.26).

One reason why these lesions can travel from one area to the other is that the periodontium communicates with the pulp tissues through many channels or pathways (apical, lateral, and accessory canals). Bacteria causative of endodontic lesions can travel in the blood vessels via the root grooves, vertical root fractures, hypoplastic cementum lesions, and root anomalies/resorptions to reach the marginal gingiva. The effects of endodontic lesions on the periodontium include severe and rapid destruction of the periodontal structures. Once the appropriate endodontic treatment is performed, the lesion should heal uneventfully without any residual defects in the periodontium.

A periodontal abscess and an endodontic abscess have similar clinical manifestations, and differ by the origin of the infection.

Note: Root perforation or root fracture during/after root canal therapy can result in an increased periodontal ligament, suppuration, and increased tooth mobility in an individual with a healthy periodontium. The principal symptoms include pain upon mastication, swelling, periodontal abscess formation, and fistula. The tooth can be vital or not and the formation of a localized deep (narrow) pocket, periodontal ligament, and widening and apical radiolucency may be present.

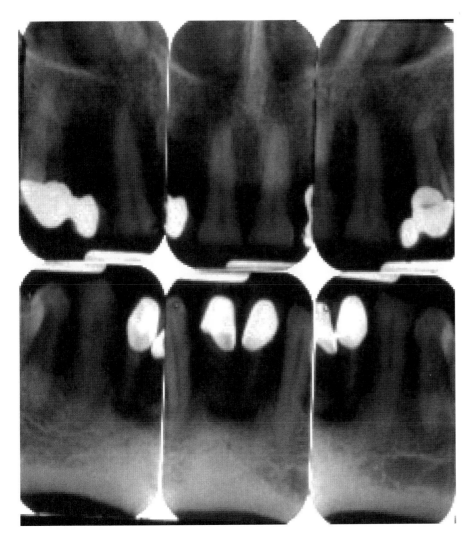

Figure 2.26. Perio-endo lesion affecting teeth number 24 and 25. There are lesions of endodontic origin as well as periodontal probings surrounding these teeth.

Periodontal pockets, furcation involvement, subgingival calculus, inflammation, deep fillings, past dental trauma, or root canal treatments must be considered to establish the correct diagnosis (Meng, 1999a,b).

VIII. DEVELOPMENTAL OR ACQUIRED DEFORMITIES AND CONDITIONS

The proposed classification is primarily based on clinical and morphologic criteria. Severity and etiologic characteristics can be used as secondary descriptors of the lesions (Pini Prato, 1999).

A. Localized tooth-related factors that modify or predispose to plaque-induced gingivitis or periodontitis (factors which favor plaque accumulation):

1. The tooth-related anatomic factors to consider may be (Matthews et al., 2004):

   — Enamel pearls and projections are related to the attachment loss in furcations of molars. They are enamel deposits located below the CEJ and extending to the furcation area, specially found on maxillary second molars

   — Tooth malposition or tooth inclination can lead to plaque accumulation and attachment loss. A tooth which is positioned more buccally on the dental arch may present a thin, bony plate leading to recession after inflammation. Trauma from abrasion can also occur more easily

   — Root proximity is a problem encountered when the volume of soft tissue and bone is reduced between the two roots of adjacent teeth, leading to more rapid destruction of periodontium during inflammation

   — Open proximal contacts resulting from defective restorations can lead to decreased deflection of food during chewing, causing food impaction interproximally

   — Root anomalies such as palato-gingival grooves are principally found on incisors. Incorrect hygiene can lead to bacterial plaque accumulation, ultimately leading to bone loss along the groove track

2. Dental restorations, appliances: A chronic inflammation or gingival recession may develop when a restoration violates the biological width around a tooth. The minimal desired space needed to preserve the health of periodontal tissues is 3 mm in total, from the crestal bone to the crown margin (Gargiulo, 1961).

3. Root fractures: Root fractures can be caused by mechanical stress from occlusion, a post, or a root canal treatment. When fractures are vertical, they are hard to distinguish if they are periodontal or endodontic lesions. These problems can lead to attachment loss due to bacterial invasion of the fracture area.

4. Cervical root resorption: Cervical root resorptions in the coronal part of the root (in contact with the oral cavity) may be involved in bacterial plaque accumulation and periodontal destruction.

B. Mucogingival deformities and conditions: The presence of mucogingival deformities often has an impact on patients in terms of esthetics and function. Mucogingival deformities may be congenital, developmental, or acquired defects and may be localized to soft tissues or associated with defects in the underlying bone. Mucogingival deformities may be classified in the following conditions (Pini Prato, 1999):

1. Gingival soft tissue recession: Gingival soft tissue recessions are noted when the free gingival margin is positioned apically to the cementoenamel junction. They can occur in two different locations:

   — Buccal or lingual surfaces

   — Interproximal surfaces

     * Etiologic factors predisposing to gingival recessions include:

       — Dehiscence or bone fenestration

       — Thin, bony plate

       — Thin or absent keratinized gingiva

       — Tooth malposition

       — Frenum traction

     * Etiological factors stimulating a recession:

       — Traumatic brushing

       — Cervical abrasion

       — Inflammation

       — Violation of biological width

       — Extraction

       — Orthodontic movement

       — Trauma due to a removable appliance, bad crown shape/margins, habit

2. Lack of keratinized gingiva: The quantity and quality of keratinized gingiva may be altered in numerous conditions. The following factors may be analyzed to establish the etiology and treatment of the condition:

   — Plaque control

   — Tooth brushing technique (toothbrush with soft bristles should be used)

— Etiological factors (frenum attachment, occlusion, prominent tooth, irritation or rubbing trauma from removable appliance)

— Age (a younger individual may be treated differently than an older one)

— Quality and quantity of attached gingiva

— Types of periodontium):

  * Type 1: 3 to 5 mm of keratinized tissue (KT), normal alveolar bone (40% of population)

  * Type 2: Less than 2 mm of KT, normal alveolar bone (10% of population)

  * Type 3: 3 to 5 mm of KT, thin alveolar bone (20% of population)

  * Type 4: Less than 2 mm of KT, thin alveolar bone (30% of population)

— Recession classification (Miller, 1985):

  * Class I: Recession doesn't pass the mucogingival junction (MCJ), no attachment loss interproximally, 100% success is expected after treatment

  * Class II: Recession at or passes MCJ, no attachment loss interproximally, 100% success is expected after treatment

  * Class III: Recession at or passes MCJ, attachment loss interproximally or unfavorable tooth position, less than 100% success is expected after treatment

  * Class IV: Recession at or passes MCJ, severe attachment loss interproximally and very unfavorable tooth position, no success is expected after treatment

3. Decreased vestibular depth

4. Aberrant frenum, muscle position

5. Gingival excess:

  a. Pseudopocket

  b. Inconsistent gingival margin

  c. Gingival excess

  d. gingival enlargement (1A3, 1B4)

C. Mucogingival deformities and conditions on the edentulous ridge:

1. Vertical and horizontal deficiency

2. Lack of gingival keratinized tissue

3. Gingival soft tissue enlargement

4. Aberrant frenum, muscle position

5. Decreased vestibular depth

6. Abnormal color

D. Occlusal trauma: A defined lesion and response of the attachment apparatus has been demonstrated in association with excessive occlusal forces, and has been termed occlusal trauma. The effect of traumatogenic occlusion on the progression of periodontitis has been associated with tooth mobility due to occlusal trauma. This creates a pathological state in which the PDL is destroyed and osteoclasts destroy alveolar bone, increasing tooth mobility. Occlusal trauma is due to the occlusal force, direct or indirect, which exceeds the resistance of the supporting tissues. It can be characterized by the following features:

— Hypermobility

— Abnormal PDL widening

— Histological analysis shows cementum tears and radicular resorption

  1. Primary occlusal trauma: Injury resulting in tissue changes from excessive occlusal forces applied to a tooth with a normal periodontal support: 1) normal bone levels, 2) normal attachment levels, and 3) excessive occlusal forces.

  2. Secondary occlusal trauma: Injury resulting in tissue changes from normal or excessive occlusal forces applied to a tooth with reduced periodontal support: 1) bone loss, 2) attachment loss, and 3) normal/excessive occlusal forces.

Indications of a traumatic occlusion may present as tooth mobility, fremitus, occlusal interference, wear facettes, tooth migration, tooth fracture, and thermal sensitivity.

Radiographs may show widened PDL space, bone loss, and radicular resorption.

BIBLIOGRAPHY

Armitage GC. 1999. Development of a classification system for periodontal diseases and conditions. *Ann Periodontol.* Dec;4(1):1–6.

Chapple ILC, Hamburger J. 2006. Periodontal Medicine: A Window on the Body. *Quintessence Publishing Co*, UK.

Charbeneau TD, Hurt WC. 1983. Gingival findings in spontaneous scurvy. A case report. *J Periodontol.* 54:694–697.

Gallagher G, Shklar G. 1987. Oral involvement in mucous membranes pemphigoid. *Clin Dermatol.* 5:18–27.

Gargiulo AW, Wentz FM, Orban B. 1961. Dimensions and relations of the dentogingival function in humans. *J Periodontol.* 32:261–267.

Gorlin RJ, Cohen MM, Levis LS. 1990. Syndromes of the head and neck. 3rd edition, New York: *Oxford University Press*. 847–855.

Greenberg MS. 1996. Herpes virus infections. *Dent Clin North Am.* 40:359–368.

Holmstrup P. 1999. Non-plaque-induced gingival lesions. *Ann Periodontol.* Dec;4(1):20–31.

Hugoson A. 1971. Gingivitis in pregnant women. A longitudinal clinical study. *Odontologisk Revy.* 22:65–84.

Kaufman AY. 1969. An oral contraceptive as an etiologic factor producing hyperplasic gingivitis and a neoplasm of the pregnancy tumor type. *Oral Surg Oral Med Oral Pathol.* 28:666–670.

Lindhe J. 2003. Clinical Periodontology and Implant Dentistry. 4th edition. *Wiley-Blackwell.*

Lozada-Nur F, Gorsky M, Silverman S Jr. 1989. Oral erythema multiforme: Clinical observation and treatment of 95 patients. *Oral Surg Oral Med Oral Pathol.* 67:36–40.

Mariotti A. 1999. Dental plaque-induced gingival diseases. *Ann Periodontol.* Dec;4(1):7–19.

Matthews DC, Tabesh M. 2000. Detection of localized tooth-related factors that predispose to periodontal infections. *Periodontol.* Vol 34;2004:136–150.

Meng HX. 1999. Periodontal abscess. *Ann Periodontol.* Dec;4(1):79–83.

Meng HX. 1999. Periodontic-endodontic lesions. *Ann Periodontol.* Dec;4(1):84–90.

Miller CS. 1996. Viral infection of the immunocompetent patient. *Dermatol Clin.* 14:225–241.

Miller CS, Redding SW. 1992. Diagnosis and management of orofacial herpes simplex virus infections. *Dent Clin North Am.* 36:879–895.

Miller PD. 1985. Root coverage using the free soft tissue autograft following Citric Acid application. III. A successful and predictable procedure in areas of deep wide recession. *Int J Periodontics Restorative Dent.* 5(2):15–37.

Neville BW, Damm DD, Allen CM, Bouquot JE. 2002. Oral and maxillofacial pathology. 2nd edition. *Saunders LTD.*

Page RC. 1985. Oral health status in the United States: prevalence of inflammatory periodontal diseases. *J Dent Educ.* 49:354–367.

Pini Prato G. 1999. Mucogingival deformities. *Ann Periodontol.* Dec;4(1):98–101.

Ranney RR. 2000. Classification of periodontal diseases. *Periodontol.* 1993;2:57–71.

Schiodt M. 1984. Oral discoid lupus erythematus II. Skin lesions and systemic lupus erythematosus in sixty-six patients with 6-year follow-up. *Oral Surg Oral Med Oral Pathol.* 57:177–180.

Sciubba JJ. 1996. Autoimmune aspect of pemphigus vulgaris in mucosal pemphigoid. *Adv Dent Res.* Apr;10(1):52-6. Review.

Sills ES, Zegarelli SJ, Hoschander MM, Strider WE. 1996. Clinical diagnosis and management of hormonally responsive oral pregnancy tumor (pyogenic granuloma). *J Reprod Med.* 41:467–470.

Stamm JW. 1986. Epidemiology of gingivitis. *J Clin Periodontol.* 13:360–366.

Sutcliffe P. 1972. A longitudinal study of gingivitis and puberty. *J Periodont Res.* 7:52–58.

Thorn JT, Holmstrup P, Rindum J, Pindborg JJ. 1988. Course of various clinical forms of oral lichen planus. A prospective follow-up study of 611 patients. *J Oral Pathol.* 17:213–218.

Chapter 3 Periodontal Risk Factors and Modification

INTRODUCTION

As a common chronic disease of the oral cavity, periodontal disease is a set of inflammatory conditions affecting the supporting structures of the dentition (Armitage, 1999). After its initiation, the disease progresses with the loss of collagen attachment to the root surface, the apical migration of the pocket epithelium, the formation of deepened periodontal pockets, and the resorption of alveolar bone. Untreated periodontal disease continues with progressive alveolar bone destruction, leading to increased tooth mobility and potential tooth loss (Page and Kornman, 1997).

Reports from epidemiological studies, analysis of tissue histology, clinical trials, and animal experiments consistently demonstrate a multi-factorial aetiology of periodontal disease. Chronic periodontitis is the most prevalent form of destructive periodontal disease (Albandar et al., 1999). Furthermore, cross-sectional and longitudinal data from epidemiological research in periodontology suggest that risk factors can be identified, and that some of these factors could be controlled to prevent the development and progression of the disease. Risk factors are part of the causal chain of a particular disease or can lead to the exposure of the host to a disease (Consensus Report, Annals of Periodontology, 1996). The presence of a risk factor implies a direct increase in the probability of a disease occurring, and if absent or modified, a reduction in that probability should occur. Risk factors are generally classified as modifiable and non-modifiable. While gender, age, and ethnicity are non-modifiable, insufficient oral hygiene or tobacco use are identified as modifiable risk factors for periodontal disease.

A risk factor may be modified by interventions, thereby reducing the probability that a particular disease will occur. However, the susceptibility to a specific disease may vary among different individuals exposed to a given risk factor over time. Additionally, cumulative interactions between both modifiable and non-modifiable risk factors, described as "complex risk factors," have been suggested (Stolk et al., 2008).

A variety of interrelated risk factors may influence both the onset of periodontal disease and its progression (Figure 3.1). The detection of periodontal disease progression remains challenging since it typically relies on the comparison of measurements made with a calibrated periodontal probe and non-standardized periapical radiographs over time. Some emphasis should be placed on the early identification of periodontal risk factors to assess the likelihood of periodontal disease progression in susceptible individuals since both methods detect periodontal breakdown only after it has occurred. The goal of this chapter is to discuss known non-modifiable and modifiable risk factors as well as their management in the dental practice to provide prevention and a careful maintenance program for the periodontal patient while following the best available evidence today.

NON-MODIFIABLE RISK FACTORS

Genetic and Hereditary Factors

Periodontal diseases are shown to be affected by genetic factors (Page and Kornman, 1997). A number of genetic disorders, such as Down syndrome, leukocyte adhesion deficiency syndrome (LADS), Papillon Lefevre syndrome, Chediak Higashi syndrome, chronic neutrophil defects, or cyclic neutropenia are associated with more or less severe periodontal conditions.

The hereditary aggregation was demonstrated in a twin study for chronic periodontitis (Michalowicz et al., 1991) and an epidemiological trial on aggressive periodontitis in a Dutch population (van der Velden et al., 1993). Following the adjustment for environmental factors such as tobacco use, it was estimated that 50% of the variance in disease may be attributed to a genetic background (Michalowicz et al., 2000).

Practical Application of Genetic Susceptibility Testing

During periodontal inflammation, inflammatory cytokines, including interleukin-1β (IL-1β) and tumor necrosis factor-α (TNF-α), activate catabolic enzymes such as matrix metalloproteinases, subsequently leading to the breakdown of connective tissue. Any gene polymorphism of such proteins potentially alters the susceptibility of the host to periodontal diseases. A single nucleotide polymorphism (SNP) is a mutation that occurs when a single nucleotide is altered within its genome due to changes in the base pair sequence.

Past periodontal diagnostic research has focused on evaluating several selected candidate gene SNPs including variations of IL-1β or TNF-α. The evidence-based perspective: Evidence from a review suggests that some polymorphisms in the genes encoding interleukins (IL)-1, Fc gamma

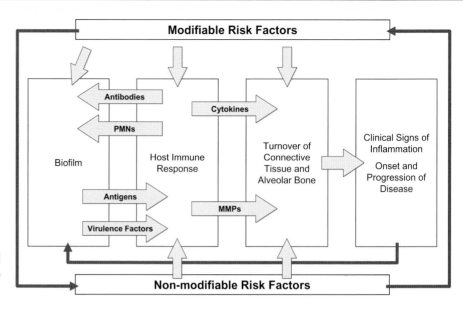

Figure 3.1. Interplay of modifiable and non-modifiable risk factors with the pathogenesis of periodontal diseases.

receptors (FcgR), IL-10, and the vitamin D receptor may be associated with periodontitis in certain ethnic groups (Loos et al., 2005). In addition, the association of the composite IL-1 genotype with periodontitis progression and/or treatment outcomes was analyzed using a systematic review approach (Huynh-Ba et al., 2007). There is limited evidence for such an association. Thus far, no specific genetic risk factor for periodontitis has been identified (Loos et al., 2005). Therefore, the clinical relevance of different commercially available genetic tests is limited.

Gender

Hormonal changes in women during menstruation, pregnancy, menopause, or therapy with pharmaceutical supplements have an impact on periodontal health. Disease susceptibility may be increased due to hormone-related alterations of the gingival blood flow (Kovar et al., 1985), the composition and flow rate of saliva (Laine, 2002), or the bone metabolism (Lerner, 2006). Additionally, data from epidemiological studies interestingly reveal that men may be at greater risk for periodontal diseases: in most clinical trials men are often found with worse periodontal health (Albandar, 2002; Meisel et al., 2007). Most often, however, these deteriorations may be explained by an increased prevalence of male tobacco use and mens' increased tendency to neglect oral hygiene (Meisel et al., 2007).

Gender-specific Practical Applications

Periodontal diseases have been associated with gender-specific complications such as an increased susceptibility for gingivitis during pregnancy (Russell and Mayberry, 2008), pre-term delivery, or low birth weight (Madianos et al., 2002). Therefore, gender-specific periodontal disease risk factors should be assessed in women by all oral health professionals (Krejci and Bissada, 2002). In pregnant women, a rigid recall

interval including oral hygiene motivation is recommended. Consequently, it is suggested that existing periodontal inflammation should be treated before pregnancy.

Factors that are increasingly investigated in recent studies include gender-specific diseases such as osteoporosis or metastatic bone disease in relation with hormone substitute therapy or bisphosphonate medication in post-menopausal women (Diel et al., 2007; Payne et al., 1999). Bisphosphonates affect osteoclast functions, leading to the inhibition of physiological bone remodeling. With both surgical and non-surgical periodontal treatment, a bisphosphonate-associated osteonecrosis of the jaws should be considered as a complication. In one prospective cohort study of osteoporotic women in early menopause, it was found that a supplementation of estrogen may be associated with reduced gingival inflammation and impaired clinical attachment loss (Reinhardt et al., 1999).

Age

The aging process itself is suggested to be an independent risk factor for periodontal diseases (Papapanou et al., 1989). In contrast, a longitudinal study involving an elderly Scandinavian population (age 75 or older) demonstrated stable periodontal conditions for five years, suggesting a limited impact of the aging process itself in otherwise relatively healthy individuals (Ajwani and Ainamo, 2001). However, the extent and severity of periodontal diseases are shown to increase with age (Albandar, 2002) as a consequence of the cumulative burden from various risk factors such as tobacco use or plaque accumulation (Albandar, 2002; Albandar et al., 1999). Additionally, metabolic disorders, including diabetes mellitus, osteoporosis, rheumatoid arthritis, or vascular diseases, are more likely to develop in the elderly and thus affect periodontal conditions (Persson, 2006).

Age-specific Practical Applications

Life expectancy has increased significantly over the past few years in industrialized countries (Holm-Pedersen et al., 2005). As compared to previous populations, the elderly population is retaining its natural dentition, potentially leading to more periodontal problems. The presence of various chronic diseases, such as diabetes mellitus or specific medications (e.g. Vitamin K antagonists), may also interact with the periodontal condition or the treatment. Thus, there is a need for multidisciplinary treatment in many cases, due to the increased likelihood of co-morbidity in the elderly (Persson, 2006). Aging is often associated with the individual's impaired mobility, probably leading to an incapacity for regular supportive periodontal treatment. A close interplay with nursing homes or public oral health care providers may be advisable. Physical or mental disorders may affect the effectiveness of supragingival plaque control. The suggestion of simple interventions, including the weekly use of chlorhexidine-containing mouth rinses in conjunction with cognitive behavioral interventions, might be useful (Hujoel et al., 1997).

MODIFIABLE RISK FACTORS

Insufficient Oral Hygiene

Today, accumulated plaque is considered to be a dental biofilm briefly defined as a complex bacterial structure adherent to wet surfaces (Socransky and Haffajee, 2002). For the therapy of periodontal diseases, it is important to consider that biofilms can protect their microorganisms, either from the host's immune response or antimicrobial agents, and thus become difficult therapeutic targets (Socransky and Haffajee, 2002). So far, only mechanical debridement was shown to be a predictable approach to successfully destruct the dental biofilm. Therefore, mechanical plaque control should be performed supragingivally by the individual on a regular basis and subgingivally, if needed, by the oral health professional.

Any factors that facilitate biofilm formation, such as plaque retention or insufficient supragingival plaque control, are common risk factors for periodontal breakdown due to their causality with gingival inflammation and possibly the onset of periodontitis. This includes several anatomic conditions, such as enamel pearls, tongues, grooves, root furcations, and concavities, as well as root proximities (Roussa, 1998; Vermylen et al., 2005). Calculus and acquired iatrogenic factors, such as insufficient restorations, additionally contribute to plaque accumulation (Lang et al., 1983; Oliver et al., 1998).

It was proven some 40 years ago by classical experiments conducted by the work group Lüe and Theilade that oral micro-organisms are relevant for the development of inflammable periodontal diseases (Theilade et al., 1966). In a lon-

gitudinal study of more than 26 years, a further research group examined the influence of plaque-induced gingival inflammation on the subsequent loss of clinical attachment in a periodontally well-maintained Scandinavian population (Schatzle et al., 2003). The supragingival plaque accumulation correlated with the degree of gingival inflammation. However, sites with bleeding on probing at every visit demonstrated about 70% more attachment loss than sites without inflammation for the duration of the study. Moreover, it was recently shown that the susceptibility of gingivitis seems to be higher among males suffering from periodontitis (Dietrich et al., 2006).

Practical Application of Microbiological Testing

A multitude of different microbiological tests, based on morphological, enzymatic, cultural, genetic, or antigenetic bacterial properties, are available for both qualitative and quantitative microbiologic risk assessment of periodontitis. In many clinical situations, however, these tests fail to provide evidence-based recommendations for therapy (Sanz et al., 2004). Nevertheless, in a few cases, microbiologic tests can support treatment planning, including cases resistant to combined mechanical-antibiotic therapies, e.g. scaling and root planing, and the prescription of metronidazole and amoxicillin.

Tobacco Use

Earlier publications confirmed tobacco consumption as a risk factor for periodontal diseases. Over the past few years, oral health research has significantly contributed to the understanding of the mechanisms leading to the deterioration of the hard and soft tissues supporting the teeth. With the recording of the number of cigarettes smoked per day, the number of years tobacco was used, and the amount of time since tobacco use cessation, a dose response relationship was established using the Comprehensive Smoking Index (Dietrich and Hoffmann, 2004).

With increased use of tobacco, patients show higher periodontal probing depths, increased clinical attachment loss, more alveolar bone resorption, a higher prevalence of gingival recessions, and a higher risk for tooth loss (Tonetti, 1998). In contrast to this, with smokers, the clinical characteristics of gingival inflammation or bleeding on periodontal probing are less established (Dietrich et al., 2004). Smokers show less positive results after conventional, surgical, and regenerative periodontal therapy. The benefits of mucogingval surgery are reduced and less successful in smokers (Erley et al., 2006). Moreover, smoking impairs the osseointegration of oral implants and is at least partly responsible for a majority of biological complications in implant dentistry, such as peri-implantitis (Strietzel et al., 2007). Based on the present understanding of periodontal diseases, the clinical findings, and the specific therapeutic outcomes with smokers, it appears to be reasonable, next to the current classification

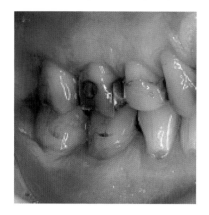
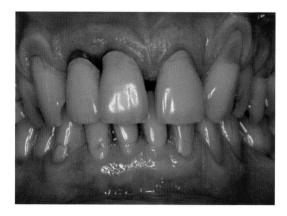
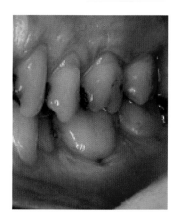
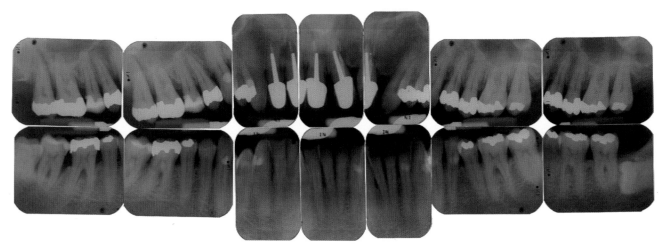

Figure 3.2. Clinical and radiographic images of a 45-year-old male smoker. Typical signs of smoker's periodontitis (20 pack years) including attachment loos, gingival recessions, and radiographic alveolar bone loss, particularly in the maxillary and mandibular front area.

of periodontal diseases, to use the term "smokers periodontitis" (Figure 3.2).

A common clinical observation is delayed wound healing after therapeutic interventions (Silverstein, 1992) (Figure 3.3).

There are various potentially significant pathogenic effects of tobacco-related substances on the periodontal tissues, immune response system, or composition of the oral flora. Periodontal destruction associated with tobacco use is caused by a wide multidimensional range of effects on different functions in cells, tissues, and organ systems. Some of these effects are diametric in nature, due to the effects of different tobacco constituents. However, when summarizing the properties of the tobacco-induced alterations in the metabolism of vasculature, connective-tissue, and bone, as well as on cell-mediated and humoral immunity, it is more than likely that tobacco use shifts the physiological balance between anabolic and catabolic mechanisms in a more destructive direction, due to an alteration of protective immune and tissue mechanisms (Johnson and Guthmiller,

2007; Palmer, 2005; Ryder, 2007). Moreover, there is evidence that tobacco consumption may change the genetically determined susceptibility for periodontal diseases (Meisel et al., 2004).

The evidence-based perspective: There is robust evidence from a systematic review (Bergstrom, 2006) that smoking is a strong risk factor for periodontal diseases. On the basis of 70 cross-sectional studies, 14 case-control studies, and 21 cohort studies, it is concluded that smoking negatively interferes with a healthy periodontal condition.

Diabetes Mellitus

Diabetes mellitus is a metabolic disorder categorized by a hyperglycemia due to impaired insulin production or insulin resistance. Insulin is a pancreatic-hormone-maintaining glucose metabolism. At least two major groups of diabetes mellitus (type 1 and type 2) are differentiated based on their pathogenesis. In addition, some diseases such as hormone-secreting tumors, conditions such as pregnancy (gestational

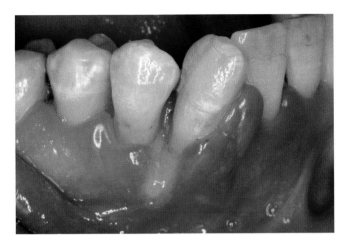

Figure 3.3. Impaired wound healing in a female smoker (age 44, 45 pack years) seven days following periodontal non-surgical debridement.

diabetes), or drugs such as corticosteroids can lead to diabetes mellitus. Treatment of diabetes mellitus primarily aims to keep blood sugar levels within a normal range. Treatment may include an interview for behavioral change for dietary adjustment, physical activity, or several drugs. They usually include oral antihyperglycemic drugs or insulin replacement therapy, as well as drugs for prevention and/or treatment of diabetes complications such as hypertension. If left untreated, serious long-term complications may occur, affecting small and large blood vessels, eyes, kidneys, nerves, or the immune system.

Diabetes mellitus has been associated with increased prevalence and severity of periodontal disease (Figure 3.4) (Emrich et al., 1991; Shlossman et al., 1990). The majority of studies demonstrate a more severe periodontal condition in diabetic adults than in adults without diabetes (Papapanou, 1996; Verma and Bhat, 2004). The type of diabetes does not affect the extent of periodontitis when the duration of diabetes is similar. However, type I diabetics develop the disease at an earlier age, and, hence, have it for longer periods, and may therefore develop a greater extent and severity of periodontitis (Oliver and Tervonen, 1994; Thorstensson and Hugoson, 1993). Well-controlled diabetics are more likely to be similar to non-diabetics in their periodontal status (Westfelt et al., 1996).

A common complication of diabetes mellitus is the increased susceptibility for microbial infections due to an impaired function of the host immune response. Diabetes mellitus may contribute to periodontal inflammation via specific mechanisms. The hyperglycemia may promote the formation of advanced glycation end products (AGE), i.e., glycated body proteins (Wautier and Guillausseau, 1998). Accumulation of AGE may have an impact on periodontal micro-vascularisation or may lead to an increased number of monocytes within the site of inflammation (Katz et al., 2005). A modification of physiologic cell functions of certain subtypes of granulocytes is also reported (Manouchehr-Pour et al., 1981a; Manouchehr-Pour et al., 1981b). Moreover, some studies suggest an alteration of pro-inflammatory mediators in gingival crevicular fluid, including tumor necrosis factor-α, prostaglandin-E2, and interleukin-1β (Engebretson et al., 2004; Salvi et al., 1997a; Salvi et al., 1997b). A further research group reported a decreased gene expression of anti-inflammatory and anti-bone-resorptive molecules such as interleukin-10 and osteoprotegerin (Duarte et al., 2007). Collagen is produced by fibroblasts and is an important molecule of the periodontium. In-vitro findings indicate a reduction of collagen synthesis in a dose-dependent fashion of glucose concentration (Willershausen-Zonnchen et al., 1991).

Interestingly, there is some evidence for periodontitis as a contributing factor in the pathogenesis of diabetes mellitus (Taylor et al., 1998). Inflammatory markers, including tumor necrosis factor-α, increase with periodontal severity and thus affect the insulin metabolism in diabetics (Engebretson et al., 2007). In contrast, their reduction occurs following antimicrobial periodontal therapy, leading to an improvement of glycemic control (Iwamoto et al., 2001).

The evidence based perspective: Evidence from a systematic review, including meta-analysis, suggests a significantly higher severity but the same extent of periodontal disease in diabetics compared with non-diabetics (Khader et al., 2006).

Stress

Stress may be caused by acute or chronic stressors. A stressor can be intrinsic or extrinsic in origin and is frequently defined as anything that causes an adaptive and non-specific neurological and physiological response in an individual. Chronic stressors are of relatively longer duration and include several "life events" such as the loss of a family member, splitting of a relationship, long-term illness, miscarriage, or "daily hassles." Events of a relative short duration, such as traffic jams, surgical interventions, dental visits, or unpleasant questions in a medical exam, on the other hand, may act as acute stressors to an individual. The physiologic response is mediated by several immune-to-brain-to-immune regulatory pathways (Breivik et al., 2006). The individual stress coping behavior depends on genetic susceptibility and environmental and developmental factors as well as gathered experiences during the course of life.

Several studies indicated an association of negative stress, depression, anxiety, or poor coping behavior with periodontal diseases (Genco et al., 1999; Hugoson et al., 2002; Wimmer et al., 2002). Negative stress may lead to an increased susceptibility to periodontitis mediated through different pathways.

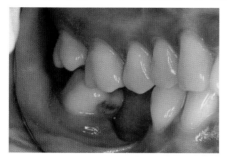 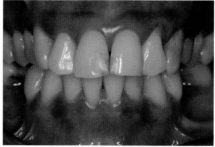 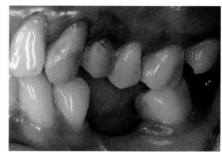

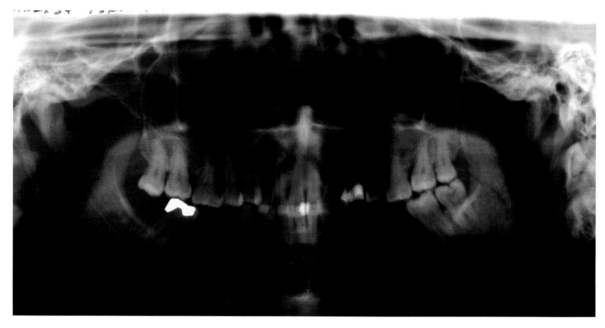

Figure 3.4. Clinical and radiographic images of a 46-year-old female patient with type II diabetes mellitus and chronic periodontitis. The metabolic disease was diagnosed in 1993 and is well controlled (level of blood sugar glucose 6, 3 mmol/l) by the physician. The patient receives oral antidiabetic drugs.

As one mechanism, it was suggested that due to stress, the oral hygiene may be limited (Deinzer et al., 2001). Additionally, academic stress was shown to cause an enhancement of interleukin-1 secretion detected in gingival crevicular fluid in a study by Deinzer and co-workers (Deinzer et al., 1999). This cytokine is a strong stimulator of osteoclasts leading to destructive bone metabolism. Interleukin-6, another inflammatory cytokine, was found to be elevated in the gingival fluid of depressed women (Johannsen et al., 2006). In addition, a prolonged reduction of the secretion of immunoglobulin A, an important salivary antibody, was observed in students participating in a major medical exam (Deinzer et al., 2000).

Cortisol and the catecholamins adrenaline and noradrenaline are the major stress hormones produced by the cortex of the suprarenal gland in response to stimulation by hypothalamus-releasing hormones. Increased levels of stress-mediated cortisol were found in the gingival crevicular fluid and in saliva (Hugo et al., 2006; Ishisaka et al., 2007; Nakajima

et al., 2006). Additionally, stress-induced hypercortisolemia was linked to elevated levels of plaque and gingivitis (Hugo et al., 2006). Moreover, evidence from animal experiments reveals changes in the periodontal tissues following stress exposure (Nakajima et al., 2006). Restraint stress was able to enhance attachment loss after challenge with the putative periodontal pathogen *Porphyromonas gingivalis*. Findings from in vitro experiments suggest an effect of catecholamines on the growth of certain oral bacteria (Roberts et al., 2002). Thus, a stress-induced increase of catecholamine levels in the gingival crevicular fluid may be able to mediate the composition of the subgingival biofilm.

HIV/AIDS

The acquired immunodeficiency syndrome (AIDS) is caused by infection with the human immunodeficiency virus (HIV), leading to a destruction of the immune system of the affected host. The CD4+ T cells as a subset of T lymphocytes are

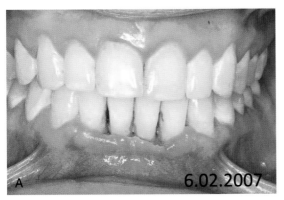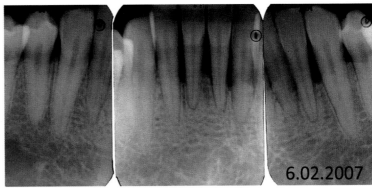
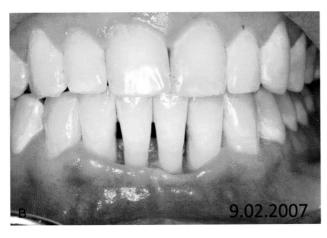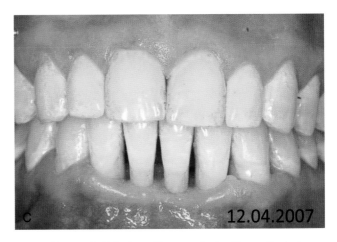

Figure 3.5. Necrotizing ulcerative periodontitis in a 26-year-old HIV-positive male (20 cigarettes per day) with medical observation for virus load and CD4 counts and no further prescription of HIV medication (HAART). A) Pre-therapeutical clinical and radiographic images, B) clinical view three days following non-surgical periodontal therapy, C) clinical view two months following therapy.

destroyed in particular. AIDS consists of various (opportunistic) infections including pulmonary and gastrointestinal infections and/or clinical manifestations including neurological and psychiatric involvement as well as tumors and other malignancies.

The current status of immunosuppression, assessed by CD4+ lymphocyte levels and viral load with HIV, are predictors of AIDS as well as HIV-associated complications in the oral cavity (Kroidl et al., 2005). A multitude of oral lesions, including Karposi's sarcoma, linear gingival erythema (LGE), necrotizing ulcerative gingivitis (NUG), and necrotizing ulcerative periodontitis (NUP), were described in individuals infected with HIV (Figure 3.5). However, the likelihood of HIV-associated oral diseases has decreased in recent years, due to advanced treatment approaches in HIV/AIDS therapy, such as highly active antiretroviral therapy (HAART) (Reichart, 2006).

HAART combines the use of several drugs, affecting or inhibiting different stages of the retrovirus life cycle, including viral entry in host cells, syntheses of viral DNA, or activity of viral proteases. A number of studies dealt with the issue of occur-

rence of periodontal disease in HIV-seropositive subjects and AIDS patients (Lamster et al., 1994; McKaig et al., 1998). After controlling for CD41 counts, HIV-infected people taking HIV-antiretroviral medication were five times less likely to suffer from periodontitis compared with those not taking such medication (McKaig et al., 1998).

The effects of taking HAART on the outcome of periodontal therapy was assessed by Jordan and co-workers (Jordan et al., 2006). Chronic periodontitis patients with HIV can be successfully treated by non-surgical scaling and root planing, followed by supportive periodontal therapy. However, a close collaboration of oral health care providers and general practitioners should become a routine procedure in HIV patients' care.

Nutrition

Possible consequences of nutrition deficiencies on oral and periodontal health have been reviewed (Dorsky, 2001). Several nutrients have been found to have a negative impact on periodontal health when not sufficiently delivered, such as vitamins, trace metals, antioxidants, and proteins (Eklund and Burt, 1994; Krall, 2001; Nishida et al., 2000a; Nishida et al., 2000b). So far, however, there are no reports in the current literature on the effect of nutrition counseling, either on the periodontal status or on the outcome of periodontal therapy.

RISK FACTOR MODIFICATION

Behavioral Change

Primary and secondary prevention oriented toward the change of inappropriate behavior is about to become a part of daily dental care. Traditional periodontal care includes the instruction of proper oral hygiene methods. Unfortunately, many health education approaches seem to be inefficient in accomplishing long-term change, potentially leading to frustration of both the patient and the clinician. Additionally, there is a shortcoming of evidence in both the dental and psychology literature on effective methods for behavior counseling in periodontal care, particularly regarding:

- Individual oral hygiene instructions for optimal oral hygiene

- Effective tobacco use prevention and cessation counseling to help abstain from tobacco

- Appropriate dietary counseling for a healthy diet

It may be necessary to apply different behavior change counseling methods to target individual behavior to get reliably effective outcomes in periodontal care. According to the best available evidence for oral hygiene instructions, the repeated demonstration of a cleaning device may be applied. For tobacco use cessation, in addition to pharmacotherapy, the method of the five A's (Ask, Advise, Assess, Assist, Arrange) may be used (Fiore, 2000). Additionally, type 2 diabetic patients may be referred to nutritionists for dietary counseling. From a practical point of view, however, it may be complicated and even discouraging to approach the periodontal patient with a variety of different methods targeting the same purpose: establishing appropriate behavior to improve the outcomes of both periodontal therapy and long-term supportive periodontal care.

Brief Motivational Interviewing (BMI)

Aiming for simplicity, it may be preferable to apply one single counseling method for behavior change in periodontal care that is shown to be effective in both primary and secondary prevention of oral diseases. Numerous behavioral research studies have confirmed the success achieved by state-of-the-art motivational interviewing (MI). MI is a patient-centered interviewing technique which was initially used as an auxiliary tool during counseling for smoking cessation and alcohol abuse (Miller and Rollnick, 2002). In the context of dentistry, a "short form" of MI known as "brief motivational interviewing" (BMI) appears to be suited for use during health behavior

interventions in dental practices. The aim of BMI is to achieve the following objectives within a short amount of time (i.e., less than five minutes):

1. To question the patient concerning her motivation to change her behavior, or

2. To give the patient the self-confidence he may need to accomplish the envisaged change of behavior, and

3. To reach an agreement to discuss behavior change at another appointment.

BMI uses a patient-driven pathway which is reflected by the acronym **OARS**:

Open-ended questions: "Yes" or "no" answers often terminate the topic of a conversation. Using "who," "what," "where," or "why" questions further allows the patient to provide more information for the counseling.

Affirm: Acknowledging the feelings of the patient offers validation and assurance that the counselor is actively listening.

Reflection: Playing back the conversation to the patient often demonstrates empathy and may also highlight ambivalent behavior.

Summarize: Providing an overview of the conversation allows confirmation of potential key points in the process of change.

For further information on communication methods for behavioral change counseling, the reader is referred to the textbook of Miller and Rollnick (Miller and Rollnick, 2002).

Supragingival Plaque Control

Proper self-performed mechanical plaque removal and compliance with needs-related recall visits are critical components of successful prevention and therapy of periodontal diseases. Both surgical and non-surgical periodontal treatment are only shown to be successful along with supragingival plaque control (Magnusson et al., 1984; Rosling et al., 1976). Additionally, periodontal therapy in combination with adequate, self-performed supragingival plaque control has been demonstrated to be effective in maintaining periodontal health for more than 20 years (Axelsson et al., 2004). Consequently, this approach has been considered as the "gold standard" for periodontal care (Figure 3.6). It is recognized that the daily removal of the bacterial biofilm represents the most important risk factor control (Figure 3.7). For the detailed instruction of supragingival plaque control for the prevention and treatment of gingivitis and periodontitis, the reader is referred to textbooks on periodontal therapy.

The evidence-based perspective: Evidence from a review suggests that an optimal level of self-performed oral hygiene

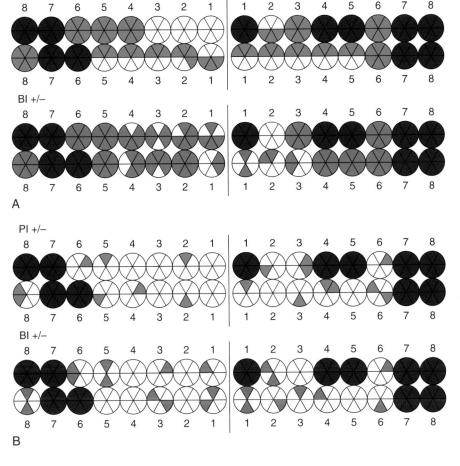

Figure 3.6. Oral hygiene motivation. Oral hygiene assessment: Visibility of supragingival plaque (PI, green) and ginigival bleeding (BI, red) are analyzed on six sites per tooth; missing teeth are colored black. The initial scores (A) indicate insufficient supragingival plaque control as well as gingival inflammation. Following oral hygiene instruction (toothbrush and interdental brushes) the plaque control improved (B).

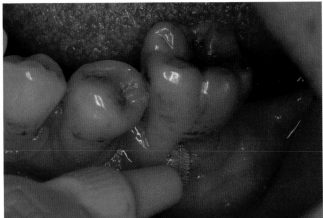

Figure 3.7. Oral hygiene aids (interdental brushes).

can have major effects on the subgingival biofilm composition and thus lead to significant therapeutic implications for the treatment of periodontal diseases (Ower, 2003).

Tobacco Use Cessation

Recent reports reveal short-term effects after quitting smoking as well as long-term results of smoking cessation on the periodontal and peri-implant status (Bergstrom, 2004) (Bain, 1996; Heasman et al., 2006). Generally, the periodontal status of former smokers is found to be intermediate between that of people who never smoked and current smokers (Bergstrom et al., 2000). Furthermore, smoking cessation has been shown to be beneficial for periodontal conditions: former smokers show less alveolar bone loss (Bergstrom et al., 2000; Bolin et al., 1993; Paulander et al., 2004) and reduced tooth loss (Krall et al., 1997) and present better outcomes after periodontal therapy (Kaldahl et al., 1996; Preshaw et al., 2005).

The potential benefit of smoking cessation is likely to be mediated through a number of different pathways. They may include shifts toward a less pathogenic subgingival flora; recovery of the gingival microcirculation; restoration of neutrophil function, metabolism, and viability; damping of the enhanced immune response; and re-establishment of any imbalance in the local or systemic production of cytokines (Heasman et al., 2006). The duration of the recovery of periodontal and peri-implant tissues following tobacco use cessation has not been determined yet. However, with the National Health and Nutrition Examination Survey (NHANES) of 12,623 patients in the USA, periodontal recovery was shown to be influenced by intensity, duration, and recency of smoking. Additionally, with this data, a half-time (50% risk reduction) of one and a half years has been computed (Dietrich and Hoffmann, 2004).

The evidence-based perspective: A review summarizing data from epidemiological, cross-sectional, and case control studies strongly suggests that smoking cessation is beneficial to patients following periodontal treatments (Heasman et al., 2006). The periodontal status of former-smokers following treatment demonstrates that quitting smoking is beneficial. However, there are only limited data from long-term longitudinal clinical trials to demonstrate unequivocally the periodontal benefit of quitting smoking. Despite the lack of data from intervention studies, these findings suggest that smoking cessation may generally result in a long-term benefit to the periodontal condition. In addition, there is no need for randomized, controlled trials of the effectiveness of smoking cessation on oral health outcomes because such trials would not be feasible and would be too costly. However, well-designed observational studies are needed to fill the knowledge gaps.

Based on this body of evidence, tobacco use cessation becomes an important factor in daily dental care. Every member of the dental practice team plays an important role in the teamwork of smoking cessation counseling. With an appropriate assignment of tasks for every team member, patients are welcomed professionally, asked regularly about their smoking status, and continuously monitored.

A comprehensive model for smoking prevention and cessation applicable for both dental and dental hygiene education has been presented by Ramseier (2003) (Figure 3.8). This tobacco use cessation strategy is based on: (1) the model "stages of change" (or transtheoretical model) (Prochaska and DiClemente, 1983); (2) the five A's using nicotine replacement therapy (NRT) (Fiore et al., 1996); and (3) the main principles of motivational interviewing techniques (Miller and Rollnick, 2002).

In brief, the model includes recording every patient's tobacco use history, followed by a brief interview of no more than five minutes. The main aim of these interviews is to help tobacco-using patients to move from pre-contemplation to contemplation, and further to preparation, action, and maintenance stages. The routine use of a tobacco use history form as well as a record sheet to monitor tobacco use intervention is suggested (Figure 3.9). Patients' tobacco use history may be recorded on this form regarding intensity, time since cessation, and duration of each period, and they may be asked about their readiness to quit. According to a number of authors, current and former tobacco users should be asked about (1) the type of tobacco used, (2) the intensity of use (quantity per day), (3) the duration of use (years), and (4) time since cessation (years) (Dietrich and Hoffmann, 2004; Ramseier, 2003).

The evidence-based perspective: Evidence from a systematic review (Carr and Ebbert, 2007) suggests that behavioral interventions for tobacco use conducted by oral health professionals incorporating an oral exam component in the dental office and community setting increase tobacco abstinence rates.

Behavioral Support

People who want to kick the smoking habit do not always take part in state-of-the-art nicotine withdrawal programs in linear fashion from start to finish. Nevertheless, simple instructions, such as those offered in the "Assist" and "Arrange" programs, can be a valuable tool for physicians supporting patients in their attempts to quit smoking.

Some smokers are so euphoric about stopping smoking that they tend to move from one step to the next in a premature, i.e., unprepared manner. Even if this approach works for some smokers, others require varying amounts of behavioral support. This behavioral support can be given in an individual manner by adopting the following steps:

1. Asking the patient to complete a tobacco use journal (Figure 3.10): Every smoker has his individual smoking habits. To pinpoint the behavioral changes required in the particular case, it is advisable to keep a tobacco use journal for several days.

2. Evaluate the tobacco use journal: Reading through the journal entries later, the patient will notice smoking patterns and assessments of which she was previously unaware. These can serve as the basis for deciding which habits she must change to give up smoking (ideally without withdrawal symptoms) and replace the old habit with new patterns of behavior. During the control period, it is advisable to reduce nicotine consumption only down to a level where the "sacrifice" is bearable.

3. Behavioral changes: The process of successfully replacing smoking habits with other activities can be difficult and time consuming. Each patient should name an action that is good for him. It might be wise to arrange additional consultations at this point so that enough time can be devoted to this important step.

Pharmacotherapy

Kotlyar and Hatsukami (2002) have reviewed the management of nicotine addiction (Kotlyar and Hatsukami, 2002). The use of nicotine replacement therapy in dental tobacco use cessation was recently reviewed by Ramseier (2003) and Christen et al. (2003) (Ramseier, 2003; Christen et al., 2003). On the quit date, the patients should be sent home from the dental practice as "former smokers." It may be worthwhile to give each individual patient a written recommendation con-

Tobacco Use Cessation (TUC) care pathway for dental practice

www.tobacco-oralhealth.net/workshop2005

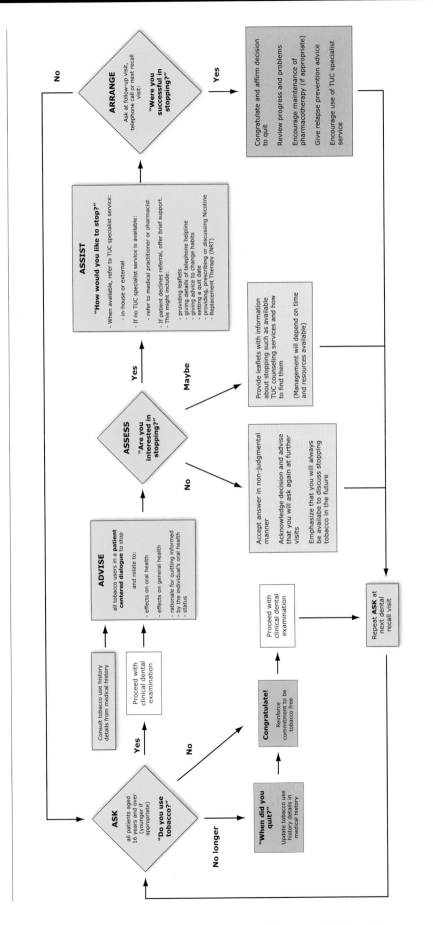

Figure 3.8. Tobacco use cessation care pathway for the dental practice.

Tobacco use history

Last / first name: _____   Date: _____

1.	Have you ever smoked more than 200 cigarettes?	☐ yes ☐ no (go on with question 6)
2.	At what age did you start to smoke regularly?	_____ years
3.	Are you currently smoking cigarettes?	☐ yes (go on with question 5) ☐ no
4.	In which year did you quit smoking?	_____
5.	How many cigarettes do you smoke per day?	_____
6.	Have you used other tobacco products regularly?	☐ no (go on with question 8) ☐ yes, the following: **Cigar** ☐ never ☐ in the past ☐ now **Pipe** ☐ never ☐ in the past ☐ now **Chewing tobacco** ☐ never ☐ in the past ☐ now **Other** ☐ never ☐ in the past ☐ now
7.	How often have you already tried quitting tobacco use?	☐ never ☐ once ☐ 2 - 4 times ☐ more than _____ times
8.	Are you currently thinking of quitting tobacco use?	☐ no ☐ yes, within the next _____ months
9.	**Personal information** a. Age b. Sex	Date of birth: _____ ☐ female ☐ male

Figure 3.9. Tobacco use history form.

TOBACCO USE JOURNAL

Date: _____

Cig.	Time	Place or activity	Accompanied by	Importance	Alternative
1					
2					
3					
3					
4					
5					
6					
7					
8					
9					
10					

Front

TOBACCO USE JOURNAL

Date: _____

Cig.	Time	Place or activity	Accompanied by	Importance	Alternative
11					
12					
13					
13					
14					
15					
16					
17					
18					
19					
20					

Back

Figure 3.10. Tobacco use journal.

cerning the use of nicotine replacement products during the next three months (Figure 3.11).

There are various nicotine replacement products on the market such as gum, patches, sublingual tablets, inhalators, and nasal sprays. For the use of each product available, the reader is referred to the manufacturers' instructions.

The evidence-based perspective: There is strong evidence from a systematic Cochrane review that different commercially available forms of NRT can help people to quit smoking (Stead et al., 2008). NRTs increase the rate of quitting by 50% to 70%. The effectiveness of NRT seems to be largely independent of the intensity of additional support provided to the individual.

Other Risk Factor Modifications

Metabolic Control

The effects of metabolic control of diabetes mellitus on the periodontal status were evaluated exclusively on the basis of cross-sectional studies and a few prospective cohort studies. To date, the results seem to be conflicting and therefore no definite conclusion can be drawn (Bridges et al., 1996; Sastrowijoto et al., 1990; Taylor et al., 1998). From a clinical perspective, it is important to note that prevalence and severity of periodontal disease vary greatly within the diabetes mellitus population, just as it does in the non-diabetic population. Some diabetics may suffer from periodontitis because of inadequate oral hygiene and tobacco use rather than their diabetic condition (Haber et al., 1993).

Recommendation for use of Nicotine Replacement Therapy

Last name: _____   First name: _____

Level of nicotine dependency:

☐ very high
☐ high
☐ moderate
☐ low

Smoking behavior:

☐ smokes regularly through the day:
    recommendations: use of patch

☐ smokes only at specific times:
    recommendations: use of gum

From Day 1 of quitting:

	Patch (mg per day)	Gum (number per day)	others (number per day)
1st month			
2nd month			
3rd month			
After month 4			

Place, Date: _____   Signature: _____

Nicotine replacement	Low nicotine dependency	Moderate nicotine dependency	High nicotine dependency	Very high nicotine dependency
Patch		■	■ in combination with another nicotine preparation	■ in combination with another nicotine preparation
Gum	■ 2 mg	■ 2 mg	■ 4 mg	■ 4 mg
Sublingual tablets	■	■	■ in combination with patch	■ in combination with patch

Figure 3.11. Recommendations for use of nicotine replacement therapy.

To appoint the risk factor diabetes mellitus and the metabolic control of blood sugar levels in a periodontitis patient seems to be important for the understanding of the pathogenesis or the outcome of periodontal treatment. Once a patient is identified to be diabetic by a medical history a close collaboration with the diabetologist is advisable (Thorstensson et al., 1996).

Stress Reduction Therapy

Recently, an interesting approach on depression-related enhanced susceptibility of periodontitis was introduced (Breivik et al., 2006). According to this approach, treatment with an anti-depressant drug inhibited periodontal bone loss in an animal model of depression. Additionally, the individual coping behavior with stress in humans is shown to interfere with periodontal conditions (Genco et al., 1999; Wimmer et al., 2005). Coping behavioral training is likely to have a positive impact on disease severity or periodontal treatment outcomes. However, meaningful longitudinal clinical studies assessing the influence of psychological stress-related therapy on the outcome of periodontal treatment are currently not available.

Both risk factors for stress and poor coping behavior must be considered to achieve positive treatment outcomes in periodontitis patients. Once a patient is identified with stress or poor coping behavior, a close collaboration with a psychiatrist or psychologist may be advisable.

SUMMARY

Clinical research data indicate that risk factors associated with periodontitis can be identified. While certain non-modifiable factors are found, modifiable factors when amended may improve both periodontal conditions and the outcome of treatment. According to recent data, it appears reasonable to suggest that second to the removal of the bacterial biofilm, smoking cessation is the most important measure in periodontitis management. Consequently, periodontal health is to be supported by appropriate behaviors such as regular self-performed supragingival plaque control, avoidance of tobacco, and consumption of a healthy diet. The dental community involved with oral health care should gain an understanding of the health effects from inappropriate behavior to successfully target prevention and disease control. As a consequence, services for primary and secondary prevention on an individual level oriented toward the change of inappropriate behavior become a professional responsibility for all oral health care providers.

REFERENCES

Ajwani S, Ainamo A. 2001. Periodontal conditions among the old elderly: five-year longitudinal study. *Spec. Care Dentist.*, 21, 45.

Albandar JM. 2002. Global risk factors and risk indicators for periodontal diseases. *Periodontol. 2000*, 29, 177.

Albandar JM, Brunelle JA, Kingman A. 1999. Destructive periodontal disease in adults 30 years of age and older in the United States, 1988-1994. *J. Periodontol.*, 70, 13.

Armitage GC. 1999. Development of a classification system for periodontal diseases and conditions. *Ann. Periodontol.*, 4, 1.

Axelsson P, Nystrom B, Lindhe J. 2004. The long-term effect of a plaque control program on tooth mortality, caries and periodontal disease in adults. Results after 30 years of maintenance. *Journal of Clinical Periodontology*, 31, 749.

Bain CA. 1996. Smoking and implant failure—benefits of a smoking cessation protocol. *Int. J. Oral Maxillofac. Implants*, 11, 756–759.

Bergstrom J. 2004. Influence of tobacco smoking on periodontal bone height. Long-term observations and a hypothesis. *J. Clin. Periodontol.*, 31, 260–266.

Bergstrom J. 2006. Periodontitis and smoking: an evidence-based appraisal. *J. Evid. Based Dent. Pract.*, 6, 33–41.

Bergstrom J, Eliasson S, Dock J. 2000. A 10-year prospective study of tobacco smoking and periodontal health. *J. Periodontol.*, 71, 1338–1347.

Bolin A, Eklund G, Frithiof L, Lavstedt S. 1993. The effect of changed smoking habits on marginal alveolar bone loss. A longitudinal study. *Swed. Dent. J.*, 17, 211–216.

Breivik T, Gundersen Y, Myhrer T, Fonnum F, Osmundsen H, Murison R, Gjermo P, von Horsten S, Opstad PK. 2006. Enhanced susceptibility to periodontitis in an animal model of depression: reversed by chronic treatment with the anti-depressant tianeptine. *J. Clin. Periodontol.*, 33, 469.

Bridges RB, Anderson JW, Saxe SR, Gregory K, Bridges SR. 1996. Periodontal status of diabetic and non-diabetic men: effects of smoking, glycemic control, and socioeconomic factors. *J. Periodontol.*, 67, 1185.

Carr AB, Ebbert JO. 2007. Interventions for tobacco cessation in the dental setting. A systematic review. *Community Dent Health*, 24, 70–74.

Christen AG, Jay SJ, Christen JA. 2003. Tobacco cessation and nicotine replacement therapy for dental practice. *Gen Dent*, 51, 525–532.

Consensus report. 1996. Periodontal diseases: epidemiology and diagnosis. *Ann. Periodontol.*, 1, 216.

Deinzer R, Forster P, Fuck L, Herforth A, Stiller-Winkler R, Idel H. 1999. Increase of crevicular interleukin 1beta under academic stress at experimental gingivitis sites and at sites of perfect oral hygiene. *J. Clin. Periodontol.*, 26, 1.

Deinzer R, Hilpert D, Bach K, Schawacht M, Herforth A. 2001. Effects of academic stress on oral hygiene—a potential link between stress and plaque-associated disease? *J. Clin. Periodontol.*, 28, 459.

Deinzer R, Kleineidam C, Stiller-Winkler R, Idel H, Bachg D. 2000. Prolonged reduction of salivary immunoglobulin A (sIgA) after a major academic exam. *Int. J. Psychophysiol.*, 37, 219.

Diel IJ, Bergner R, Grotz KA. 2007. Adverse effects of bisphosphonates: current issues. *J. Support. Oncol.*, 5, 475.

Dietrich T, Bernimoulin JP, Glynn RJ. 2004. The effect of cigarette smoking on gingival bleeding. *J. Periodontol*, 75, 16–22.

Dietrich T, Hoffmann K. 2004. A comprehensive index for the modeling of smoking history in periodontal research. *J. Dent. Res.*, 83, 859–863.

Dietrich T, Kaye EK, Nunn ME, Van DT, Garcia RI. 2006. Gingivitis susceptibility and its relation to periodontitis in men. *J. Dent. Res.*, 85, 1134.

Dorsky R. 2001. Nutrition and oral health. *Gen. Dent.*, 49, 576–582.

Duarte PM, Neto JB, Casati MZ, Sallum EA, Nociti Jr. FH. 2007. Diabetes modulates gene expression in the gingival tissues of patients with chronic periodontitis. *Oral Dis.*, 13, 594.

Eklund SA, Burt BA. 1994. Risk factors for total tooth loss in the United States; longitudinal analysis of national data. *J. Public Health Dent.*, 54, 5–14.

Emrich LJ, Shlossman M, Genco RJ. 1991. Periodontal disease in non-insulin-dependent diabetes mellitus. *J. Periodontol.*, 62, 123.

Engebretson S, Chertog R, Nichols A, Hey-Hadavi J, Celenti R, Grbic J. 2007. Plasma levels of tumour necrosis factor-alpha in patients with chronic periodontitis and type 2 diabetes. *J. Clin. Periodontol.*, 34, 18.

Engebretson SP, Hey-Hadavi J, Ehrhardt FJ, Hsu D, Celenti RS, Grbic JT, Lamster IB. 2004. Gingival crevicular fluid levels of interleukin-1beta and glycemic control in patients with chronic periodontitis and type 2 diabetes. *J. Periodontol.*, 75, 1203.

Erley KJ, Swiec GD, Herold R, Bisch FC, Peacock ME. 2006. Gingival recession treatment with connective tissue grafts in smokers and non-smokers. *J. Periodontol.*, 77, 1148–1155.

Fiore MC. 2000. US public health service clinical practice guideline: treating tobacco use and dependence. *Respir. Care*, 45, 1200–1262.

Fiore MC, Bailey WC, Cohen SJ. 1996. *Smoking cessation: clinical practice guideline, No. 18*. Rockville, MD: U.S. Department for Health Care Policy and Research.

Genco RJ, Ho AW, Grossi SG, Dunford RG, Tedesco LA. 1999. Relationship of stress, distress and inadequate coping behaviors to periodontal disease. *J. Periodontol.*, 70, 711.

Haber J, Wattles J, Crowley M, Mandell R, Joshipura K, Kent RL. 1993. Evidence for cigarette smoking as a major risk factor for periodontitis. *J. Periodontol.*, 64, 16.

Heasman L, Stacey F, Preshaw PM, McCracken GI, Hepburn S, Heasman PA. 2006. The effect of smoking on periodontal treatment response: a review of clinical evidence. *J. Clin. Periodontol.*, 33, 241–253.

Holm-Pedersen P, Vigild M, Nitschke I, Berkey DB. 2005. Dental care for aging populations in Denmark, Sweden, Norway, United kingdom, and Germany. *J. Dent. Educ.*, 69, 987.

Hugo FN, Hilgert JB, Bozzetti MC, Bandeira DR, Goncalves TR, Pawlowski J, de Sousa ML. 2006. Chronic stress, depression, and cortisol levels as risk indicators of elevated plaque and gingivitis levels in individuals aged 50 years and older. *J. Periodontol.*, 77, 1008.

Hugoson A, Ljungquist B, Breivik T. 2002. The relationship of some negative events and psychological factors to periodontal disease in an adult Swedish population 50 to 80 years of age. *J. Clin. Periodontol.*, 29, 247.

Hujoel PP, Powell LV, Kiyak HA. 1997. The effects of simple interventions on tooth mortality: findings in one trial and implications for future studies. *J. Dent. Res.*, 76, 867.

Huynh-Ba G, Lang NP, Tonetti MS, Salvi GE. 2007. The association of the composite IL-1 genotype with periodontitis progression and/or treatment outcomes: a systematic review. *J. Clin. Periodontol.*, 34, 305–317.

Ishisaka A, Ansai T, Soh I, Inenaga K, Yoshida A, Shigeyama C, Awano S, Hamasaki T, Sonoki K, Takata Y, Takehara T. 2007. Association of salivary levels of cortisol and dehydroepiandrosterone with periodontitis in older Japanese adults. *J. Periodontol.*, 78, 1767.

Iwamoto Y, Nishimura F, Nakagawa M, Sugimoto H, Shikata K, Makino H, Fukuda T, Tsuji T, Iwamoto M, Murayama Y. 2001. The effect of antimicrobial periodontal treatment on circulating tumor necrosis factor-alpha and glycated hemoglobin level in patients with type 2 diabetes. *J. Periodontol.*, 72, 774.

Johannsen A, Rylander G, Soder B, Asberg M. 2006. Dental plaque, gingival inflammation, and elevated levels of interleukin-6 and cortisol in gingival crevicular fluid from women with stress-related depression and exhaustion. *J. Periodontol.*, 77, 1403.

Johnson GK, Guthmiller JM. 2007. The impact of cigarette smoking on periodontal disease and treatment. *Periodontol. 2000*, 44, 178–194.

Jordan RA, Gangler P, Johren HP. 2006. Clinical treatment outcomes of periodontal therapy in HIV-seropositive patients undergoing highly active antiretroviral therapy. *Eur. J. Med. Res.*, 11, 232–235.

Kaldahl WB, Johnson GK, Patil KD, Kalkwarf KL. 1996. Levels of cigarette consumption and response to periodontal therapy. *J. Periodontol.*, 67, 675–681.

Katz J, Bhattacharyya I, Farkhondeh-Kish F, Perez FM, Caudle RM, Heft MW. 2005. Expression of the receptor of advanced glycation end products in gingival tissues of type 2 diabetes patients with chronic periodontal disease: a study utilizing immunohistochemistry and RT-PCR. *J. Clin. Periodontol.*, 32, 40.

Khader YS, Dauod AS, El-Qaderi SS, Alkafajei A, Batayha WQ. 2006. Periodontal status of diabetics compared with nondiabetics: a meta-analysis. *J. Diabetes Complications*, 20, 59–68.

Kotlyar M, Hatsukami DK. 2002. Managing nicotine addiction. *J. Dent. Educ.*, 66, 1061–1073.

Kovar M, Jany Z, Erdelsky I. 1985. Influence of the menstrual cycle on the gingival microcirculation. *Czech. Med.*, 8, 98.

Krall EA. 2001. The periodontal-systemic connection: implications for treatment of patients with osteoporosis and periodontal disease. *Ann. Periodontol.*, 6, 209–213.

Krall EA, Dawson-Hughes B, Garvey AJ, Garcia RI. 1997. Smoking, smoking cessation, and tooth loss. *J. Dent. Res.*, 76, 1653–1659.

Krejci CB, Bissada NF. 2002. Women's health issues and their relationship to periodontitis. *J. Am. Dent. Assoc.*, 133, 323.

Kroidl A, Schaeben A, Oette M, Wettstein M, Herfordt A, Haussinger D. 2005. Prevalence of oral lesions and periodontal diseases in HIV-infected patients on antiretroviral therapy. *Eur. J. Med. Res.*, 10, 448–453.

Laine MA. 2002. Effect of pregnancy on periodontal and dental health. *Acta Odontol. Scand.*, 60, 257.

Lamster IB, Begg MD, Mitchell-Lewis D, Fin, JB, Grbic JT, Todak GG, el-Sadr W, Gorman JM, Zambon JJ, Phelan JA. 1994. Oral manifestations of HIV infection in homosexual men and intravenous drug users. Study design and relationship of epidemiologic, clinical, and immunologic parameters to oral lesions. *Oral Surg. Oral Med. Oral Pathol.*, 78, 163–174.

Lang NP, Kiel RA, Anderhalden K. 1983. Clinical and microbiological effects of subgingival restorations with overhanging or clinically perfect margins. *J. Clin. Periodontol.*, 10, 563.

Lerner UH. 2006. Inflammation-induced bone remodeling in periodontal disease and the influence of post-menopausal osteoporosis. *J. Dent. Res.*, 85, 596.

Loos BG, John RP, Laine ML. 2005. Identification of genetic risk factors for periodontitis and possible mechanisms of action. *J. Clin. Periodontol.*, 32 Suppl 6, 159.

Madianos PN, Bobetsis GA, Kinane DF. 2002. Is periodontitis associated with an increased risk of coronary heart disease and preterm and/or low birth weight births? *J. Clin. Periodontol.*, 29 Suppl 3, 22.

Magnusson I, Lindhe J, Yoneyama T, Liljenberg B. 1984. Recolonization of a subgingival microbiota following scaling in deep pockets. *J. Clin. Periodontol.*, 11, 193.

Manouchehr-Pour M, Spagnuolo PJ, Rodman HM, Bissada NF. 1981a. Comparison of neutrophil chemotactic response in diabetic patients with mild and severe periodontal disease. *J. Periodontol.*, 52, 410.

Manouchehr-Pour M, Spagnuolo PJ, Rodman HM, Bissada NF. 1981b. Impaired neutrophil chemotaxis in diabetic patients with severe periodontitis. *J. Dent. Res.*, 60, 729.

McKaig RG, Thomas JC, Patton LL, Strauss RP, Slade GD, Beck JD. 1998. Prevalence of HIV-associated periodontitis and chronic periodontitis in a southeastern US study group. *J. Public Health Dent.*, 58, 294–300.

Meisel P, Reifenberger J, Haase R, Nauck M, Bandt C, Kocher T. 2007. Women are periodontally healthier than men, but why don't they have more teeth than men? *Menopause.* 2008 Mar–Apr;15(2), 270–5.

Meisel P, Schwahn C, Gesch D, Bernhardt O, John U, Kocher T. 2004. Dose-effect relation of smoking and the interleukin-1 gene polymorphism in periodontal disease. *J. Periodontol*, 75, 236–242.

Michalowicz BS, Aeppli D, Virag JG, Klump DG, Hinrichs JE, Segal NL, Bouchard Jr. TJ, Pihlstrom BL. 1991. Periodontal findings in adult twins. *J. Periodontol.*, 62, 293–299.

Michalowicz BS, Diehl SR, Gunsolley JC, Sparks BS, Brooks CN, Koertge TE, Califano JV, Burmeister JA, Schenkein HA. 2000. Evidence of a substantial genetic basis for risk of adult periodontitis. *J. Periodontol.*, 71, 1699–1707.

Miller WR, Rollnick S. 2002. *Motivational Interviewing*. New York, Guilford Press.

Nakajima K, Hamada N, Takahashi Y, Sasaguri K, Tsukinoki K, Umemoto T, Sato S. 2006. Restraint stress enhances alveolar bone loss in an experimental rat model. *J. Periodontal Res.*, 41, 527.

Nishida M, Grossi SG, Dunford RG, Ho AW, Trevisan M, Genco RJ. 2000a. Calcium and the risk for periodontal disease. *J. Periodontol.*, 71, 1057–1066.

Nishida M, Grossi SG, Dunford RG, Ho AW, Trevisan M, Genco RJ. 2000b. Dietary vitamin C and the risk for periodontal disease. *J. Periodontol.*, 71, 1215–1223.

Oliver RC, Brown LJ, Loe H. 1998. Periodontal diseases in the United States population. *J. Periodontol.*, 69, 269.

Oliver RC, Tervonen T. 1994. Diabetes—a risk factor for periodontitis in adults? *J. Periodontol.*, 65, 530.

Ower P. 2003. The role of self-administered plaque control in the management of periodontal diseases: I. A review of the evidence. *Dent. Update*, 30, 60–64, 66, 68.

Page RC, Kornman KS. 1997. The pathogenesis of human periodontitis: an introduction. *Periodontol. 2000*, 14, 9.

Palmer RM. 2005. Should quit smoking interventions be the first part of initial periodontal therapy? *J. Clin. Periodontol.*, 32, 867–868.

Papapanou PN. 1996. Periodontal diseases: epidemiology. *Ann. Periodontol.*, 1, 1.

Papapanou PN, Wennstrom JL, Grondahl K. 1989. A 10-year retrospective study of periodontal disease progression. *J. Clin. Periodontol.*, 16, 403.

Paulander J, Wennstrom JL, Axelsson P, Lindhe J. 2004. Some risk factors for periodontal bone loss in 50-year-old individuals. A 10-year cohort study. *J Clin Periodontol*, 31, 489–496.

Payne JB, Reinhardt RA, Nummikoski PV, Patil KD. 1999. Longitudinal alveolar bone loss in postmenopausal osteoporotic/osteopenic women. *Osteoporos. Int.*, 10, 34.

Persson GR. 2006. What has ageing to do with periodontal health and disease? *Int. Dent. J.*, 56, 240–249.

Preshaw PM, Heasman L, Stacey F, Steen N, McCracken GI, Heasman PA. 2005. The effect of quitting smoking on chronic periodontitis. *J. Clin. Periodontol.*, 32, 869–879.

Prochaska JO, DiClemente CC. 1983. Stages and processes of self-change of smoking: toward an integrative model of change. *J. Consult. Clin. Psychol.*, 51, 390–395.

Ramseier CA. 2003. Smoking prevention and cessation. *Oral Health Prev. Dent.*, 1 Suppl 1, 427–439; discussion 440–422.

Reichart P. 2006. US1 HIV—changing patterns in HAART era, patients' quality of life and occupational risks. *Oral Dis.*, 12 Suppl 1, 3.

Reinhardt RA, Payne JB, Maze CA, Patil KD, Gallagher SJ, Mattson JS. 1999. Influence of estrogen and osteopenia/osteoporosis on clinical periodontitis in postmenopausal women. *J. Periodontol.*, 70, 823.

Roberts A, Matthews JB, Socransky SS, Freestone PP, Williams PH, Chapple IL. 2002. Stress and the periodontal diseases: effects of catecholamines on the growth of periodontal bacteria in vitro. *Oral Microbiol. Immunol.*, 17, 296.

Rosling B, Nyman S, Lindhe J. 1976. The effect of systematic plaque control on bone regeneration in infrabony pockets. *J. Clin. Periodontol.*, 3, 38.

Roussa E. 1998. Anatomic characteristics of the furcation and root surfaces of molar teeth and their significance in the clinical management of marginal periodontitis. *Clin. Anat.*, 11, 177.

Russell SL, Mayberry LJ. 2008. Pregnancy and oral health: a review and recommendations to reduce gaps in practice and research. *MCN. Am. J. Matern. Child Nurs.*, 33, 32–37.

Ryder MI. 2007. The influence of smoking on host responses in periodontal infections. *Periodontol. 2000*, 43, 267–277.

Salvi GE, Collins JG, Yalda B, Arnold RR, Lang NP, Offenbacher S. 1997a. Monocytic TNF alpha secretion patterns in IDDM patients with periodontal diseases. *J. Clin. Periodontol.*, 24, 8.

Salvi GE, Yalda B, Collins JG, Jones BH, Smith FW, Arnold RR, Offenbacher S. 1997b. Inflammatory mediator response as a potential risk marker for periodontal diseases in insulin-dependent diabetes mellitus patients. *J. Periodontol.*, 68, 127.

Sanz M, Lau L, Herrera D, Morillo JM, Silva A. 2004. Methods of detection of Actinobacillus actinomycetemcomitans, Porphyromonas gingivalis and Tannerella forsythensis in periodontal microbiology, with special emphasis on advanced molecular techniques: a review. *J. Clin. Periodontol.*, 31, 1034.

Sastrowijoto SH, Abbas F, Abbraham-Inpijn L, van der Velden U. 1990. Relationship between bleeding/plaque ratio, family history of diabetes mellitus and impaired glucose tolerance. *J. Clin. Periodontol.*, 17, 55.

Schatzle M, Loe H, Burgin W, Anerud A, Boysen H, Lang NP. 2003. Clinical course of chronic periodontitis. I. Role of gingivitis. *J. Clin. Periodontol.*, 30, 887.

Shlossman M, Knowler WC, Pettitt DJ, Genco RJ. 1990. Type 2 diabetes mellitus and periodontal disease. *J. Am. Dent. Assoc.*, 121, 532.

Socransky SS, Haffajee AD. 2002. Dental biofilms: difficult therapeutic targets. *Periodontol. 2000*, 28, 12.

Stead LF, Perera R, Bullen C, Mant D, Lancaster T. 2008. Nicotine replacement therapy for smoking cessation. *Cochrane Database Syst. Rev.*, CD000146.

Stolk RP, Rosmalen JG, Postma DS, de Boer RA, Navis G, Slaets JP, Ormel J, Wolffenbuttel BH. 2008. Universal risk factors for multifactorial diseases: LifeLines: a three-generation population-based study. *Eur. J. Epidemiol.*, 23, 67.

Strietzel FP, Reichart PA, Kale A, Kulkarni M, Wegner B, Kuchler I. 2007. Smoking interferes with the prognosis of dental implant treatment: a systematic review and meta-analysis. *J. Clin. Periodontol.*, 34, 523–544.

Taylor GW, Burt BA, Becker MP, Genco RJ, Shlossman M. 1998. Glycemic control and alveolar bone loss progression in type 2 diabetes. *Ann. Periodontol.*, 3, 30.

Theilade E, Wright WH, Jensen SB, Loe H. 1966. Experimental gingivitis in man. II. A longitudinal clinical and bacteriological investigation. *J. Periodontal Res.*, 1, 1.

Thorstensson H, Hugoson A. 1993. Periodontal disease experience in adult long-duration insulin-dependent diabetics. *J. Clin. Periodontol.*, 20, 352.

Thorstensson H, Kuylenstierna J, Hugoson A. 1996. Medical status and complications in relation to periodontal disease experience in insulin-dependent diabetics. *J. Clin. Periodontol.*, 23, 194.

Tonetti MS. 1998. Cigarette smoking and periodontal diseases: etiology and management of disease. *Ann. Periodontol.*, 3, 88–101.

van der Velden U, Abbas F, Armand S, de Graaff J, Timmerman MF, van der Weijden GA, van Winkelhoff AJ, Winkel E. 1993. The effect of sibling relationship on the periodontal condition. *J. Clin. Periodontol.*, 20, 683–690.

Verma S, Bhat KM. 2004. Diabetes mellitus—a modifier of periodontal disease expression. *J. Int. Acad. Periodontol.*, 6, 13.

Vermylen K, De Quincey GN, Wolffe GN, van 't Hof MA, Renggli HH. 2005. Root proximity as a risk marker for periodontal disease: a case-control study. *J. Clin. Periodontol.*, 32, 260.

Wautier JL, Guillausseau PJ. 1998. Diabetes, advanced glycation end-products and vascular disease. *Vasc. Med.*, 3, 131.

Westfelt E, Rylander H, Blohme G, Jonasson P, Lindhe J. 1996. The effect of periodontal therapy in diabetics. Results after 5 years. *J. Clin. Periodontol.*, 23, 92.

Willershausen-Zonnchen B, Lemmen C, Hamm G. 1991. Influence of high glucose concentrations on glycosaminoglycan and collagen synthesis in cultured human gingival fibroblasts. *J. Clin. Periodontol.*, 18, 190.

Wimmer G, Janda M, Wieselmann-Penkner K, Jakse N, Polansky R, Pertl C. 2002. Coping with stress: its influence on periodontal disease. *J. Periodontol.*, 73, 1343.

Wimmer G, Kohldorfer G, Mischak I, Lorenzoni M, Kallus KW. 2005. Coping with stress: its influence on periodontal therapy. *J. Periodontol.*, 76, 90.

Chapter 4 Scaling and Root Planing

INTRODUCTION

Ever since Loe demonstrated the role that plaque plays in the development of gingivitis (Loe et al., 1965; Theilade et al., 1966) there has been an emphasis on plaque removal as the primary goal of non-surgical periodontal therapy. With the confirmation that microorganisms are involved in the initiation and progression of periodontal infections, studies have examined the efficacy of various modalities of treatment to eliminate or suppress these microorganisms and reverse the inflammatory changes or damage to the periodontium. Manual scaling and root planing (SRP) are considered the basis of periodontal treatment and as such are often the control to which other modalities are compared. This chapter provides an evidence-based understanding of what can and cannot be achieved with scaling and root planing and how its effectiveness can be optimized.

Scaling refers to the removal of hard and soft deposits from the crown and root surfaces. Root planing denotes the removal of cementum and dentin that is rough or impregnated with bacteria, endotoxins, and calculus to produce a root surface that is smooth and hard. SRP can be performed as either a closed or open procedure. An open procedure differs from a closed one in that it denotes reflection of the gingival tissues, allowing direct visualization of the root surface—this is also known as surgical scaling.

The general purpose of SRP is to reduce or eliminate plaque-associated gingival inflammation (Figure 4.1). Specifically, this is achieved by mechanical instrumentation of the affected root surfaces. The result of this instrumentation is a reduction of bacterial plaque via disruption and/or removal of the microbial biofilm, the removal of accretions from the root surface, and ultimately a shift in the ecology of the pocket from one that favors disease to one that is conducive to health.

Instruments that can be used for scaling can be either manual or power-driven. Power-driven types can be sonic or ultrasonic, rotating instruments such as fine-grained diamonds, reciprocating instruments represented by the Profin Directional System, or lasers. The most commonly used and studied instruments for mechanical debridement are manual scalers and sonic or ultrasonic scalers.

INSTRUMENTATION

Manual Scalers

All manual instruments have three sections: (1) the handle, (2) the shank, which can have bends, and (3) the working end or blade (Figure 4.2). The various scalers differ primarily in the number and angle of bends at the shank, and the shape, curvature, and number of cutting edges at the blade. There are five major classifications: sickle, curette, file, hoe, and chisel. The most commonly used are the sickle and curette. The design of a sickle scaler enables it to be used effectively for supragingival calculus removal, while curettes are better suited for subgingival application.

The working end of a sickle scaler is triangular in cross-section, coming to a point at the tip. The blade faces up and is angled 90 degrees to the terminal shank with cutting edges on both sides of the face. This shape facilitates removal of heavy calculus and access to the area associated with the gingival embrasure and the proximal contact, which can be quite narrow. It is also very useful as an initial instrument to remove large, heavy deposits of supragingival calculus, thus improving access to the subgingival areas with the curettes. While sickle-type scalers are very effective at supragingival sites, they are not designed to be used at subgingival sites because the sharp tip can easily traumatize gingival tissues and gouge the root surface. Furthermore, the blade shape does not adapt well against the often concave, subgingival root anatomy (Figure 4.3).

Accessing the complex subgingival anatomy and minimizing damage to the delicate sulcular tissues is better achieved with curettes. Curettes are subdivided into two types, universal and Gracey. The main difference is that Gracey curettes are area specific; this specificity is realized via differences in the working ends. Gracey curettes have bends in the shank to facilitate access to either of the four sides of a tooth: mesial, distal, oral, or facial. In addition, the face of the blade is angled down 120 degrees to the terminal shank and only the lower side of the blade is sharpened. Thus, the Gracey 11/12 curette is designed to scale only the mesial surfaces of molars and premolars, while the Gracey 13/14 is specific to the distal surfaces (Figure 4.4). On the other hand, the universal curettes are not area-specific; the same instrument

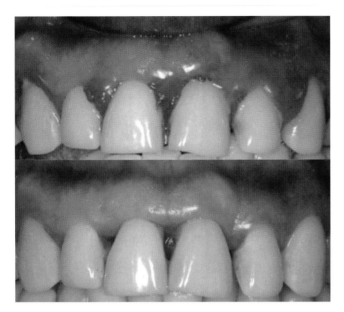

Figure 4.1. One month follow-up demonstrating resolution of gingival inflammation after scaling and root planing.

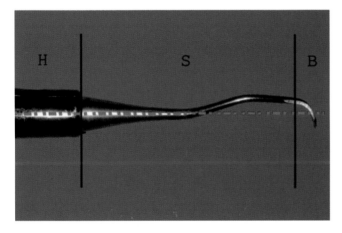

Figure 4.2. Scaler design. H: handle, S: shank, B: blade. Note that the blade is centered to the handle for ideal force transmission.

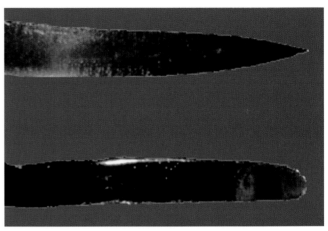

Figure 4.3. Contrast between the sharp tip of a sickle scaler (above) and the rounded toe of a curette (below).

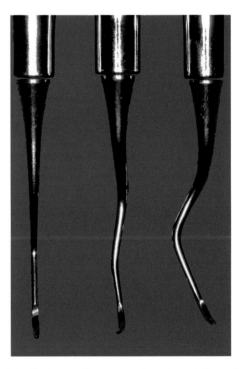

Figure 4.4. Series of Gracey scalers from left to right: 1/2 (anteriors), 11/12 (mesial of posteriors), and 13/14 (distal of posteriors). Note the increasing angle of bends in the shank to allow access to more posterior sites.

can be used anteriorly or posteriorly and for any of the four sides of the tooth. This is because both sides of the blade are sharpened and the angle of the face to the terminal shank is 90 degrees (Figure 4.5). Neither is objectively better than the other and thus operator preference based on an understanding of the instrument's design and the dental anatomy being scaled determines which instrument is best for any particular circumstance.

Power-driven Scalers

Power-driven scalers are classified as either sonic or ultrasonic; the ultrasonic variety are sub-classified as magnetostrictive or piezoelectric. They are broadly distinguished according to the type of tip movement and tip vibration frequency. The sonic scalers operate at low frequencies ranging from 3,000 to 8,000 cycles per second (Cps) with a tip movement that is generally orbital, while both types of ultrasonic scalers operate at much higher frequencies. The magnetostrictive range is from 18,000 to 45,000 Cps with an elliptical tip movement, while piezoelectric units have a Cps in the 25,000 to 50,000 range and a tip movement that is generally linear.

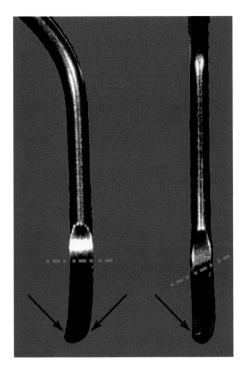

Figure 4.5. Key differences in blade design between universal and Gracey curettes. Universal: the face of the blade is 90 degrees to the shank (red dotted line) with both sides sharpened (arrows). Gracey: the face is angled 120 degrees to the shank (red dotted line) with only the lower side of the blade sharpened (arrow).

Sonic and ultrasonic instruments were originally only used for supragingival plaque, calculus, and stain removal. They were found to leave an uneven root surface, and thus it was thought that manual root planing was required following ultrasonic scaling to smooth the root surface. Over the years, there have been many modifications in the instruments, including smaller tip diameters, longer working lengths, different angles, and diamond coatings. These developments, along with a better, evidence-based understanding of the root surface alterations, has allowed powered scalers to be used safely and effectively in deep subgingival probing depths and difficult anatomy such as furcations, without having to be supplemented with subsequent manual instrumentation.

It should be noted that manual and sonic/ultrasonic scalers are used in a very different manner. The blade of a curette is inserted within the sulcus apical to the deposit at the base of the pocket. The calculus is then engaged and removed as the scaler is pulled coronally out of the sulcus. On the other hand, sonic and ultrasonic scalers engage the deposit at its coronal extent. The instrument is inserted within the pocket like a dental probe, with the working end parallel to the root surface and the tip pointing into the sulcus. Calculus is removed with multiple, light apically directed strokes. It is beyond the scope of this chapter to discuss how each instru-

ment is used and maintained. However, it should be understood that all scalers are technique sensitive. It is critical that the clinician be fully aware of an instrument's design and its proper use because incorrect application of a scaler will result in poor calculus removal and damage to the root surface or gingival tissues.

Manual vs. Power-driven Scalers

The advances in ultrasonic and sonic instrument design and the expansion of their use to subgingival sites has resulted in a body of literature that compares their effectiveness with hand scalers. These studies have examined the efficacy of the debridement to bring about improvements in clinical endpoints such as probing depth and bleeding on probing, as well as shifts in the microbiological profile of the sulcus. Researchers have also considered alterations to the root surface and whether there is any advantage with powered scalers in accessing difficult anatomy or reducing the time required to effect this debridement.

Clinical Endpoints

Generally, the studies show that there is no statistical difference in clinical endpoints such as reduction in bleeding on probing, pocket depth reduction, attachment level gain, and reduction in sites with plaque (Loos et al., 1987; Badersten et al., 1984; Copulos et al., 1993; Boretti et al., 1995; Laurell and Pettersson, 1998). The reduction in probing depths with sonic or ultrasonic instruments ranges from 1.2 mm to 2.7 mm (Drisco et al., 1996). This compares favorably with the reductions achieved with manual scalers of 1.29 mm to 2.16 mm (Cobb, 1996). The microbiological changes are related to the clinical outcomes. Here, as well, there does not appear to be a clear difference between the two types of debridement; both treatments result in similar shifts in the microbial flora (Baehni et al., 1992; Oosterwaal et al., 1987).

Access to the Base of the Pocket or Difficult Anatomy

In relation to the similarity in clinical and microbiological endpoints achieved, it should be noted that in their systematic review, Tunkel et al. point out that most studies comparing powered and manual scaling are either done on single-rooted teeth or they group the results of single- and multi-rooted teeth, and that more research is required to assess the efficacy of powered instrumentation on multi-rooted teeth (Tunkel et al., 2002). In this regard there is evidence that suggests that ultrasonic instruments have an advantage over hand scalers for the debridement of furcations (Leon et al., 1987; Oda et al., 1989). These studies have found that both types of instruments are equally efficacious in Class I furcations, but in Class II and III situations the ultrasonic scalers are more effective. If one considers that anatomical studies have found that the entrance to a furcation is often smaller

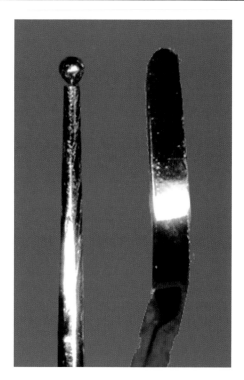

Figure 4.6. The smaller tip size of an ultrasonic scaler (left), designed for access into a furcation, contrasted with a curette (right).

than the width of a curette (Bower, 1979), then it is not surprising that specialized ultrasonic tips with widths of 0.55 mm or less would have an advantage (Figure 4.6).

Other modifications of ultrasonic tips are designed to allow improved penetration into the base of deep pockets. These tips, which are slimmer and probe-like in shape, can reach closer to the base of the pocket (0.78 mm) than manual curettes (1.25 mm) (Dragoo, 1992). This result was confirmed recently by Barendregt et al., who also found that ultrasonic tips penetrated deeper, particularly in moderate (4 mm to 6 mm) and severe (≥7 mm) pockets (Barendregt et al., 2008).

In both of these papers, the greater penetration depth for ultrasonic scalers was on untreated periodontitis patients. The relevance of this point is highlighted by the Barendregt paper, which found that unlike the results observed for the periodontitis group, the maintenance group (less inflamed gingival tissue) showed equal penetration depth for manual curettes and ultrasonic instruments. It is likely that in the periodontitis group some of the greater depth reached by the ultrasonic scaler could be explained as ingress of the ultrasonic tip through the epithelial attachment and into the connective tissue. This has been observed when using a periodontal probe to measure pocket depth in inflamed tissues where the difference in probing depths between treated and untreated pockets amounted to approximately 1.2 mm (Fowler et al., 1982). Even if all of the deeper access

cannot be explained by connective tissue invasion, it has yet to be established if greater penetration translates to improved calculus and plaque removal.

Where studies have shown clear differences is in the time required to clean the root surface. A review of the evidence indicates that manual instrumentation takes 20% to 50% longer to achieve the same clinical results as with powered scaling (Cobb, 1996).

Surface Roughness and Cementum Removal

Since the introduction of sonic/ultrasonic instruments there have been investigations to determine if these instruments remove less or more root surface than hand scalers, as well as the smoothness of the resultant surface. Recent evidence suggests that ultrasonic scalers remove less cementum (Vastardis et al., 2005; Ritz et al., 1991) but leave a rougher surface than curettes (Kocher et al., 2001; Schlageter et al., 1996). However, as will be discussed later, the clinical significance of a rougher surface has yet to be elucidated. Irrespective, sonic and ultrasonic instrumentation can result in excessive cementum removal if used improperly. Increasing instrument pressure, contact time, or tip to tooth angle can all cause more root damage. In this regard it has been suggested that the ultrasonic scaler be used at low or medium power with multiple, *light* overlapping strokes and with the tip angled parallel to the root surface (Flemmig et al., 1997). The importance of light strokes is underlined by a study which found that increasing the application force from 0.3 N to 0.7 N resulted in a twofold increase in root surface loss (Jespen et al., 2004).

Summary

In general, studies have found that a comparison of clinical endpoints shows manual and power-driven instruments to be equally effective. Thus, if the desired therapeutic outcome is reduction in inflammation, reduction in probing depth, and removal of root surface accretion, then either manual or powered instruments can be used. Despite these findings, powered scalers demonstrate some advantages, particularly with respect to time efficiency and access to challenging root anatomy. It remains to be seen if continued advances in tip design and ultrasonic energy generators will further improve the efficacy of these instruments.

SCALING AND ROOT PLANING

Objectives

As indicated above, effective scaling and root planing can be achieved by either powered or manual instrumentation. Although advances in technology may engender advantages to one instrument or the other, the focus of the therapy remains constant: the primary objective of mechanical non-surgical therapy is the removal of bacterial plaque from the tooth surface. This is affected by removal of the soft microbial biofilm on the root surface as well as the hard accretions or calculus that harbor bacteria within their structure. With this mechanical reduction or disturbance of the microbial community, we expect resolution of the inflammatory changes in the tissues of the periodontium, which in turn precipitate a change in the local environment of the sulcus from one that supports inflammatory destruction to one that is conducive to the maintenance of periodontal health.

To gain a holistic understanding of mechanical non-surgical therapy we need to consider not only the response of the periodontium to our hygiene efforts but also the factors that modify this response. In this way we can better optimize our results as well as understand the limits of and limitations on this form of therapy.

Changes in Clinical Endpoints

The most common endpoints used to evaluate the clinical outcome of mechanical therapy are probing pocket depth and clinical attachment level. Although there is only a weak correlation between bleeding on probing and continued disease activity (Lang et al., 1990), decreases in the percentage of bleeding sites continue to be considered a surrogate indicator for the resolution of gingival inflammation. In this regard it is useful to note that collectively, studies investigating all forms of mechanical therapy show reductions in gingival inflammation by 45% in 4-mm to 6.5-mm pockets (Cobb, 2002). In addition, this resolution of inflammation is affected largely by subgingival instrumentation, with supragingival plaque control alone providing little or no benefit (Cobb, 2002).

Many researchers have investigated the effect of scaling and root planing on probing depth and clinical attachment level. Cobb conducted a review of these papers and presented the results of the collective data reported in these studies (Figure 4.7). He found that in sites with initial probing depths of 1 mm to 3 mm there was a pocket depth reduction of 0.03 mm with a loss in clinical attachment of 0.34 mm. At sites measuring 4 mm to 6 mm the probing depth reduction was 1.3 mm with a gain of 0.55 mm in the clinical attachment level. The greatest improvements were gained at pocket depths ≥7 mm with probing depth reductions of 2.16 mm and gains in the clinical attachment level of 1.19 mm (Cobb, 1996). A systematic review by Van der Weijden reported that in sites measuring ≥5 mm the reduction in probing depth was 1.18 mm with an attachment gain of 0.64 mm (Van der Weijden et al., 2002). Both studies found that the effect of treatment on clinical outcome measures was related to the initial pocket depth; improvements in sites with initially deeper probing depths were greater than in those that were initially shallower. They

Initial PPD	Δ PD	Δ CAL
1–3	-0.03	-0.34
4–6	-1.3	+ 0.55
≥7	-2.16	1.19

Δ: change PD: pocket depth CAL: clinical attachment level

all measurements in millimeters   *adapted from Cobb 1996*

Figure 4.7. Summary of pocket depth and attachment level changes following SRP.

also found that half of the decrease in probing depth could be attributed to attachment gain and thus the remaining decrease was the result of a change in the gingival margin position.

As a caveat, it should be noted that in many of the classic scaling studies very proficient clinicians spent 10 minutes or more per tooth. Thus, the gains achieved represent an ideal result rather than the usual clinical reality, in which considerably less time is spent and possibly with less proficient operators. Additionally, most studies group molar and non-molar sites. There is limited evidence to suggest that the improvements obtained at multi-rooted furcation involved teeth with probing depths measuring ≥4 mm are less than those achieved at single-rooted teeth (Kalkwarf et al., 1988; Claffey et al., 1990; Loos et al., 1989). In these studies pocket depth changes at moderately deep sites (4 mm to 6 mm) ranged from 0 to 1.02 mm, and at deep (≥7 mm) sites the range was 0 to 1.52 mm, which is considerably less than the 2.16-mm decrease observed when all teeth are grouped.

Microbiological Changes

In general, studies show that subgingival debridement results in a decrease in gram-negative microbes with an accompanying increase in the numbers of gram-positive cocci and rods. This shift in the composition of subgingival plaque from one with many pathogenic bacteria to one dominated by beneficial species usually results in a decrease in gingival inflammation, resulting in an improvement in clinical outcome measures such as pocket depth and bleeding on probing (Cobb, 2002).

Cugini et al., in a recent study using DNA probe counts, found that SRP resulted in decreased prevalence and levels of *Porphyromonas gingivalis*, *Tannerella forsythensis*, and *Treponema denticola*. This decrease in pathogenic species was concomitant with an increase in prevalence and levels of beneficial species such as *Actinomyces* species,

Fusobacterium nucleatum subspecies, *Streptococci* species, and *Veillonella parvula*. It should be noted, however, that while SRP appeared to be effective in lowering the numbers of selected periodontal pathogens, none of these species was completely eliminated from any subject by this therapy. Another important observation is that SRP was only effective in reducing a specific subset of the subgingival microflora. Specifically, reductions in pocket depth were most strongly associated with decreases in *Tannerella forsythensis*, which suggests that individuals with non-susceptible (to scaling) species or low numbers of susceptible pathogenic species would experience limited benefits from non-surgical mechanical treatment (Cugini et al., 2000). This finding correlates well with a number of other studies (Mombelli et al., 2000; Haffajee et al., 1997; van Winkelhoff et al., 1988; Shiloah et al., 1994) that have found that *Actinomyces Actinomycetemcomitans* and *Porphyromonas gingivalis* are more resistant to removal by non-surgical mechanical means and that the persistence of these bacteria has been associated with poor response to scaling and root planing.

To better understand these findings it is useful to know that bacteria exist at three areas within the pocket: the tooth surface, on and within the gingival tissues of the sulcus wall, and in planktonic form in the pocket space between the tooth and sulcus wall. It may be that the ability of particular bacteria to invade the gingival tissues allows them to evade removal by mechanical means.

Another limitation in microbiological changes is pre-treatment pocket depth. Haffajee et al. found that although the greatest reduction in counts of periodontal pathogens was found at deep (greater than 6 mm) sites, the counts at all time points (three, six, nine, and 12 months) were always higher in deep sites than at the shallow sites (less than 4 mm). Deep sites continue, even after treatment, to be an environment conducive to certain pathogenic bacteria (Haffajee et al., 1997). Thus, gingival health does not necessarily follow thorough debridement. In this regard, Haffajee et al. reported that mechanical non-surgical therapy resulted in improving clinical parameters only 68% of the time and that 32% of the time there was no benefit.

Additionally, it should be noted that the shifts in the microbial flora are transient, particularly in pockets with residual probing depths of ≥6 mm, with reestablishment of a pathogenic microflora at varied time points depending largely on the frequency of supportive periodontal therapy and proficiency of oral hygiene. Various mechanisms have been proposed for the transient character of this shift, including re-colonization from other intra-oral niches such as tongue and mucosa (Quirynen et al., 1999), re-colonization from tissue-invading bacteria, particularly *Actinomyces Actinomycetemcomitans* and to a lesser extent *Porphyromonas gingivalis* (Cugini et al., 2000), high post-treatment plaque levels due to incomplete

eradication of the pathogenic bacteria (Sbordone et al., 1990), and the level of patient oral hygiene (Sbordone et al., 1990).

Efficacy of Plaque and Calculus Removal

A review of the literature indicates that although scaling and root planing is effective for the reduction of plaque and calculus, it cannot affect the complete removal of deposits. Rather, what we find is varying degrees of success in producing calculus-free teeth depending on a variety of factors. Variables that have been investigated are: (1) initial probing depth, (2) surgical access, (3) furcation involvement, (4) level of operator training, and (5) manual vs. machine-driven scalers.

The most significant limitations on the residual amount of plaque or calculus following mechanical therapy are the depth of the pocket and furcation involvement. Although studies demonstrate a wide range of residual calculus left on roots, from 5% to 80%, the general trend is that as probing depth increases the effectiveness of mechanical debridement diminishes. In probing depths measuring 3 mm or less there is a good chance of removing all of the subgingival plaque. But in pocket depths ranging from 3 mm to 5 mm, the chance of failure to completely debride the root exceeds the chance of success. Furthermore, in pockets measuring 5 mm or more, failure becomes the dominant result (Stambaugh et al., 1981; Rabbani et al., 1981).

Studies investigating the concept of visualizing the root surface to improve the efficacy of scaling and root planing have found that surgical (open) access allows the operator to be much more effective in achieving calculus-free teeth but only in ≥4 mm depths. In shallow pockets of less than 4 mm, non-surgical debridement is as effective or only slightly less effective than surgical debridement (Brayer et al., 1989; Buchanan et al., 1987; Caffesse et al., 1986). Nevertheless, even with direct visualization, scaling efficacy was reduced with increasing pocket depth. Furthermore, most of the residual calculus was found in grooves, fossae, and furcations (Caffesse et al., 1986). Together, these observations suggest that root anatomy has a significant influence on the thoroughness of debridement.

The effect of anatomy on treatment results was also investigated by Wylam et al., who found that although the effectiveness of scaling and root planing on multi-rooted teeth was significantly improved with open access over closed (54.3% vs. 33%), if the results were restricted to an examination of the furcation areas there remained heavy residual calculus regardless of the type of access. In addition, increased time spent did not correlate with improved calculus removal (Wylam et al., 1993). Fleischer also found that even with open access difficult areas such as furcations often had more residual calculus than other surfaces after scaling and root planing (Fleischer, 1989).

These finding are not surprising when one considers that the width of a molar furcation is often not large enough to allow insertion of a standard Gracey curette. Bower observed that 58% of molar furcation entrances had a width of less than 0.75 mm and 81% were less than 1 mm, while an average curette was 0.75 mm to 1.1 mm wide (Bower, 1979). It should be noted that both the Wylam and Fleischer papers used manual instruments, and while the Fleischer study did use ultrasonic instrumentation, it was with a P-10 tip, which is indicated for supragingival use. Their results are not transferable to powered scalers using tips designed for subgingival and furcation sites. In fact, it is in these areas that ultrasonic instruments with tips measuring .55 mm or less have shown an advantage (Oda et al., 1989).

Operator experience also appears to play a role in the efficacy of root surface debridement. Studies have found that inexperienced dentists (Kocher et al., 1997) and periodontists in training (Brayer et al., 1989; Fleischer et al., 1989) left residual calculus on a greater number of root surfaces than trained periodontists. These studies also found that experienced periodontists took more time to scale, suggesting either a better understanding of the time required to scale teeth or a more sensitive tactile endpoint.

An interesting finding was that use of ultrasonic instead of hand instruments does not improve results for inexperienced operators, and thus the ultrasonic scaler should not be considered an instrument for less skilled operators.

Summary

Regardless of the variables affecting the efficacy of mechanical therapy, complete debridement of the root surface does not appear to be a realizable goal. Even surgical access only makes a slight improvement, and thus it seems a likely inference from all of the studies that the limitations on the effectiveness of scaling are related only in part to operator experience, instrument type, and direct visualization, and that ultimately efforts to completely remove calculus are hampered by difficulty in accessing both the macroscopic anatomy such as furcations, concavities, and grooves, and the microscopic anatomy such as erosions and porosities. In any event, healing following scaling and root planing is a clinical reality, which raises questions regarding which aspects of mechanical debridement are important to success. It may be that all are required, at least in the short term, to cause a disturbance of a pathogenic subset of the microbial biofilm or achieve an as yet undetermined threshold of debridement, and that thoroughness of debridement is more relevant to long-term maintenance of the initial resolution of inflammation.

ROOT SURFACE SMOOTHNESS

Another aspect of scaling and root planing that has been explored is post-treatment root surface changes and their effect on plaque accumulation and resolution of inflammation. A smooth root surface is often used as a clinical endpoint for thorough debridement. At a microscopic level it has been found that the different root planing instruments achieve varying degrees of root surface smoothness. Although these differences cannot be detected clinically, they have been investigated for their effect on rate of plaque accumulation and ultimately tissue healing.

It is generally agreed that rougher surfaces promote and increase the rate of plaque accumulation (Leknes et al., 1994; Quirynen et al., 1995). However, with respect to root surface smoothness following root planing, no instrument leaves behind a smooth surface. An in vivo study on root surface roughness following scaling by various instruments found that 15 µm rotating diamonds and Gracey curettes left the smoothest surface followed by the piezoelectric, 75 µm diamond and sonic scalers with roughness values (R_a) ranging from 1.64 µm to 2.1 µm (Schlageter et al., 1996). The point of the paper that is relevant to this discussion is that all of the tested instruments left a root surface that was eight to 13 times rougher than the smoothness threshold of 0.2 µm, which was determined in a literature review to be the R_a value above which plaque accumulation is facilitated (Quirynen et al., 1995). Thus, it appears that even if we accept that the rate of biofilm formation decreases with smoother surfaces, the root surface roughness subsequent to scaling, regardless of instrument choice, will always facilitate plaque accumulation.

Furthermore, despite the correlation between surface smoothness and plaque accumulation, it has not been established that a rougher surface is significant for healing. An early study using closed scaling failed to find an effect on gingival inflammation (Rosenberg and Ash, 1974) and later, in vivo studies using direct visualization (surgical access) failed to find differences in healing after flap surgery between root surfaces that were smoothed after being cleaned and those that were intentionally roughened with a diamond (Khatiblou and Ghodossi, 1983; Oberholzer et al., 1996).

These findings reinforce a point previously made, that healing subsequent to SRP is not dependent on complete removal of plaque but rather a disruption of the biofilm sufficient to change a pathogenic microbial profile to one that is conducive to periodontal health.

FULL-MOUTH DEBRIDEMENT

An area that has received recent attention is the difference in clinical and microbiological results when standard therapy—defined as four quadrants of root planing, each separated by one or two—is compared to full-mouth root planing, whereby all four quadrants are scaled within 24 hours. The philosophy behind this alternative treatment regimen is that it prevents re-colonization of instrumented sites by bacteria from non-instrumented sites. It is also claimed that multiple scalings within 24 hours can stimulate an immune response, supplementing the mechanical effect of debridement on plaque.

A number of papers from a group of researchers based out of the Catholic University of Leuven, Belgium, have demonstrated additional gains in pocket depth reduction of about 1 mm at moderately deep pockets (4 mm to 6 mm) and 1.6 mm to 1.9 mm at deep (≥7 mm) sites. In addition, these studies found greater reductions in proportions of spirochetes and motile rods, although these differences were no longer statistically significant after two months (Quirynen et al., 1999; Mongardini et al., 1999; De Soete et al., 2001). In contrast, studies from other centers have all failed to find any statistically significant differences (Apatzidou et al., 2004; Jervoe-Storm et al., 2006; Nagata et al., 2001). Thus, although the concept behind full-mouth scaling may seem reasonable, conflicting results have been reported in the literature. Regardless, both treatment regimens seem to provide at least comparable gains and thus the choice of modality may be better based on practical concerns for the patient such as convenience, comfort, and financial considerations.

PRACTICAL ASPECTS

Given the plethora of instruments on the market, with new ones being continually introduced, it is imperative to use the literature to make educated practical decisions regarding both instrument selection and their correct application. Taking the studies collectively, it appears that the most important factors influencing complete debridement are instrument access and dental anatomy. Root concavities and grooves, the cementoenamel junction, interproximal areas, deep pockets, and furcations all complicate the debridement process and are the sites most likely to exhibit residual calculus.

Many advances in scaling instrument design are intended to improve access to the complex root anatomy that impedes calculus removal. Thus, maximizing the quality of debridement requires both an understanding of an instrument's design and an intimate knowledge of root anatomy. Knowing the physical characteristics of the working end of a scaler enables the practitioner to choose the instrument most appropriate for the anatomy being scaled. For example, when scaling a root groove or through a constricted entrance in class II and III furcation involvements, the narrow tip of an ultrasonic scaler would be more efficacious than a curette. There may also be an advantage of ultrasonics in deep,

narrow pockets. Here the thin, probe-like shape can provide less traumatic calculus removal than the larger blade of curettes. Because there is individual variation in root shape, even among similar teeth, an experienced tactile sense also plays an important part.

Considering that manual instrumentation requires more complex hand movements (with respect to firm, stable fulcrums and specific blade angulations against the root surface), increased chair time, and greater stamina, it may be that ultrasonic scalers will become the instrument of choice. Nevertheless, whether the clinician prefers manual or powered scalers, a dogmatic adherence to one type of scaler limits the armamentarium of the clinician. An integrated approach with both powered and manual scalers enables the clinician to approach each tooth individually and use the advantages of any instrument to reach the desired endpoint.

As discussed, increasing pocket depth greatly diminishes the efficacy of debridement, and although surgical access is not immune to the variable of pocket depth, it does nevertheless significantly enhance results over closed scaling in pocket depths measuring greater than 4 mm. An interesting twist is introduced into our decision-making process when a paper by Lindhe is considered. Lindhe et al. looked at the surgical modality from the perspective of critical probing depth, defined as the pocket depth above which there was an improvement in clinical attachment level for surgical over non-surgical scaling. The value was 4.5 mm for molars, compared to 6 mm to 7 mm for incisors and premolar teeth; a shallower depth was required for molars before surgery provided a better result (Lindhe et al., 1982). These results can be understood in the context of access and root anatomy, both of which are generally more complicated at molar teeth. Thus, when considering improving visualization with surgery, the pocket depth must be considered in the context of the tooth with which it is associated.

A final important practical aspect is the matter of how one determines if a root surface has been adequately debrided. Originally, roots were scaled and planed aggressively to a hard, glossy finish. This was intended to completely remove plaque, calculus, and cementum contaminated by bacteria and their endotoxins. This practice has recently been called into question due to observations that endotoxins form a superficial layer on cementum that can be removed with gentle scaling (Cheetham et al., 1988) or ultrasonic debridement (Smart et al., 1990). In 1996, the consensus report of the World Workshop in Periodontics stated that the removal of cementum for the purposes of endotoxin removal was no longer considered prudent (Cobb, 1996). However, it is still relevant to plane roots to some degree because short of using endoscopy or surgical visualization, without smoothing roots we cannot evaluate the completeness of calculus removal. Although scaling is certainly indicated for the removal of plaque and calculus, root planing should be used judiciously to avoid unnecessary and excessive removal of root substance.

In this respect it is advantageous to use ultrasonic scalers for the bulk of the debridement because although manual scalers produce a smoother surface than sonic/ultrasonic scalers, they do so at the expense of greater root substance removal. One may consider the difference to be small (in the order of microns) and not of clinical consequence, but years of repeated root planing at regular maintenance visits will add up to a clinically significant amount.

CONCLUSION

Although it is well accepted that plaque biofilms are the main etiologic factor for periodontal disease, we now understand that there are other considerations that need to be taken into account if we are to fully understand the pathogenesis of periodontal disease. Genetic, environmental, and host systemic factors all play an important role in modulating the progression of periodontal disease and the response to periodontal therapy. Nevertheless, scaling and root planing remains the primary therapy for dealing with periodontal infections. Mechanical debridement can affect the composition of the bacterial plaque directly, affect the host response to bacteria, or alter the habitat; alterations of any of these factors can have an impact on the remaining factors in this triad.

To successfully use scaling and root planing in the armamentarium to combat periodontal disease, the trained professional must gain a thorough understanding of the evidence for what can be realistically achieved, how one can optimize those gains, and what factors can limit the efficacy of this modality of treatment. As discussed, due to microbial, environmental, or anatomical limitations, mechanical debridement alone is not always successful in controlling periodontal disease or its progression. Thus, although scaling and root planing is the predominant form of periodontal therapy, it should be understood from the outset that it is to be regarded as a component of an overall treatment plan and, if required, may be supplemented by other forms of non-surgical therapy such as local or systemic antimicrobials or surgical means. The determination can be made on a patient-by-patient basis at the re-evaluation appointment or at subsequent maintenance visits.

When considering the evidence on the benefits of scaling and root planing we must take into account the endpoints being evaluated. Most commonly our attention is directed toward clinical changes in inflammation, probing depth, and attachment level. As important as these changes are, a holistic approach to patient care must also take into account other factors including efficiency, costs, compliance issues, and a host of others. Thus, when planning treatment, consideration should be given not only to the expected gains from scaling and root planing but also to what more may be required to maintain any gains or prevent the initiation of disease in new sites or its progression in existing sites.

REFERENCES

Anderson GB, Palmer JA, Bye FL, Smith BA, Caffesse RG. 1996. Effectiveness of subgingival scaling and root planing. Single versus multiple episodes of instrumentation. *J. Periodontol.* 67(4), 367–373.

Apatzidou DA, Kinane DF. 2004. Quadrant root planing versus same-day full-mouth root planing. I. Clinical findings. *J. Clin. Periodontol.* 31(2), 132–140.

Apatzidou DA, Kinane DF. 2004. Quadrant root planing versus same-day full-mouth root planing. II. Microbiological findings. *J. Clin. Periodontol.* 31(2), 141–148.

Badersten A, Nilveus R, Egelberg J. 1984. Effect of nonsurgical periodontal therapy. II. Severely advanced periodontitis. *J. Clin. Periodontol.* 11(1), 63–76.

Baehni P, Thilo B, Chapuis B, Pernet D. 1992. Effects of ultrasonic and sonic scalers on dental plaque microflora in vitro and in vivo. *J. Clin. Periodontol.* 19(7), 455–459.

Barendregt DS, van der Velden U, Timmerman MF, van der Weijden F. 2008. Penetration depths with an ultrasonic mini insert compared with a conventional curette in patients with periodontitis and in periodontal maintenance. *J. Clin. Periodontol.* 35(1), 31–36.

Boretti G, Zappa U, Graf H, Case D. 1995. Short-term effects of phase I therapy on crevicular cell populations. *J. Periodontol.* 66(3), 235–240.

Bower RC. 1979. Furcation morphology relative to periodontal treatment. Furcation entrance architecture. *J. Periodontol.* 50(1), 23–27.

Brayer WK, Mellonig JT, Dunlap RM, Marinak KW, Carson RE. 1989. Scaling and root planing effectiveness: the effect of root surface access and operator experience. *J. Periodontol.* 60(1), 67–72.

Buchanan SA, Robertson PB. 1987. Calculus removal by scaling/root planing with and without surgical access. *J. Periodontol.* 58(3), 159–163.

Caffesse RG, Sweeney PL, Smith BA. 1986. Scaling and root planing with and without periodontal flap surgery. *J. Clin. Periodontol.* 13(3), 205–210.

Cheetham WA, Wilson M, Kieser JB. 1988. Root surface debridement—an in vitro assessment. *J. Clin. Periodontol.* 15(5), 288–292.

Claffey N, Nylund K, Kiger R, Garrett S, Egelberg J. 1990. Diagnostic predictability of scores of plaque, bleeding, suppuration and probing depth for probing attachment loss. 3.5 years of observation following initial periodontal therapy. *J. Clin. Periodontol.* 17(2), 108–114.

Cobb CM. 1996. Non-surgical pocket therapy: mechanical. *Ann. Periodontol.* 1, 443–490.

Cobb CM. 2002. Clinical significance of non-surgical periodontal therapy: an evidence-based perspective of scaling and root planing. *J. Clin. Periodontol.* 29(Suppl 2), 6–16.

Copulos TA, Low SB, Walker CB, Trebilcock YY, Hefti AF. 1993. Comparative analysis between a modified ultrasonic tip and hand instruments on clinical parameters of periodontal disease. *J. Periodontol.* 64(8), 694–700.

Cugini MA, Haffajee AD, Smith C, Kent Jr. RL, Socransky SS. 2000. The effect of scaling and root planing on the clinical and microbiological parameters of periodontal diseases: 12-month results. *J. Clin. Periodontol.* 27(1), 30–36.

De Soete M, Mongardini C, Peuwels M, Haffajee A, Socransky S, van Steenberghe D, Quirynen M. 2001. One-stage full-mouth disinfection. Long-term microbiological results analyzed by checkerboard DNA-DNA hybridization. *J. Periodontol.* 72(3), 374–382.

Dragoo MR. 1992. A clinical evaluation of hand and ultrasonic instruments on subgingival debridement. Part 1. With unmodified and modified ultrasonic inserts. *Int. J. Periodontics Restorative Dent.* 12(4), 310–323.

Drisko CL, Lewis L. 1996. Ultrasonic instruments and antimicrobial agents in supportive periodontal treatment and retreatment of recurrent or refractory periodontitis. *Periodontol. 2000.* 12, 90–115.

Fleischer HC, Mellonig JT, Brayer WK, Gray JL, Barnett JD. 1989. Scaling and root planing efficacy in multirooted teeth. *J. Periodontol.* 60(7), 402–409.

Flemmig TF, Petersilka GJ, Mehl A, Rüdiger S, Hickel R, Klaiber B. 1997. Working parameters of a sonic scaler influencing root substance removal in vitro. *Clin. Oral Invest.* 1(2), 55–607.

Fowler C, Garrett S, Crigger M, Egelberg J. 1982. Histologic probe position in treated and untreated human periodontal tissues. *J. Clin. Periodontol.* 9(5), 373–385.

Haffajee AD, Cugini MA, Dibart S, Smith C, Kent Jr RL, Socransky SS. 1997. The effect of SRP on the clinical and microbiological parameters of periodontal diseases. *J. Clin. Periodontol.* 24(5), 324–334.

Haffajee AD, Ricardo PT, Socransky SS. 2006. The effect of periodontal therapy on the composition of the subgingival microbiota. *Periodontol. 2000.* 42, 219–258.

Jervoe-Storm PM, Semaan E, AlAhdab H, Engel S, Fimmers R, Jepsen S. 2006. Clinical outcomes of quadrant root planing versus full-mouth root planing. *J. Clin. Periodontol.* 33(3), 209–215.

Jespen S, Ayna M, Hedderich J, Eberhard J. 2004. Significant influence of scaler tip design on root substance loss resulting from ultrasonic scaling: a laserprofilometric in vitro study. *J. Clin. Periodontol.* 31(11), 1003–1006.

Kalkwarf KL, Kaldahl WB, Patil KD. 1988. Evaluation of furcation region response to periodontal therapy. *J. Periodontol.* 59(12), 794–804.

Khatiblou FA, Ghodossi A. 1983. Root surface smoothness or roughness in periodontal treatment. A clinical study. *J. Periodontol.* 54, 365–367.

Kocher T, Ruehling A, Momsen H, Plagmann HC. 1997. Effectiveness of subgingival instrumentation with power-driven instruments in the hands of experienced and inexperienced operators. A study on manikins. *J. Clin. Periodontol.* 24(7), 498–504.

Kocher T, Rosin M, Langenbeck N, Bernhardt O. 2001. Subgingival polishing with a teflon-coated sonic scaler insert in comparison to conventional instruments as assessed on extracted teeth (II). Subgingival roughness. *J. Clin. Periodontol.* 28(8), 723–729.

Lang NP, Adler R, Joss A, Nyman S. 1990. Absence of bleeding on probing. An indicator of periodontal stability. *J. Clin. Periodontol.* 17(10), 714–721.

Laurell L, Pettersson B. 1988. Periodontal healing after treatment with either the Titan-S sonic scaler or hand instruments. *Swed. Dent. J.* 12(5), 187–192.

Leknes KN, Lie T, Wikesjö UM, Bogle GC, Selvig KA. 1994. Influence of tooth instrumentation roughness on subgingival microbial colonization. *J. Periodontol.* 65(4), 303–308.

Leon LE, Vogel RI. 1987. A comparison of the effectiveness of hand scaling and ultrasonic debridement in furcations as evaluated by differential dark-field microscopy. *J. Periodontol.* 58(2), 86–94.

Lindhe J, Nyman S, Socransky SS, Haffajee AD, Westfelt E. 1982. "Critical probing depth" in periodontal therapy. *J. Clin. Periodontol.* 9, 323–336.

Loe H, Theilade E, Jensen S. 1965. Experimental gingivitis in man. *J. Periodontol.* 36, 177–187.

Loos B, Kiger R, Egelberg J. 1987. An evaluation of basic periodontal therapy using sonic and ultrasonic scalers. *J. Clin. Periodontol.* 14(1), 29–33.

Loos B, Nylund K, Claffey N, Egelberg J. 1989. Clinical effects of root debridement in molar and non-molar teeth. A 2-year follow-up. *J. Clin. Periodontol.* 16(8), 498–504.

Mombelli A, Schmid B, Rutar A, Lang NP. 2000. Persistence patterns of Porphyromonas gingivalis, Prevotella intermedia/nigrescens, and Actinobacillus actinomycetemcomitans after mechanical therapy of periodontal disease. *J. Periodontol.* 71(1), 14–21.

Mongardini C, van Steenberghe D, Dekeyser C, Quirynen M. 1999. One state full- versus partial-mouth disinfection in the treatment of chronic adult or generalized early-onset periodontitis. I. Long-term clinical observations. *J. Periodontol.* 70(6), 632–645.

Nagata MJH, Anderson GB, Bonaventura GT. 2001. Full-mouth disinfection versus standard treatment of periodontitis: A clinical study. *J. Periodontol.* 72(11), 1636.

Oberholzer R, Rateitschak KH. 1996. Root cleaning or root smoothing. An in vivo study. *J. Clin. Periodontol.* 23(4), 326–330.

Oda S, Ishikawa I. 1989. In vitro effectiveness of a newly-designed ultrasonic scaler tip for furcation areas. *J. Periodontol.* 60(11), 634–639.

Oosterwaal PJ, Matee MI, Mikx FH, van 't Hof MA, Renggli HH. 1987. The effect of subgingival debridement with hand and ultrasonic instruments on the subgingival microflora. *J. Clin. Periodontol.* 14(9), 528–533.

Quirynen M, Bollen CM. 1995. The influence of surface roughness and surface-free energy on supra- and subgingival plaque formation in man. A review of the literature. *J. Clin. Periodontol.* 22(1), 1–14.

Quirynen M, Mongardini C, Pauwels M, Bollen CM, Van Eldere J, van Steenberghe D. 1999. One-stage full- versus partial-mouth disinfection in the treatment of chronic adult or generalized early-onset periodontitis. II. Long-term impact on microbial load. *J. Periodontol.* 70(6), 646–656.

Rabbani GM, Ash Jr MM, Caffesse RG. 1981. The effectiveness of subgingival scaling and root planing in calculus removal. *J. Periodontol.* 52(3), 119–123.

Ritz L, Hefti AF, Rateitschak KH. 1991. An in vitro investigation on the loss of root substance in scaling with various instruments. *J. Clin. Periodontol.* 18(9), 643–647.

Rosenberg RM, Ash Jr MM. 1974. The effect of root roughness on plaque accumulation and gingival inflammation. *J. Periodontol.* 45(3), 146–150.

Sbordone L, Ramaglia L, Gulletta E, Iacono V. 1990. Recolonization of the subgingival microflora after scaling and root planing in human periodontitis. *J. Periodontol.* 61(9), 579–584.

Schlageter L, Rateitschak-Pluss EM, Schwarz JP. 1996. Root surface smoothness or roughness following open debridement. An in vivo study. *J. Clin. Periodontol.* 23(5), 460–464.

Shiloah J, Patters MR. 1994. DNA probe analysis of the survival of selected periodontal pathogens following scaling, root planing, and intra-pocket irrigation. *J. Periodontol.* 65(6), 568–575.

Smart GJ, Wilson M, Davies EH, Kieser JB. 1990. The assessment of ultrasonic root surface debridement by determination of residual endotoxin levels. *J. Clin. Periodontol.* 17(3), 174–178.

Stambaugh R, Dragoo M, Smith D, Carasali L. 1981. The limits of subgingival scaling. *Int. J. Periodontics Restorative Dent.* 1(5), 30–41.

Theilade E, Wright WH, Jensen SB, Loe H. 1966. Experimental gingivitis in man II. A longitudinal clinical and bacteriological investigation. *J. Periodontal. Res.* 1, 1–13.

Tunkel J, Heinecke A, Flemmig TF. 2002. A systematic review of efficacy of machine-driven and manual subgingival debridement in the treatment of chronic periodontitis. *J. Clin. Periodontol.* 29(Suppl 3), 72–81.

Van der Weijden GA, Timmerman MF. 2002. A systematic review on the clinical efficacy of subgingival debridement in the treatment of chronic periodontitis. *J. Clin. Periodontol.* 29(Suppl 3), 55–71.

van Winkelhoff AJ, Van der Velden U, de Graaff J. 1988. Microbial succession in recolonizing deep periodontal pockets after a single course of supra- and subgingival debridement. *J. Clin. Periodontol.* 15(2), 116–122.

Vastardis S, Yukna RA, Rice DA, Mercante D. 2005. Root surface removal and resultant surface texture with diamond-coated ultrasonic inserts: an in vitro and SEM study. *J. Clin. Periodontol.* 32(5), 467–473.

Wylam JM, Mealey BL, Mills MP, Waldrop TC, Moskowicz DC. 1993. The clinical effectiveness of open versus closed scaling and root planing on multi-rooted teeth. *J. Periodontol.* 64(11), 1023–1028.

Chapter 5 Occlusion

INTRODUCTION

Concepts of occlusion in the early twentieth century were based primarily on the rehabilitation of totally edentulous patients with complete dentures. At the time, a relatively large segment of the population was edentulous, in part because of the wide-spread acceptance of the focal infection theory (Goymerac and Woollard, 2004). Complete mouth extraction was commonly prescribed by physicians for patients with systemic diseases in an attempt to eliminate any oral infections that were assumed to act as focal infections and cause the systemic disease.

CENTRIC RELATION AND CENTRIC OCCLUSION

Concepts of centric relation evolved as dentists refined their treatment methods for edentulous patients (Hanau, 1929). It was observed by many dentists that the mandible of an edentulous patient could be guided upward and backward to a stable, repeatable position. In this position, the mandible appeared to hinge or rotate about an axis (Figure 5.1). Because these dentists assumed that each condyle was centered in its respective glenoid fossa when the mandible reached this position, the position was referred to as centric relation (Hanau, 1929). Many dentists believed that the condyles were in the most retruded position when the mandible was in centric relation (Thompson, 1946), and by the latter half of the twentieth century, most definitions of centric relation described it as the most retruded mandibular position. It was also assumed, at the time, that the condyles were in centric relation when a dentate patient brought together the maxillary and mandibular opposing teeth (Niswonger, 1934); therefore, the position with the opposing teeth fitting together was referred to as centric occlusion. Posselt's (1952) research on mandibular movements clearly demonstrated that, with most patients, the condyles were not in centric relation when the teeth fit together best. He suggested the term intercuspal position (ICP) to designate the best fit of the teeth, rather than centric occlusion.

American dentists ignored Posselt's suggestion and continued to use the term centric occlusion to designate the ICP. Finally, in 1987, the *Glossary of Prosthodontic Terms*, fifth edition (Academy of Prosthodontics, 1987), introduced the term maximum intercuspal position (MIP) (later modified to maximal intercuspal position in a subsequent edition of the *Glossary*) as the designation for the best fit of the teeth.

The term centric occlusion was not abandoned but was redefined as "the occlusion of opposing teeth when the mandible is in centric relation" (Academy of Prosthodontics, 1987), a position that may or may not coincide with MIP. In that fifth edition of the *Glossary*, centric relation was also redefined as, "the maxillomandibular relationship in which the condyles articulate with the thinnest avascular portion of their respective disks with the complex in the anterior-superior position against the slopes of the articular eminences. This position is independent of tooth contact. This position is clinically discernible when the mandible is directed superiorly and anteriorly. It is restricted to a purely rotary movement about the transverse horizontal axis." This definition was based on a new understanding of the physiology of the temporomandibular joint (Figure 5.2). Centric relation was not relocated; it was redefined. In 1995, McDevitt et al. conducted a magnetic resonance imaging study of a group of patients and confirmed the validity of the new definition.

It has become universally accepted that the MIP for a totally edentulous patient should coincide with centric relation. This concept was later applied to patients with natural teeth. Many dentists believed that a natural MIP that did not coincide with the centric relation position was a malocclusion, while others disagreed.

BALANCED ARTICULATION

Developing an MIP that coincides with centric relation provides denture stability in MIP; however, mastication is not restricted to pure hinge movement. Mastication involves lateral, protrusive, and retrusive three-dimensional movements. Arranging the artificial teeth of complete dentures to allow simultaneous contact of the teeth in eccentric positions can enhance denture stability, uniformly distribute the forces directed to the edentulous ridges, and improve masticatory performance and patient comfort (Ohguri et al., 1999; Khamis et al., 1998; Sutton and McCord, 2007) (Figure 5.3). Dentists noticed, empirically, that if the artificial teeth for complete dentures were set to balanced articulation (cross-arch, cross-tooth balance, whereby all teeth contact without interferences in all eccentric positions), there appeared to be less resorption of the edentulous ridges, and the dentures were more stable during mastication. Balanced articulation became the gold standard for complete denture occlusion.

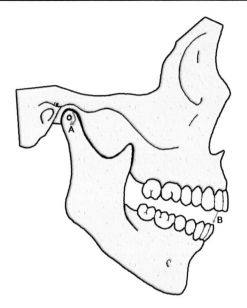

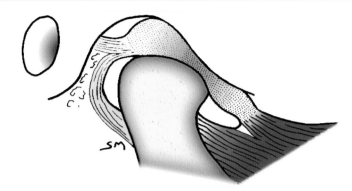

Figure 5.2. The current definition of centric relation describes condyles as articulating with the thinnest avascular portion of their respective disks with the complex in the anterior-superior position against the slopes of the articular eminencies.

Figure 5.1. When the mandible is in centric relation it rotates about an axis.

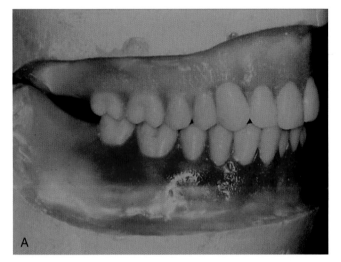

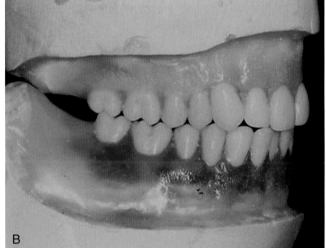

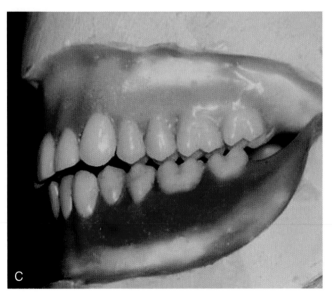

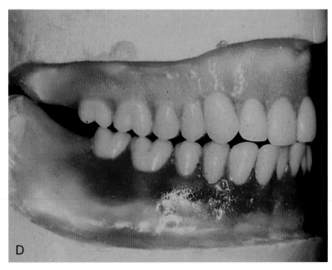

Figure 5.3. Thirty-degree anatomical teeth have been arranged in wax with balanced articulation. A, MIP; B, working side contacts; C, nonworking side (balancing-side) contacts; D, contacts in protrusion.

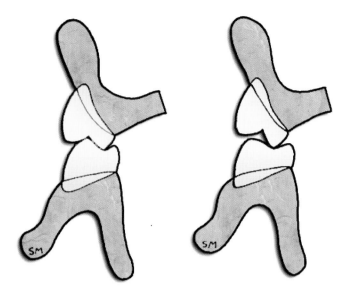

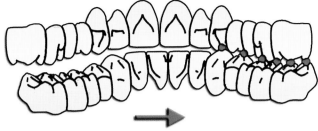

● **Working contacts**

Figure 5.6. Group function or unilateral balance.

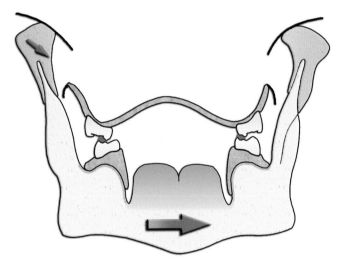

Figure 5.4. Left, classical balanced articulation; right, lingualized occlusion.

Figure 5.5. With lingualized occlusion, there is cross-arch balance but no cross-tooth balance.

A modified form of balanced articulation was described by Payne in 1941. Payne suggested an arrangement of the artificial teeth with cross-arch balance, but not cross-tooth balance (Figures 5.4, 5.5). The term lingualized occlusion was later used to describe this method of developing an artificial occlusion (Pound, 1970). This occlusal concept has become popular and is commonly advocated for implant-supported removable prosthodontics. Clinical and in vitro studies have shown that balanced lingualized occlusion can be as effective as classical balanced articulation (Ohguri et al., 1999; Khamis et al., 1988; Sutton and McCord, 2007).

OCCLUSAL CONCEPTS FOR CONVENTIONAL FIXED PROSTHODONTICS

With advances in materials and techniques in the 1930s and 1940s, it became possible to rehabilitate a natural dentition with fixed restorations. Early attempts to provide complete-mouth rehabilitation with fixed prosthodontics used occlusal concepts that were established for complete denture prosthodontics; i.e., balanced articulation was prescribed. It is understandable that dentists would attempt to mimic an occlusal scheme that was highly successful for edentulous patients. It was obvious that balanced articulation resulted in dentures that did not loosen; also, with occlusal balance, there appeared to be less bone resorption beneath the dentures. At the time, the cause of periodontal disease was obscure. The term dental plaque did not exist. Many dentists assumed that bone loss around natural teeth was the result of occlusal overload. Balancing the occlusion was assumed to be a method to uniformly distribute the forces of occlusion and avoid occlusal overload.

Developing balanced articulation with dentate patients required very sophisticated instrumentation. An articulator that could precisely mimic eccentric jaw movements (a fully adjustable instrument) was necessary, and much of the efforts of prosthodontists in the 1930s and 1940s were directed toward developing tracing devices and articulators that could transfer a patient's 3D jaw movements to an articulator that could be adjusted to reproduce these movements.

In the late 1950s and early 1960s the concept of developing balanced articulation for fixed prosthodontics was challenged. Two primary philosophical approaches were suggested. Unilateral balance, later referred to as group function, was advocated by Schuyler (1963) (Figure 5.6). Stuart (1964) suggested eliminating all posterior tooth contacts in eccentric positions. This occlusal scheme has been described as mutually protected occlusion because the posterior teeth act as vertical stops (closure stoppers) and prevent excessive

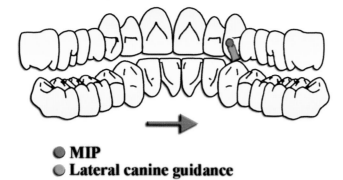

● **MIP**
◐ **Lateral canine guidance**

Figure 5.7. Mutually protected occlusion with lateral canine guidance.

contact of the anterior teeth in MIP, and the anterior teeth disengage the posterior teeth in eccentric positions to protect the posterior teeth from lateral forces (Figure 5.7). Another term that has been used to describe this occlusal scheme is anterior disclusion (anterior teeth discluding the posterior teeth in eccentric positions). If the canine alone (without involvement of the incisors) discludes the posterior teeth in lateral eccentric positions, the mutually protected occlusal scheme is described as canine disclusion.

ANTERIOR DISCLUSION (CANINE DISCLUSION) AND GROUP FUNCTION

Throughout the 1960s and 1970s there was considerable controversy concerning the best eccentric occlusal scheme for a fixed prosthodontic oral rehabilitation. Group function was considered optimal by some dentists, primarily periodontists, because empirically it appeared that simultaneous contact of all teeth on the working side in a lateral occlusal position would uniformly distribute forces among all teeth. Nevertheless, most prosthodontists were advocating anterior disclusion or canine disclusion. Some periodontists felt that anterior disclusion or canine disclusion would cause occlusal overload of the anterior teeth, trauma from occlusion, and eventual hypermobility of the anterior teeth; however, prosthodontists were commonly prescribing this occlusal arrangement with good results.

Arguments ensued for at least two decades concerning the optimal eccentric occlusal scheme, but definitive research by Gibbs and Lundeen (1982) shed new light on the physiology of mastication and quelled the arguments. Gibbs and Lundeen reported three distinct adult chewing patterns. They described these as good occlusion, malocclusion, and worn occlusion.

Patients with good occlusion had an arrangement of the dentition whereby the anterior teeth prevented contact of the

posterior teeth in eccentric positions. These patients chewed with smooth, repeatable strokes. During mastication, tooth gliding contacts occurred while the mandible was entering MIP. However, these contacts occurred at the very end of the closing stroke, and they were of short duration and low magnitude when compared with the forces generated in MIP. The investigators tracked the envelope of motion or border envelope (Posselt, 1952) and the envelope of function with superimposed tracings. It was clear from these tracings (Figure 5.8) that the maxillary and mandibular anterior teeth passed very close to each other during mastication, without contacting. It was the tactile sensation and tactile memory, or proprioception (Crum and Loiselle, 1972) of the teeth, as governed by the periodontal ligaments, that appeared to guide the chewing strokes for these patients with good occlusion, always returning to MIP without long gliding contacts on the anterior teeth.

A different chewing stroke was observed with patients whose anterior teeth did not prevent contact of the posterior teeth in eccentric positions. These patients lacked repeatable strokes. Chewing was erratic with long, gliding contacts. This group of patients was designated as having malocclusion.

A third type of chewing stroke was observed in patients with worn occlusal and incisal surfaces. These patients lacked overlap of the anterior teeth and chewed with broad side-to-side strokes. This group was described by the investigators as having a worn occlusion.

The results of these studies by Gibbs and Lundeen confirmed the desirability of anterior disclusion or canine disclusion for the restoration of a dentition with fixed prosthodontics (Figure 5.9.) The results also refuted the contention that a patient's natural MIP must coincide with centric relation. In Gibbs and Lundeen's studies, patients always returned to the MIP during mastication because of the tactile memory and tactile sensation of the teeth. Therefore, when a patient has a normal, healthy MIP and a functional anterior guidance (vertical and horizontal overlap of the anterior teeth), the dentist should preserve this occlusal relationship when placing several crowns or a short-span fixed partial denture (FPD). If the MIP is dysfunctional and cannot be preserved because it will be destroyed with crown preparations (as with complete-mouth oral rehabilitation), or does not exist (as with a patient edentulous in one or both jaws), centric relation would be the treatment position. It is interesting to note that Gibbs and Lundeen found only a small difference when condylar positions in MIP and centric relation were compared. The mean anterior-posterior difference was 0.13 mm and the mean superior-inferior difference was less than 0.5 mm. These findings suggest that restoring a dentition by developing an MIP coincidental with CR is physiologically sound

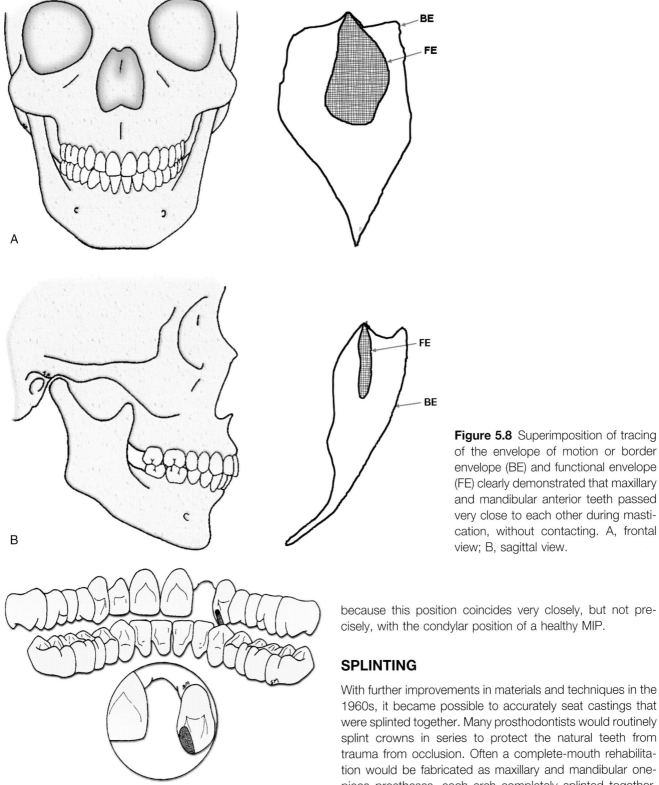

Figure 5.8 Superimposition of tracing of the envelope of motion or border envelope (BE) and functional envelope (FE) clearly demonstrated that maxillary and mandibular anterior teeth passed very close to each other during mastication, without contacting. A, frontal view; B, sagittal view.

Figure 5.9. The patient will receive three-unit fixed partial denture to replace a missing lateral incisor. The canine relationship of natural teeth should be preserved in the final restoration to ensure canine disclusion.

because this position coincides very closely, but not precisely, with the condylar position of a healthy MIP.

SPLINTING

With further improvements in materials and techniques in the 1960s, it became possible to accurately seat castings that were splinted together. Many prosthodontists would routinely splint crowns in series to protect the natural teeth from trauma from occlusion. Often a complete-mouth rehabilitation would be fabricated as maxillary and mandibular one-piece prostheses, each arch completely splinted together. Splinting of natural teeth is no longer advocated. Splinting makes it more difficult to fabricate the prosthesis. An occlusal interference on one splinted crown will be transmitted to all teeth and the interfering tooth cannot move away from the interference (Figure 5.10). A problem with one tooth or one crown can jeopardize the prognosis of the entire prosthesis. Complete-arch splinting is especially undesirable in the mandible because of the phenomenon of mandibular flexure (Fischman, 1976) (Figure 5.11). Splinting of implant-supported crowns in series is often advocated and is discussed below.

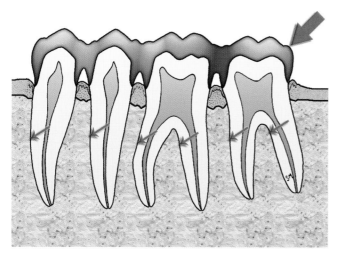

Figure 5.10. Occlusal interference on one splinted crown will be transmitted to all teeth and the interfering tooth cannot move away from the interference.

IMPLANT-SUPPORTED ARTIFICIAL OCCLUSION

Perceptions of occlusion vary with different dental specialties. Orthodontists are interested in moving teeth to develop an Angle Class I occlusal relationship because the maxillary and mandibular teeth tend to fit together best with this arrangement. Prosthodontists are concerned with fabricating dental prostheses in a laboratory on an articulator, and then delivering the prostheses to restore esthetics, phonetics, and function with favorable biomechanics. Traditionally, periodontists were primarily concerned with controlling trauma from occlusion in the natural dentition; however, the contemporary periodontist devotes a considerable amount of time to surgically placing dental implants. Implant dentistry is planned from the crown down; i.e., the prosthodontist or restorative dentist determines the required location and contour of the planned artificial tooth or teeth with a wax trial arrangement of an artificial tooth or teeth, and the implant is then planned to permit this required position of the tooth or teeth (Figure 5.12). To do this effectively, the periodontist must have more background related to occlusal biomechanics.

Fixed Implant-supported Restorations

Gibbs and Lundeen's research highlighted the importance of proprioceptive input from the periodontal ligaments for fine motor control of the masticatory stroke. Because osseointe-

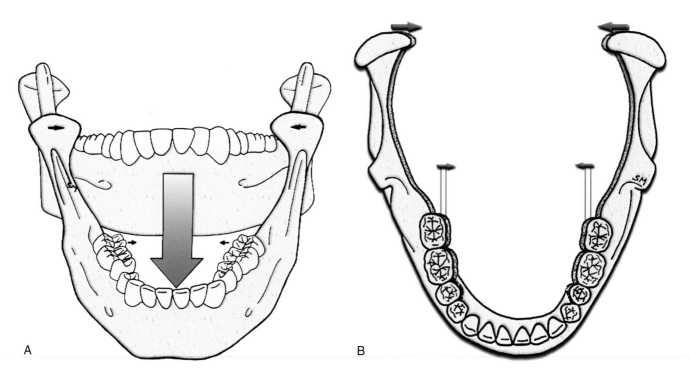

Figure 5.11. A, Because of the medial pull of the lateral pterygoid muscles, with maximal opening, the condyles are pulled medially. B, The result is flexure of the mandible and contraction of the mandibular arch. Splinting teeth from last molar to last molar in the mandible can create unfavorable stresses.

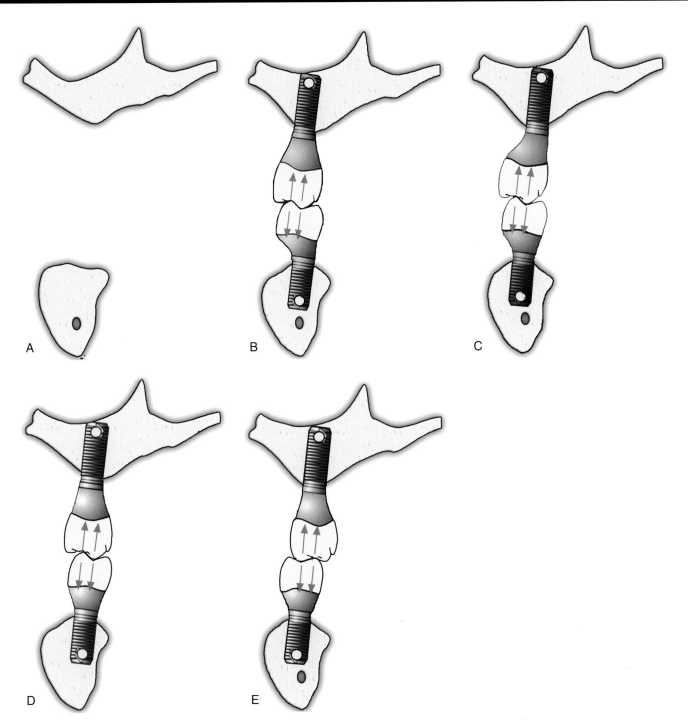

Figure 5.12. A, Resorbed maxillary and mandibular edentulous ridges. It is impossible to accurately place implants without prosthetic planning. B, Forces on the maxillary crown are compressive (favorable), but unfavorable torquing forces exist with the mandibular crown. C, Improved force distribution. D, Optimal force distribution. E, Sometimes optimal forces require a cross-bite occlusal relationship due to the pattern of bone resorption.

grated implants lack a periodontal ligament, the sensation generated from occlusal contacts is completely different from the sensation experienced with natural teeth (Figure 5.13). A clinical study by Jacobs and van Steenberghe (1993) on passive tactile sensation of natural teeth and implant-supported prostheses reported a threshold that is 50 times greater with implant-supported prostheses when compared with natural teeth. This marked difference in sensation suggests that a patient could easily, and without awareness, overload an implant-supported restoration.

Careful control of biomechanics is essential to the long-term serviceability of implant-supported fixed prostheses. Poor placement can lead to biomechanical overload, which can manifest itself as chronic screw loosening, screw fracture, implant fracture, or loss of osseointegration (Figure 5.14). A retrospective study by Eckert et al. (2000) of fractured implants reported that screw loosening preceded implant fracture for the majority of the implants, suggesting that screw loosening can be a sign of occlusal overload.

When a single missing tooth is replaced with an implant-supported crown, the differences in displaceability of the natural teeth and single implant must be considered. The tooth can be displaced within its socket, but the implant is, for all practical purposes, non-displaceable (Figure 5.15). When the patient occludes lightly on a single implant-supported crown, shim stock (a Mylar strip, 8 μm in thickness) should easily pass through the occlusal surfaces of the implant-supported crown and opposing natural tooth. When the patient occludes with heavy force, the implant-supported crown should not hold the shim stock any tighter than the adjacent teeth hold a shim stock (Figure 5.16).

The method of implant support will also influence the biomechanics. A finite element analysis (Morgano and Geramy, 2004) of a mandibular single molar supported by a 3.75-mm diameter implant, a 5-mm diameter implant, and two implants reported a reduction of approximately 50% in micro-motion of the crown with the 5-mm diameter implant and the double implant support (Figure 5.17). Micro-motion is an important

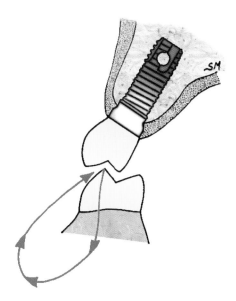

Figure 5.13. Fine motor control of the envelope of function depends on tactile sensation and tactile memory from receptors within periodontal ligaments of teeth; however, osseointegrated implants lack a periodontal ligament.

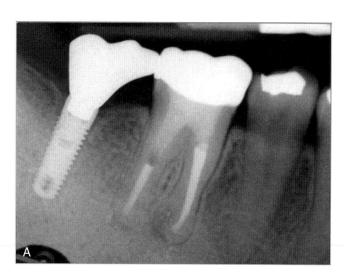
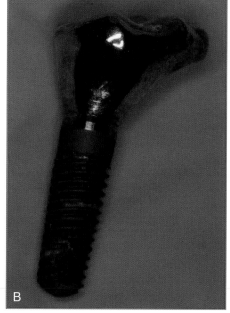

Figure 5.14. A, The implant was placed too far distally, resulting in an artificial crown with poor biomechanics. B, The result was loss of osseointegration.

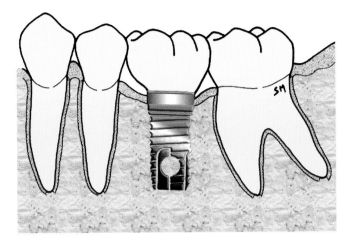

Figure 5.15. Differences in displaceability of natural teeth, which are surrounded by periodontal ligaments, and a single implant must be considered when adjusting occlusion.

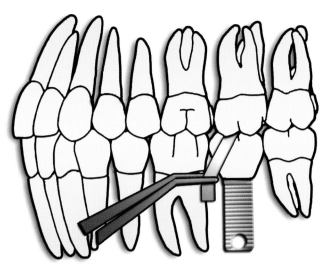

Figure 5.16. A shim stock is used to adjust occlusion.

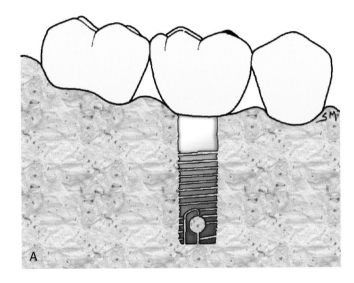

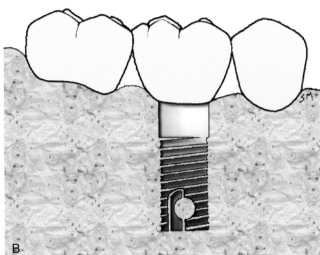

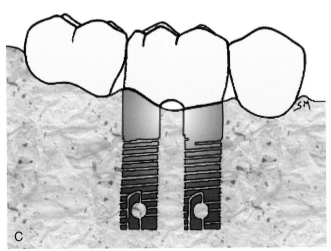

Figure 5.17. A finite element analysis by Morgano and Geramy (2004) of a mandibular single molar supported by A, a 3.75-mm diameter implant, B, a 5-mm diameter implant, and C, two implants reported approximately 50% reduction in micromotion of the crown with the 5-mm diameter implant and the double implant design.

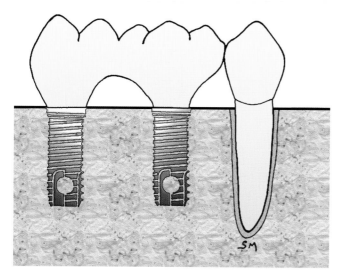

Figure 5.18. In vitro evidence suggests that splinting implants together can distribute forces more uniformly and improve biomechanics.

consideration in implant prosthodontics because it has been reported to produce various clinical problems for implant-supported crowns, including soft tissue complications (Dixon et al., 1995), bone loss (Hermann et al., 2001), and mechanical problems, such as fracture and loosening of screws (Gratton, 2001). A strain gauge study (Seong et al., 2000) with a similar design to the study by Morgano and Geramy reported similar results. Also, when implants are in a series, splinting them together helps distribute forces more uniformly and improve the biomechanics (Guichet et al., 2002) (Figure 5.18).

Implant-supported Removable Prosthodontics (Overdentures)

The application of osseointegrated implants to support and retain complete dentures has the potential to improve the quality of life for totally edentulous patients (Awad et al., 2003). However, it is important to appreciate that implant-supported restorations are not trouble free (Goodacre et al., 2003). One important consideration is occlusal stability (Kohavi, 1993). The acrylic resin teeth commonly used with conventional complete dentures tend to wear rapidly with implant-supported overdentures because of the amount of force the patient can generate. The use of porcelain artificial teeth or custom metal occlusal surfaces should be seriously considered, especially for patients with strong musculature.

With implant-supported overdentures, classical balanced articulation or balanced lingualized occlusion should be used to ensure favorable force distribution and masticatory efficiency. Lingualized occlusion has become very popular with implant-supported overdentures because of the improved lever balance. Lever balance was first described by Ortman

(1977), and relates to directing the forces of occlusion over the supporting area of a complete denture, thus reducing unfavorable leverage. Because the maxillary palatal cusp is the only intercuspating cusp with lingualized occlusion, it is easier to centralize forces over the supporting implants with lingualized occlusion.

ARTICULATORS

An articulator, which has several functions, is used when restoring a dentition. An articulator must serve as a holding instrument for the maxillary and mandibular casts and ensure a positive centric lock. It is desirable for an articulator to accept a face-bow to transfer the patient's opening and closing axis to the instrument. Adjustable condylar guidances are also important features.

Rehabilitation with Fixed Prosthodontics

Mutually protected occlusion is commonly prescribed when rehabilitating a dentition with conventional fixed prosthodontics. Because the goal of mutually protected occlusion is the disclusion of all posterior teeth in eccentric positions, this type of occlusal scheme can be achieved with the use of a semi-adjustable articulator (Lundeen, 1979). A semi-adjustable articulator can be programmed for positive or negative error. If an eccentric tooth contact on the articulator is an interference in the mouth, it is described as positive error. If an eccentric tooth contact on the articulator discludes in the mouth, it is negative error (Figure 5.19).

Setting the horizontal condylar guidance below the normal range found in clinical studies will result in negative error in protrusion and in a non-working (mediotrusive) movement because the separation of the posterior teeth on the articulator will be less than the separation that occurs in the mouth. Therefore, if the posterior teeth disclude in protrusion and non-working movements in the articulator, they will disclude by more in the mouth.

With a working-side movement, the setting of the Bennett angle (angle of the progressive side shift) on the articulator can be used to produce negative error. The amount of progressive lateral movement is determined by the Bennett angle (the wider the Bennett angle, the greater the progressive lateral movement). Therefore, setting the Bennett angle on the articulator wider than what has been reported in clinical studies will allow the articulator to move laterally a greater amount than can occur in the mouth. As a consequence, posterior teeth on the working side will disclude in the mouth with a separation greater than what occurred on the articulator.

The range of the protrusive angle has been reported as 25 degrees to 65 degrees, and the Bennett angle has been

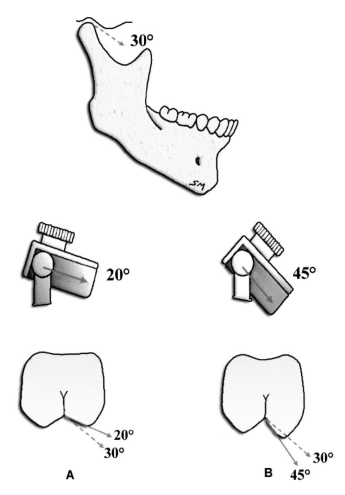

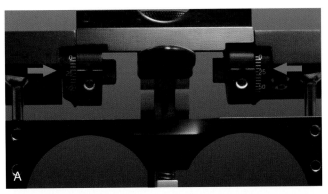

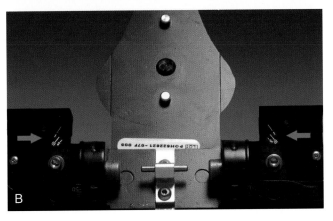

Figure 5.20. If a semi-adjustable articulator is set with A, a protrusive angle of 20 degrees and B, a Bennett angle of 15 degrees, it will be programmed for negative error, ensuring anterior disclusion.

Figure 5.19. An articulator can be programmed for negative or positive error. A patient's natural condylar guidance is 30 degrees (dotted line). A, The articulator has been set with a 20-degree condylar inclination. What contacted on the articulator (solid line) missed in mouth (dotted line)—negative error. B, The articulator has been set with a 45-degree condylar inclination. What contacted on the articulator (solid line) became interference in the mouth (dotted line)—positive error.

reported as 7 degrees to 8 degrees (Lundeen and Wirth, 1973; Lundeen, 1979). If a semi-adjustable articulator is set with a protrusive angle of 20 degrees and a Bennett angle of 15 degrees, it will be programmed for negative error (Figure 5.20).

Rehabilitation with Complete Dentures

With complete denture prosthodontics, balanced articulation is desired, whereby the posterior teeth contact simultaneously in the right and left lateral occlusal positions and in protrusion. Harmonious eccentric occlusal contacts firmly seat the denture(s) and distribute the occlusal load, promoting denture stability and masticatory efficiency (Figure 5.21). Because posterior eccentric contacts are desirable, the

concept of negative error cannot be used. A protrusive record is made to set the protrusive angle on the articulator. Lateral check records can be made to set the Bennett angles; however, the variability in the Bennett angles of edentulous patients is very small. Langer and Michman (1970) reported that the Bennett angle for edentulous patients was approximately twice the values reported for dentate patients ±2 degrees. Therefore, commonly, the Bennett angle is set arbitrarily at 15 degrees for edentulous patients.

AUTHORS' VIEWS/COMMENTS

Early principles of occlusion were empiric concepts designed for complete dentures that were almost entirely mechanical. Centric relation was used as the treatment position for the MIP of the dentures, and the occlusion was designed with eccentric balance. This balanced arrangement of the teeth was used to promote denture stability and uniformly distribute forces. Dentists learned that a single interceptive occlusal contact could disturb the position of the denture bases on the mucosa, thus promoting instability, poor retention, tissue

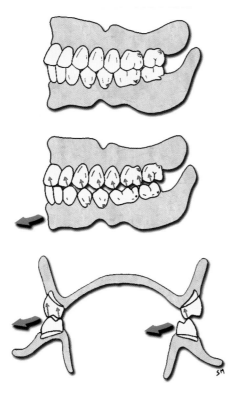

Figure 5.21. Balanced articulation firmly seats the dentures and distributes the occlusal load, promoting denture stability and masticatory efficiency.

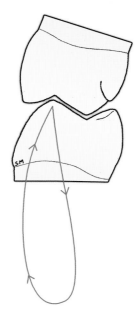

Figure 5.22. Relatively steep overlap of the anterior teeth (anterior guidance) produces a vertical chewing stroke, protecting posterior teeth from lateral forces.

trauma, soreness, and accelerated bone resorption. Several clinical studies have reported improved performance with complete dentures when classical balanced articulation or lingualized occlusion was used.

Attempts to apply this mechanical approach to complete mouth rehabilitation with fixed prosthodontics were unsuccessful. The concepts of occlusion for fixed prosthodontics gradually moved from a mechanical approach to a biomechanical approach. Current scientific knowledge suggests that mutually protected occlusion is a biomechanically sound approach to designing the occlusal scheme for a fixed prosthodontic rehabilitation. With a complete-mouth rehabilitation, the MIP will be destroyed because of the tooth preparations, so the treatment position for the newly created MIP would be centric relation.

There is no evidence to suggest that a stable, healthy MIP that does not coincide with centric relation should be altered. Most patients have a slight discrepancy between the condylar positions when the condyle is in centric relation and when the teeth are in MIP. Simple restorations that involve a few teeth should be made to harmonize with the existing MIP.

The masticatory function of natural teeth depends on feedback from the receptors in the periodontal ligaments of the teeth. Because implants are not surrounded by periodontal ligaments, the sensation from implants is different from that of natural teeth. The dentist must be cognizant of this difference in the sensation when designing the occlusal scheme for implants. Steep vertical overlap of natural anterior teeth is considered desirable because the receptors in the periodontal ligaments of the anterior teeth will guide the mandible through the 3D space with a relatively vertical chewing stroke. This vertical stroke helps to protect the posterior teeth from lateral forces (mutually protected occlusion) (Figure 5.22). Because implant-supported anterior crowns lack periodontal ligaments, the sensation is also lacking. Steep anterior vertical overlap is likely to cause chipping of porcelain. An implant-supported fixed rehabilitation should be developed with very shallow anterior guidance, shallow cusps, and narrowed occlusal tables (for improved lever balance). Group function occlusion is also an option. A functionally generated path recording can be used to develop group function with the use of a semi-adjustable articulator (Meyer, 1959).

The occlusion for implant-supported overdentures should mimic the occlusion for conventional complete dentures—either classic balanced articulation or balanced lingualized occlusion. Special attention should be directed toward ensuring occlusal stability by preventing excessive wear of the occlusal surfaces of the posterior teeth (Figure 5.23).

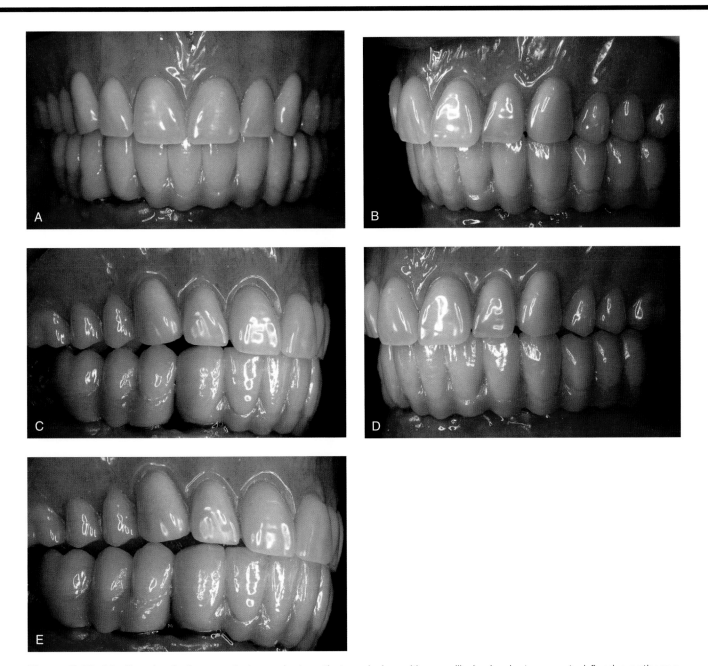

Figure 5.23. Maxillary implant-supported overdenture that occludes with mandibular implant-supported fixed prostheses. Lingualized occlusion has been used, with porcelain posterior artificial teeth in overdenture and porcelain occlusal surfaces on mandibular metal-ceramic fixed partial dentures. A and B, MIP; C, right nonworking; D, left working (note the lack of contact of buccal cusps); E, protrusion. Courtesy of Dr. Dmitri Svirsky, Toronto, Ontario, Canada.

REFERENCES

Academy of Prosthodontics. 1987. Glossary of Prosthodontic Terms. 5th ed. *J. Prosthet. Dent.* 58, 725.

Awad MA, Lund JP, Shapiro SH, Locker D, Klemetti E, Chehade A, Savard A, Feine JS. 2003. Oral health status and treatment satisfaction with mandibular implant overdentures and conventional dentures: a randomized clinical trial in a senior population. *Int. J. Prosthodont.* 16, 390–6.

Crum RJ, Loiselle RJ. 1972. Oral perception and proprioception: A review of the literature and its significance to prosthodontics. *J. Prosthet. Dent.* 28, 215–30.

Dixon DL, Breeding LC, Sadler JP, McKay ML. 1995. Comparison of screw loosening, rotation, and deflection among three implant designs. *J. Prosthet. Dent.* 74, 270–8.

Eckert SE, Meraw SJ, Cal E, Ow RK. 2000. Analysis of incidence and associated factors with fractured implants: a retrospective study. *Int. J. Oral Maxillofac. Implants.* 15, 662–7.

Fischman BM. 1976. The influence of fixed splints on mandibular flexure. *J. Prosthet. Dent.* 35, 643–7.

Gibbs CH, Lundeen HL. 1982. Jaw movements and forces during chewing and swallowing and their clinical significance. In Gibbs CH, Lundeen HL. eds. Advances in Occlusion. John Wright PSG, Inc., Boston. pp. 2–50.

Goodacre CJ, Guillermo B, Rungcharassaeng K, Kan JYK. 2003. Clinical complications with implants and implant prostheses. *J. Prosthet. Dent.* 90, 121–32.

Goymerac B, Woolard G. 2004. Focal infection: a new perspective on an old theory. *Gen. Dent.* 52, 357–61.

Gratton DG, Aquilino SA, Stanford CM. 2001. Micro-motion and dynamic fatigue properties of the dental-implant interface. *J. Prosthet. Dent.* 85, 47–52.

Guichet DL, Yoshinobu D, Caputo AA. 2002. Effect of splinting and interproximal contact tightness on load transfer by implant restorations. *J. Prosthet. Dent.* 87, 528–35.

Hanau RH. 1929. Occlusal changes in centric relation. *J. Am. Dent. Assoc.* 16, 1903–15.

Hermann JS, Schoolfield JD, Schenk RK, Buser D, Cochran DL. 2001. Influence of the size of the microgap on crestal bone changes around titanium implants. A histometric evaluation of unloaded non-submerged implants in the canine mandible. *J. Periodontol.* 72, 1372–83.

Jacobs R, van Steenberghe D. 1993. Comparison between implant-supported prostheses and teeth regarding passive threshold level. *Int. J. Oral Maxillofac. Implants.* 8, 549–54.

Khamis MM, Zaki HS, Rudy TE. 1998. A comparison of the effect of different occlusal forms in mandibular implant overdentures. *J. Prosthet. Dent.* 79, 422–9.

Kohavi D. 1993. Complications in the tissue integrated prostheses components: clinical and mechanical evaluation. *J. Oral. Rehabil.* 20, 413–22.

Langer A, Michman J. 1970. Evaluation of lateral tracings of edentulous subjects. *J. Prosthet. Dent.* 23, 381–6.

Lundeen HC, Wirth CG. 1973. Condylar movement patterns engraved in plastic blocks. *J. Prosthet. Dent.* 30, 866–75.

Lundeen HC. 1979. Mandibular movement recordings and articulator adjustments simplified. *Dent. Clin. North Am.* 23, 231–41.

McDevitt WE, Brady AP, Stack JP, Hobdell MH. 1995. A magnetic resonance imaging study of centric maxillomandibular relation. *Int. J. Prosthodont.* 8, 377–91.

Meyer FS. 1959. The generated path technique in reconstruction dentistry. Part II. Fixed partial dentures. *J. Prosthet. Dent.* 9, 432–40.

Morgano SM, Geramy A. 2004. Finite element analysis of three designs of an implant-supported molar crown. *J. Prosthet. Dent.* 92, 434–40.

Niswonger MF. 1934. The rest position of the mandible and centric relation. *J. Am. Dent. Assoc.* 21, 1572–82.

Ohguri T, Kawano F, Ichikawa T, Matsumoto N. 1999. Influence of occlusal scheme on the pressure distribution under a complete denture. *Int. J. Prosthodont.* 12, 353–8.

Ortman HR. 1977. Complete denture occlusion. *Dent. Clin. North. Am.* 21, 299–320.

Payne SH. 1941. A posterior set-up to meet individual requirements. *Dent. Digest.* 47, 20–2.

Posselt U. 1952. Studies in the mobility of the human mandible, *Acta Odont. Scandinav.* 10, 19–160, Suppl. 10.

Pound E. 1970. Utilizing speech to simplify a personalized denture service. *J. Prosthet. Dent.* 24, 586–600.

Schuyler CH. 1963. The function and importance of incisal guidance in oral rehabilitation. *J. Prosthet. Dent.* 13, 1011–29.

Seong WJ, Korioth TW, Hodges JS. 2000. Experimentally induced abutment strains in three types of single-molar implant restorations. *J. Prosthet. Dent.* 84, 318–26.

Stuart CE. 1964. Good occlusion for natural teeth. *J. Prosthet. Dent.* 14, 716–724.

Sutton AF, McCord JF. 2007. A randomized clinical trial comparing anatomic, lingualized, and zero-degree posterior occlusal forms for complete dentures. *J. Prosthet. Dent.* 97, 292–8.

Thompson JR. 1946. The rest position of the mandible and its significance to dental science. *J. Am. Dent. Assoc.* 33, 151–80.

Chapter 6 Systemic and Local Drug Delivery of Antimicrobials

INTRODUCTION

The recognition of the importance of bacteria as etiologic agents of periodontal disease and the seminal studies of previous decades which identified key pathogens have led to numerous investigations into the role of antibiotics in periodontal treatment. Unfortunately, due to differences of these studies in design, duration, antibiotic class and dosage, concomitant mechanical treatment, and disease classification, the extrapolation of concise conclusions is not easy, as several authors in the field have noted. In addition, during the last two decades, advances in laboratory technology have provided new insight about the structure and properties of the subgingival biofilm and its resistance to antimicrobials and raised questions about their efficacy. The above-mentioned parameters combined with the emerging global threat of antimicrobial resistance and the well known side effects or adverse reactions during antibiotic administration have developed a trend among clinicians for more cautious prescription of this class of drugs.

Knowledge of the disadvantages of systematic administration of antibiotics and difficulties in patient compliance (especially in long-term regimens) have also prompted researchers to develop several local delivery systems in periodontology, i.e., antimicrobial agents embodied in excipients for direct placement and action in periodontal pockets. Due to advanced material technology, several compounds are available for clinicians and a number of studies have evaluated their effects on periodontal conditions.

This chapter focuses on evidence-based systemic and local administration of antibiotics in periodontology and provides guidelines for their indications, according to current evidence and documentation.

EVIDENCE-BASED OUTCOMES

Current major issues of concern among clinicians include the following: Can antibiotics be considered as a sole therapy for periodontal diseases? Are there adjunctive benefits to conventional mechanical treatment or periodontal surgery? Can antibiotics enhance periodontal regeneration or treat acute periodontal conditions? In this section, we review current evidence which should guide clinicians to indications and methods of delivery.

The issue of using antibiotics as monotherapy to treat periodontal disease has been addressed in several studies.

Current data regarding biofilm structure and resistance to antimicrobials show that subgingival biofilms can be more effectively controlled when they are mechanically disrupted. When their dense structure has been altered and the huge number of bacteria diminished, the antimicrobials have the potential to better diffuse and eliminate the microbial target (Socransky and Haffajee, 2002). In addition, antimicrobial activity has been shown to be more effective in "young" and not well organized biofilms. In the Sixth European Workshop on Periodontology, in 2008, Herrera and coworkers addressed the question of whether systemic antimicrobials can be efficacious if the biofilm is not disrupted. The authors reviewed the existing literature and concluded, in agreement with previous position papers and systematic reviews (AAP, 1996; Haffajee et al., 2003), that clinicians should not consider antibiotics as a sole therapy for periodontal diseases and that antibiotics should be combined with mechanical means of disrupting or removing biofilms in gingival sulci and pockets. Therefore, currently, clinicians should act based on good medical practice and administer systemic antibiotics as adjuncts rather than as the main and sole therapy.

As mentioned above, although numerous studies have tested the role of systematic administration of antimicrobials in patients with chronic, aggressive, and refractory periodontitis, several discrepancies among them preclude the comparison and classification of their results and the extrapolation of guidelines. Although as many as 1,300 reports in the literature refer to systemic antibiotics in periodontology, fewer than 30 fulfilled the scientifically sound criteria set by Herrera et al. (2002) for the Fourth European Workshop and Haffajee et al. (2003) for the World Workshop to be included in meta-analysis.

For further comprehensive presentation and comparison of the various studies, the reader is referred to the above mentioned two recent reports, to excellent relevant reviews (Slots and Rams, 1990; van Winkelhoff et al., 1996, Slots and Ting, 2002; Slots 2002a,b, 2004), the previous reports of the American Academy of Periodontology (1996), and previous Workshops of the European Federation of Periodontology (van Winkelhoff et al., 1993).

Today, scientifically sound clinical studies should be designed as randomized clinical trials (RCTs) with the inclusion of controls, a duration of at least six months, and in accordance with strictly defined criteria and statistical analysis as described in the Consolidated Standards for Reporting Trials

(CONSORT) statement (Altman et al., 2001). Therefore, clinicians are encouraged to thoroughly examine the design of scientific trials on antibiotics before considering their conclusions.

Historically, clinical studies regarding the benefits of the systematic administration of antimicrobials in periodontology began in the late 1970s and initially referred to patients with localized juvenile periodontitis (LJP), a disease which partially coincides with localized aggressive periodontitis. In the classical studies of the 1980s and '90s, both in the U.S. and Scandinavia, it has been shown that in LJP patients, systemic administration of antibiotics (the tetracyclines and metronidazole) can improve clinical parameters and decrease the pathogenic subgingival microflora, especially *Aggregatibacter* (*Actinobacillus*) *actinomycetemcomitans* (Slots and Rosling, 1983; Saxen et al., 1990; Saxen and Asikainen, 1993). The efficiency of the combined systemic administration of metronidazole and amoxicillin in LJP patients was investigated by van Winkelhoff et al. (1989), who have shown an improvement of clinical parameters and elimination of *A. actinomycetemcomitans* for at least nine months and therefore introduced this regimen in other classes of periodontal diseases.

For chronic periodontitis patients, who make up the majority in clinical practice, practitioners should currently comply with the most recent reports and meta-analyses, which generally and under confinements suggest benefits from the systematic administration of antimicrobials in chronic periodontitis, using as clinical evaluation the index probing attachment level (PAL). The Herrera et al. (2002) and Haffajee et al. (2003) reports concluded that the administration of antibiotics improves the mean attachment level in patients with chronic periodontitis when used as adjuncts to scaling and root planing. In both reports, at that time, it was stated that existing data precluded their ability to configure guidelines for clinicians concerning the most efficient antibiotic regimen and the appropriate time for administration (before, during, or after the initial treatment phase).

Current data concerning the impact of the quality of debridement and the sequence of antibiotic usage on clinical parameters were also analyzed in the recent report of the Sixth European Workshop on Periodontology (Herrera et al., 2008). After combining evidence in the literature, the authors suggest that if antibiotics are to be used as adjuncts, there is indirect evidence that they should be administered on the day of completion of debridement, which preferably should be performed in a short time and be of adequate quality to optimize clinical benefits for patients. Therefore, according to existing evidence, when treating chronic periodontitis patients, a meticulous debridement by a highly skilled operator should be performed in less than a week, preferably, and antibiotics—if administered—should be prescribed immediately

afterward. Both strategies aim at avoiding the reorganization of the disrupted biofilm and achieving a shift in the subgingival microflora compatible with periodontal health. The results of this combined treatment include a reduction of prevalence, levels, and proportions of pathogenic species such as *Porphyromonas gingivalis, Tannerella forsythia,* and *Treponema denticola*; members of the "red complex" and gram-negative anaerobic species; and members of the "orange complex" described by Socransky et al. (1998), as well as an increase of *Streptococcus* and *Actinomyces* spp.

The report by Haffajee et al. (2006) describes the effect of various periodontal therapies (including antibiotic use) on the subgingival microflora. Data from more than 400 periodontal patients who participated in longitudinal studies conducted over a decade by the Department of Periodontology at the Forsyth Institute were combined to evaluate clinical and microbiological effects of therapies adjunctive to scaling and root planing for up to 24 months. The analysis of more than 10,000 subgingival samples for 40 bacterial species by "checkerboard" DNA-DNA hybridization developed by Socransky and coworkers (1994) in the same department provides very significant insight into the changes of the subgingival habitat induced by various treatments, including periodontal surgery and antibiotic administration. Data from this important report have shown, among others, that the addition of various systemic antibiotics enhanced clinical and microbiological effects of mechanical treatment for up to 24 months. These benefits have been attributed by the authors to several factors, including the reduction of the total bacterial load in the oral cavity and thus the possibility of reinfection, as well as the reduction of specific periodontal pathogens in the pocket environment. Although the main microbiological outcome in this report appears to be the reduction of levels, proportions, and percentages of sites colonized by important periodontal pathogens, they are seldom eliminated and can regrow over time, especially without maintenance care.

After reviewing the literature, the evidence referring to antibiotic effects on patients diagnosed with early-onset or rapidly progressive periodontitis (earlier studies) or aggressive periodontitis (newer studies) is more solid. These patients generally seem to gain further clinical and/or microbiological benefits by the systematic administration of several antimicrobials (metronidazole, tetracyclines, clindamycin, a combination of metronidazole and amoxicillin). These conclusions have been shown in both the Herrera et al. (2002) and the Haffajee et al. (2003) reports after meta-analysis of well-designed studies and in newer RCTs (Guerrero et al., 2005; Xajigeorgiou et al., 2006).

Combining the above findings, it appears that in patients with a diagnosis of aggressive periodontitis, where the genetic background and immunity factors predispose for severe periodontal destruction, optimum control of the bacterial load and periodontal pathogens is extremely important, and from this point of view administration of antimicrobials is indicated for patients in this category.

The results of clinical studies concerning the systematic administration of antimicrobials in combination with periodontal surgery to eliminate the pockets or to achieve periodontal regeneration are contradictory. It is known that antimicrobials can be useful for preventing post-surgical complications. In this case, antibiotic coverage usually targets bacteria that can cause transfections, although for periodontal surgery there are no studies confirming the necessity of antimicrobial administration. It is suggested that sterile conditions and antiseptic mouthwashes can be efficient in preventing complications (Newman and van Winkelhoff, 2001; Konstantinidis, 2007).

Findings concerning the clinical benefits of the combined use of antimicrobials with surgical periodontal treatment are controversial. Based on the limited data in the literature, both the Haffajee et al. (2003) and Herrera et al. (2008) reports suggest marginal or insufficient evidence for additional clinical benefits from periodontal surgery when combined with systemic antimicrobials.

The combination of guided tissue regeneration (GTR) with the administration of several antimicrobial regimens also does not appear to uniformly offer stable beneficial clinical outcomes, neither to efficiently prevent bacterial colonization nor to prevent complications (Demolon et al., 1993; Zuchelli et al., 1999; Vest et al., 1999; Loos et al., 2002). The recent relevant report of the Sixth European Workshop states that there is no sufficient evidence to support the administration of antibiotics during regenerative procedures.

At this point, it should be emphasized, the microflora of patients with deep periodontal pockets, especially after the repeated administration of antimicrobials, can include non-oral gram-negative species such as enteric rods and *Pseudomonas* spp., where the administration of other classes of antimicrobials such as the quinolones are indicated (Slots et al., 1990; Rams et al., 1992). In this group of patients the administration of a combination of metronidazole and ciprofloxacin appears to provide additional clinical improvement. Antimicrobials also have been administrated for acute inflammatory conditions of the periodontal tissues, such as periodontal abscess, necrotizing ulcerative gingivitis (NUG) or periodontitis (NUP), and peri-implantitis.

In the previous century, antiseptics were used for the treatment of NUG, while in the 1960s it was confirmed that the systematic administration of penicillin or metronidazole could contribute to the management of the acute phase of inflammation, especially when systemic manifestations such as fever, malaise, and lymphadenitis are present (Fletcher and Plant, 1966; Collins, 1970). Clinical cases without these symptoms can be adequately managed with no antimicrobials (Holmstrup and Westergaard, 2003).

The frequent occurrence of NUG in patients who are HIV-positive raised the question about the necessity of administration of antimicrobials in this patient category. According to the latest findings there is no need for antimicrobial coverage of this group if generalized symptoms are absent. In addition, the possibility of *Candida* spp. infection as a side effect of systemic antimicrobial administration suggests that antibiotics should be prescribed with caution and after consulting the physician (Konstantinidis, 2007).

There is insufficient or contradictory evidence in the literature to document the necessity of antimicrobial administration for treatment of acute periodontal abscess. Existing studies are usually case reports and there are no comparative studies that demonstrate adjunctive benefits from systemic antimicrobials. Generally, in the case of acute periodontal abscess, antimicrobials are considered necessary when the abscess is very extended, diffused, and accompanied by intense pain and/or coexisting compromising medical conditions and systemic manifestations. The combination of drainage with systemic administration of penicillin, hydrochloric tetracycline, or metronidazole was found efficient for the management of the acute conditions, while the combination of amoxicillin/clavulanic and the newer macrolide azithromycin resulted in recovery from acute symptoms without the simultaneous initial drainage of the abscess (Palmer, 1984; Smith and Davies, 1986; Genco, 1991; Herrera et al., 2000a). In any event, according to good medical practice, the initial drainage or surgical fission of the periodontal abscess is considered the necessary first step for managing its acute phase (AAP, 2000; Herrera, 2000b).

Limited documentation also exists about the use of antimicrobials in peri-implantitis, an infection in which there are no established treatment protocols. Existing data from animal and human studies support a positive contribution of the systemic administration of antimicrobials, especially nitroimidazoles or the combination of amoxicillin and metronidazole (Mombelli and Lang, 1998; Mombelli, 2002).

In addition, there is insufficient scientific documentation about administering antimicrobials to prevent complications during dental implant surgery. Two relative studies present controversial results. The Swedish study questions the need for antimicrobial use to prevent post-surgical complications (Gynther et al., 1998), while the American study indicates that the administration of antimicrobials is related to lower percentages of implant failures (Laskin et al., 2000). Nevertheless, because there are no RCTs on this issue, in everyday practice, clinicians usually prescribe antibiotics for implant placement based on the possibility of a complication and less on scientific documentation.

It should be pointed out that the above-mentioned data refer to systemically healthy individuals, whereas the approach for medically compromised subjects is modified. In addition, certain medical conditions require antimicrobial prophylaxis for all periodontal procedures, as will be described in the indications and technique sections below.

Data in the literature regarding evidence-based outcomes of local delivery systems in periodontology are far more limited. Most of the existing systems were originally tested in split-mouth models as monotherapy and compared to scaling and root-planing or no treatment and then as adjuncts to mechanical treatment, mainly in chronic periodontitis patients. These systems were usually applied at the initial treatment phase or during supportive treatment. A systematic review by Hanes and Purvis (2003) has evaluated existing evidence concerning pharmacological agents applied locally in chronic periodontitis patients. They reported that after meta-analysis of 19 studies, the adjunctive use of minocycline gel, minocycline in microspheres, chlorhexidine chip, and doxycycline gel results in significant probing depth reduction and probing attachment level gain compared to mechanical treatment alone, and therefore carefully concluded that in some populations these sustained-release systems, but not irrigations, can reduce probing depth and bleeding on probing equivalent to scaling and root planing.

INDICATIONS

The indications for prescribing systemic antibiotics in periodontology are listed in Table 6.1 and are guided by combining current data and evidence in the literature and the current trend in the medical community to limit antibiotic use under the global threat of antimicrobial resistance. Clinicians are encouraged to constantly review the literature

Table 6.1. Evidence-based indications for systemic antibiotics in periodontology.

Chronic periodontitis	— Advanced chronic periodontitis
	— Refractory
	— Generalized recurrence during supportive treatment
Aggressive periodontitis	— Localized or generalized
	— Refractory
	— Generalized recurrence during supportive treatment
Acute periodontal abscess	When generalized symptoms are present
Necrotizing gingivitis	When generalized symptoms are present
Necrotizing periodontitis	
Peri-implantitis	

for updated information on this important aspect of periodontal therapy.

For all periodontal procedures (including periodontal charting) in medically compromised individuals, clinicians should carefully review the subject's medical history and consult with the physician. Specific medical conditions require antibiotic prophylaxis and practitioners should comply with revised, periodically issued guidelines from scientific societies. The British Society for Antimicrobial Chemotherapy (2006) and the American Heart Association (2007) have revised their guidelines for antimicrobial chemoprophylaxis during dental procedures after carefully reviewing evidence about the correlation of dental procedures with infective endocarditis (Gould et al., 2006; Wilson et al., 2007). Both scientific societies have limited the cardiological conditions requiring chemoprophylaxis but increased the spectrum of dental procedures in which antibiotics should be prescribed. These indications, the dental procedures, and the recommended regimens are presented in Tables 6.2 and 6.3. Regarding local delivery systems, the main indication currently remains residual or recurrent pockets during supportive periodontal therapy, according to existing data in the literature.

TECHNIQUES

The antibiotic regimens usually prescribed in periodontology for indications listed above are presented in Table 6.4. It should be noted that differences exist between various countries, according to the manufacturing company. Regarding local delivery systems, clinicians should be aware of advantages of their use as presented in Table 6.5.

Other factors to be considered by clinicians when choosing a local delivery system include the antimicrobial agent that it contains, the initial concentration and pharmacokinetics of this agent in the periodontal pocket environment, and the form, structure, and chemical properties of the excipient which regulate the time and rate of delivery of the antimicrobial (Goodson, 1996). It must remembered that the initial efforts to deliver antimicrobials by subgingival irrigations (Rams and Slots, 1996) had limited clinical results, while the incorporation of antimicrobial substances in polymers ensured a more stable rate of diffusion and release and therefore a more predictable presence of active concentration of the antimicrobials for efficient time in the subgingival environment. The anatomy of the pocket region and the restriction of antimicrobial activity in a confined area of the body are favorable for these systems but the continuous flow of the gingival crevicular fluid is a major challenge to be overcome by the biomaterials technology and, more recently, nanotechnology (Goodson, 2003).

The most widely known local delivery systems are presented in Table 6.6. Tetracycline fibers, the only system with zero

Table 6.2. Dental procedures and cardiac conditions for which antibiotic prophylaxis is required.

Dental procedures for which endocarditis prophylaxis is recommended for patients	Cardiac conditions associated with the highest risk of adverse outcome from endocarditis for which prophylaxis with dental procedures is recommended
All dental procedures that involve manipulation of gingival tissue or the periapical region of teeth or perforation of the oral mucosa.*	• Prosthetic cardiac valve • Previous infective endocarditis • Congenital heart disease (CHD)[†] • Unrepaired cyanotic CHD, including palliative shunts and conduits • Completely repaired congenital heart defect with prosthetic material or device, whether placed by surgery or by catheter intervention, during the first six months after the procedure[‡] • Repaired CHD with residual defects at the site or adjacent to the site of a prosthetic patch or prosthetic device (which inhibits endothelialization) • Cardiac transplantation recipients who develop cardiac valvulopathy

*The following procedures and events do not need prophylaxis: routine anaesthetic injections through noninfected tissue, taking dental radiographs, placement of removable prosthodontic or orthodontic appliances, adjustment of orthodontic appliances, placement of orthodontic brackets, shedding of primary teeth, and bleeding from trauma to the lips or oral mucosa.

[†] Except for the conditions listed above, antibiotic prophylaxis is no longer recommended for any other form of CHD.

[‡] Prophylaxis is recommended because endothelialization of prosthetic material occurs within six months after the procedure.

Wilson W, Taubert KA, Gewitz M, and colleagues. Prevention of infective endocarditis: Guidelines from the American Heart Association. JADA 2007;138(6):739–60. Copyright © 2007 American Dental Association. All rights reserved. Reprinted by permission.

Table 6.3. Regimens for a dental procedure.

Situation	Agent	Regimen: Single dose 30 to 60 minutes before procedure	
		Adults	**Children**
Oral	Amoxicillin	2 g	50 mg/kg
Unable to take oral medication	Ampicillin OR	2 g IM* or IV[†]	50 mg/kg IM or IV
	cefazolin or ceftriaxone	1 g IM or IV	50 mg/kg IM or IV
Allergic to penicillins or ampicillin oral	Cephalexin[‡§] OR	2 g	50 mg/kg
	clindamycin OR	600 mg	20 mg/kg
	azithromycin or clarithromycin	500 mg	15 mg/kg
Allergic to penicillins or ampicillin and unable to take oral medication	Cefazolin or ceftriaxone OR	1 g IM or IV	50 mg/kg IM or IV
	Cephalexin[‡§]	600 mg IM or IV	20 mg/kg IM or IV

*IM: Intramuscular.

[†] IV: Intravenous.

[‡] Or other first- or second-generation oral cephalosporin in equivalent adult or pediatric dosage.

[§] Cephalosporins should not be used in a person with a history of anaphylaxis, angioedema, or urticaria with penicillins or ampicillin.

Wilson W, Taubert KA, Gewitz M, and colleagues. Prevention of infective endocarditis: Guidelines from the American Heart Association. JADA 2007;138(6):739–60. Copyright © 2007 American Dental Association. All rights reserved. Reprinted by permission.

Table 6.4. Antibiotic regimens for periodontal conditions (when indicated).

A. Periodontitis

Antimicrobial	Dosage
Metronidazole	500 mgr/8 hours for 7 days
Tetracycline	250 mgr/6 hours for 21 days
Doxycycline	200 mgr the first day
	100 mgr/24 hours for 21 days
Minocycline	200 mgr the first day
	100 mgr/24 hours for 21 days
Clindamycin	100 mgr/12 hours for 21 days
Metronidazole and ciprofloxacin	500 mgr each/8 hours for 7 days
Metronidazole and amoxicillin	500 mgr each/8 hours for 7 days

B. Periodontal abscess (a), necrotic ulcerative gingivitis (b), peri-implantitis (c)

Antimicrobial	Dosage
Metronidazole (a, b, c)	500 mgr/8 hours for 7 days
Amoxicillin (a)	500 mgr/6 hours for 7 days
Amoxicillin and clavulanic acid (a)	625 mgr/12 hours for 7 days
Clarithromycin (a)	250 mgr/12 hours for 7 days
Metronidazole and amoxicillin (c)	500 mgr each/8 hours for 7 days

Table 6.5. Advantages of local delivery antimicrobial systems.

Release rate of antimicrobials that ensures therapeutic results
Reduction of toxicity and side effects of systematic delivery
Difficulty in antimicrobial agent decomposition
Patient compliance
(Possibly) lower cost and lower waste of antimicrobials

order kinetics and thus with stable concentration of the antibiotic for the 10 days that they remain in the pocket environment, are not currently available on the market and they are the only system that requires physical removal of the system, since they are non-degradable. All of the other systems listed in the table are degradable and user-friendly because they are applied subgingivally either with a blunt needle that is provided or with a blunt instrument in the case of periochip.

AUTHOR'S VIEWS/COMMENTS

Therapeutic planning in contemporary periodontology should be driven by scientific evidence. The use of antibiotics, especially systemic ones, has been a matter of debate and contradictory findings for several years. Clinicians should be aware that currently only results from well organized randomized clinical trials should be taken into consideration. Periodically issued systematic reviews and meta-analyses provide data and guidelines useful for clinical practice. The current trend in the medical and dental community to confine the use of antimicrobial agents should also apply to contemporary periodontology and therefore, they should be considered as adjuncts and not substitutes for proper mechanical treatment. Because specific clinical situations or certain microbiological profiles appear to benefit from adjunctive antimicrobials, in the future, a personalized antibiotic regimen, preferably after microbial analysis, could be a desirable target.

REFERENCES

Altman DG, Schulz KF, Moher D, Egger M, Davidoff F, Elbourne, D, Gøtzsche PC, Lang T. 2001. The Revised CONSORT Statement for Reporting Randomized Trials: Explanation and Elaboration. *Annals of Internal Medicine*, 13, 663–694.

American Academy of Periodontology. 1996. Systemic Antibiotics in Periodontics. *Journal of Periodontology*, 67, 831–866.

American Academy of Periodontology. 2000 Parameters on acute periodontal diseases. *Journal of Periodontology*, 71, 863–866.

Collins JF. 1970. Antibiotic therapy in the treatment of acute necrotizing ulcerative gingivitis. *Journal of Oral Medicine*, 25, 3–6.

Demolon IA, Persson GR, Moncla BJ, Johnson RH, Ammons WF. 1993. Effects of antibiotic treatment on clinical conditions and bacterial growth with guided tissue regeneration. *Journal of Periodontology*, 64, 609–616.

Table 6.6. Local delivery systems in periodontology.

System	Antimicrobial	Form	Initial concentration in GCF	Biodegradability
Actisite	Chlortetracycline	Fiber	1,300 μgr/ml	–
Elyzol	Metronidazole	Gel	461 μgr/ml	+
Periochip	Chlorhexidine	Chip	500 ppm	+
Atridox	Doxycycline	Gel	148 μgr/ml	+
Arestin	Minocycline	Microspheres	340 μgr/ml	+

Fletcher JP, Plant CG. 1966. An assessment of metronidazole in the treatment of acute ulcerative pseudomembranous gingivitis (Vincent's disease). *Oral Surgery, Oral Medicine and Oral Pathology*, 22, 729–736.

Genco RJ. 1991. Using antimicrobial agents to manage periodontal diseases. *The Journal of the American Dental Association*, 122, 30–38.

Goodson JM. 1996. Principles of pharmacologic intervention. *Journal of Clinical Periodontology*, 23, 268–272.

Goodson JM. 2003. Gingival crevice fluid flow. *Periodontology* 2000, 31, 43–54.

Gould FK, Elliott TS, Foweraker J, Malford M, Perry JD, Roberts GJ, et al. 2006. Guidelines for the prevention of endocarditis report of the Working Party of the British Society for Antimicrobial Chemotherapy. *Journal of Antimicrobial Chemotherapy*, 57, 1035–1042.

Guerrero A, Griffiths G, Nibali L, Suvan J, Moles DR, Laurell L, Tonetti MS. 2005. Adjunctive benefits of systemic amoxicillin and metronidazole in non surgical treatment of generalized aggressive periodontitis: Randomized placebo-controlled clinical trial. *Journal of Clinical Periodontology*, 32, 1096–1107.

Gynther GW, Kondell PA, Moberg LE, Heimdahl A. 1998. Dental implant installation without antibiotic prophylaxis. *Oral Surgery, Oral Medicine, Oral Pathology, Oral Radiology, and Endodontics*, 85, 509–511.

Haffajee AD, Socransky SS, Gunsolley JC. 2003. Systemic anti-infective periodontal therapy. A systematic review. *Annals of Periodontology*, 8, 115–181.

Haffajee AD, Teles RP, Socransky SS. 2006. The effect of periodontal therapy on the composition of the subgingival microbiota. *Periodontology* 2000, 42, 219–258.

Hanes PJ, Purvis JP. 2003. Local anti-infective therapy: pharmacological agents. A systematic review. *Annals of Periodontology*, 8, 79–98.

Herrera D, Alonso B, León R, Roldán S, Sanz M. 2008. Antimicrobial therapy in periodontitis: the use of systemic antimicrobials against the subgingival biofilm. *Journal of Clinical Periodontology*, 35, (S. 8), 45–66.

Herrera D, Roldan S, Connor A, Sanz M. 2000a. The periodontal abscess (II). Short-term clinical and microbiological efficacy of 2 systemic antibiotic regimes. *Journal of Clinical Periodontology*, 27, 395–404.

Herrera D, Roldan S, Sanz M. 2000b. The periodontal abscess: a review. *Journal of Clinical Periodontology*, 27, 377–386.

Herrera D, Sanz M, Jepsen S, Needleman I, Roldan S. 2002. A systematic review on the effect of systemic antimicrobials as an adjunct to scaling and root planing in periodontitis patients. *Journal of Clinical Periodontology*, 29, 136–159.

Holmstrup P, Westergaard J. 2003. Necrotizing Periodontal Disease. In: Lindhe J, Carring T, Lang N, eds. Clinical Periodontology and Implant Dentistry, 4th ed. Blackwell-Munksgaard. pp. 243–259.

Konstantinidis AB. 2007. Periodontology, Second Volume, pp. 1397–1433.

Laskin DM, Dent CD, Morris HF, Ochi S, Olson JW. 2000. The influence of preoperative antibiotics on success of endosseous implants at 36 months. *Annals of Periodontology*, 5, 166–174.

Loos BG, Louwerse PHG, Van Winkelhoff AJ, Burger W, Gilijamse M, Hart AAM, van der Velden U. 2002. Use of barrier membranes and systemic antibiotics in the treatment of intraosseous defects. *Journal of Clinical Periodontology*, 29, 910–921.

Mombelli A, Lang NP. 1998. The diagnosis and treatment of peri-implantitis. *Periodontology* 2000, 17, 63–76.

Mombelli A. 2002. Microbiology and antimicrobial therapy of peri-implantitis. *Periodontology* 2000, 28, 177–189.

Newman MG, van Winkelhoff AJ. 2001. Antibiotic and antimicrobial use in dental practice, *Quintessence Publishing,* Second Edition.

Palmer RM. 1984. Acute lateral periodontal abscess. *British Dental Journal*, 157, 311–312.

Rams TE, Slots J. 1996. Local delivery of antimicrobial agents in the periodontal pocket. *Periodontology* 2000, 10, 139–159.

Rams TE, Feik D, Young V, Hammond BF, Slots J. 1992. *Enterococci* in human periodontitis. *Oral Microbiology and Immunology*, 7, 249–252.

Saxen L, Asikainen S. 1993. Metronidazole in the treatment of localized juvenile periodontitis. *Journal of Clinical Periodontology*, 20, 166–171.

Saxen L, Asikainen S, Kanervo A, Kari K, Jousimies S. 1990. The long-term efficacy of systemic doxycycline medication in the treatment of localized juvenile periodontitis. *Archives of Oral Biology*, 35 Suppl, 227S–229S.

Slots J. 2002a. Selection of antimicrobial agents in periodontal therapy. *Journal of Periodontal Research*, 37, 389–398.

Slots J. 2002b. The search for effective, safe and affordable periodontal therapy. *Periodontology* 2000, 28, 9–11.

Slots J, Rams TE. 1990. Antibiotics in periodontal therapy: advantages and disadvantages. *Journal of Clinical Periodontology*, 17, 479–493.

Slots J, Rosling BG. 1983. Suppression of the periodontopathic microflora in localized juvenile periodontitis by systemic tetracycline. *Journal of Clinical Periodontology*, 10, 465–486.

Slots J, Ting M. 2002. Systemic antibiotics in the treatment of periodontal disease. *Periodontology* 2000, 28, 106–176.

Slots J, Feik D, Rams TE. 1990. Prevalence and antimicrobial susceptibility of *Enterobacteriaceae, Pseudomonadaceae* and *Acinetobacter* in human periodontitis. *Oral Microbiology and Immunology*, 5, 149–154.

Slots J. 2004. Systemic antibiotics in periodontics. *Journal of Periodontology*, 75, 1553–1565.

Smith RG, Davies RM. 1986. Acute lateral periodontal abscesses. *British Dental Journal*, 161, 176–178.

Socransky SS, Haffajee AD. 2002. Dental biofilms: difficult therapeutic targets. *Periodontology* 2000, 28, 12–55.

Socransky S, Haffajee AD, Cugini MA, Smith C, Kent Jr. R. 1998. Microbial complexes in subgingival plaque. *Journal of Clinical Periodontology*, 25, 134–144.

Socransky S, Smith C, Martin L, Paster BJ, Dewhirst FE, Levin AE. 1994. Checkerboard DNA-DNA hybridization. *Biotechniques*, 17, 788–792.

Van Winkelhoff AJ, Pavicic MJ, de Graaf J. 1993. Antibiotics in periodontal therapy. In: Lang NP, Karring T, eds. Proceedings of the 1st European Workshop on Periodontics, London: Quintessence, pp. 258–273.

Van Winkelhoff AJ, Rodenburg JP, Goene RJ, Abbas F, Winkel EG, de Graaff J. 1989. Metronidazole plus amoxycillin in the treatment of *Actinobacillus actinomycetemcomitans* associated periodontitis. *Journal of Clinical Periodontology*, 16, 128–131.

Van Winkelhoff AJ, Rams TE, Slots J. 1996. Systemic antibiotic therapy in periodontics. *Periodontology 2000*, 10, 45–78.

Vest TM, Greenwell H, Drisko C, Wittwer JW, Bichara J, Yancey J, Goldsmith J, Rebitski G. 1999. The effect of postsurgical antibiotics and a bioabsorbable membrane on regenerative healing in Class II furcation defects. *Journal of Periodontology*, 70, 878–887.

Wilson W, Taubert K, Gewitz M, Lockhart PB, Baddour LM, Levison M. et al. 2007. Prevention of infective endocarditis. Guidelines from the American Heart Association. *Journal of American Dental Association*, 138(6), 739–760.

Xajigeorgiou C, Sakellari D, Slini T, Baka A, Konstantinidis A. 2006. Clinical and microbiological effects of different antimicrobials on generalized aggressive periodontitis. *Journal of Clinical Periodontology*, 33, 254–264.

Zucchelli G, Sforza, NM, Clauser C, Cesari C, De Sanctis M. 1999. Topical and systemic antimicrobial therapy in guided tissue regeneration. *Journal of Periodontology*, 70, 239–247.

Chapter 7 Periodontal Osseous Resective Surgery

INTRODUCTION

Successful treatment of periodontal disease can be achieved today through a number of surgical and nonsurgical procedures, each aiming to control infection and inflammation and reduce pocket depth. Periodontal surgery can still be considered a keystone in the treatment of periodontitis. Osseous resective surgery is defined as a means of changing the diseased tissue contour to reproduce a more physiologic anatomy. Knowledge of the pathogenetic mechanisms of the disease process and identification of the defect characteristics enable the clinician to select the appropriate surgical therapy to correct the deformity and establish a healthy environment.

The degree of destruction of periodontal tissues involving bone, periodontal ligament, cementum, and connective tissue depends on several factors such as type of bacteria, host response, teeth anatomy, hard and soft tissue biotypes, and so forth. Once the lesion has progressed apically, a discrepancy between the gingival margin and bone contour is established, resulting in a pocket. The characteristics of this pocket are determined by gingival biotype, morphology of the osseous crest, and teeth anatomy and location. As the inflammation caused by the periodonto-pathogens moves apically in the periodontal apparatus, a change in the anatomy of the zone takes place. If the bone is thick enough, a funnel-shaped defect is created while the surrounding bone not involved in the demineralization process maintains the gingival tissue in the same position. In the case of thin bone, such as buccal bone or interproximal bone between mandibular incisors, a horizontal pattern of resorption usually takes place, and depending on the soft tissue thickness, a recession or a suprabony pocket is formed.

INDICATIONS AND ENDPOINTS

The goal of osseous resective surgery is to establish minimal or physiologic probing depth and create a gingival contour compatible with good self-performed oral hygiene (Barrington, 1981). Even if regeneration of the lost periodontal apparatus is considered to be the ideal form of treatment, this can be successfully applied only to a limited number of defects according to their infraosseous depth and morphology. There is a clear indication in the literature that regenerative principles should be applied to those defects with an intraosseous component greater than or equal to 4 mm. Therefore, osseous resection is indicated in a number of clinical situations whenever the infra-osseous defect depth is in the 3-mm range or whenever a one-wall defect is present (Ochsenbein, 1986).

Bone re-contouring should be carried out to achieve the so-called positive architecture. This term refers to the physiologic morphology of the alveolar bone that is located in a more coronal position interproximally compared to the radicular buccal and palatal/lingual aspect of the teeth (Figure 7.1). The bone contour follows the cementoenamel junction of the teeth and may be more or less concave, according to the tooth type and genetic biotype (Becker et al., 1997). Therefore, the alveolar crest architecture would have a more pronounced scalloping around incisors and canines, while that toward the molar region would progress in a more flat profile (Figure 7.2).

In a healthy condition, the gingival margin follows the bone architecture so that a consistency between the two entities can be recorded (Matherson, 1988). This is considered during surgical correction of osseous defects to avoid excessive or inappropriate remodelling of the osseous crest. Another field of application for osseous resective surgery is in the case of pre-prosthetic applications. Exposing sound tooth structure, re-establishing a biologic space between alveolar bone and the restoration margin, or correcting an un-esthetic gingival contour can be achieved through osseous resective surgery. In those instances the surgical approach is best known as a crown lengthening procedure (Ingber et al., 1977).

PHYSIOLOGIC AND PATHOLOGIC ALVEOLAR BONE ANATOMY

Unaltered alveolar bone morphology is characterized by the following conditions:

- The interproximal bone peaks are located at a more coronal position compared to the buccal or palatal bone. This is identified as a positive architecture. A negative architecture is considered whenever, due to the effect of periodontal disease, the position of the interdental bone is apical to the one of the buccal or palatal/lingual side. A flat type of architecture is identified whenever interproximal and buccal or palatal bone contour lie on the same line. This can be an effect of periodontal disease or the result of a surgical treatment if an ideal osseous recontouring cannot be achieved.

- The buccal or palatal/lingual bone architecture follows the cementoenamel junction (CEJ) of the related tooth. Therefore, the concavity may be more or less accentuated according to the tooth anatomy. The bone crest appears to be more scalloped at the single-rooted teeth compared to the molars, which present a more flat contour.

- The interproximal bone anatomy reflects the position and root anatomy of the proximal teeth. In the anterior areas, because of the reduced interproximal embrasure and the more or less conical anatomy of the root of the adjacent teeth, this morphology has a knife-edge contour. On the contrary, in the molar area the embrasure is wider and the roots have a more complex anatomy with concavity and convexity leading to a flatter morphology.

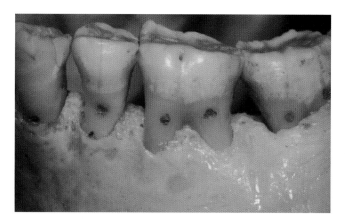

Figure 7.1. An example of positive architecture is shown in this human dry mandible. The buccal alveolar bone is apical to the interproximal crest. Courtesy of Dr. Hyman Smukler, Brookline, MA, USA.

These differences also have an impact from a histologic point of view. A thin knife edge interproximal area usually includes only cortical bone with minimal or no cancellous component (Figure 7.3). This is true, as demonstrated by Tal (1984), any time the distance between two adjacent roots is less than 3 mm. In this case, around 1 mm on each tooth side of the inter-radicular space is occupied by the periodontal ligament and only about 1 mm is left for the alveolar crest that would be made of only cortical bone. In a molar area the embrasure is usually wider and therefore the inter-radicular bone may include both cortical and cancellous bone compartments (Figure 7.4). These above-mentioned anatomical features play a significant role in the pathogenesis of an infra-osseous defect. The inflammatory process, in the case of a narrow interproximal space with a mainly cortical interdental bone, usually determines a horizontal pattern of resorption. Conversely, in the case of a wider embrasure, with thicker cortical and cancellous bone, an infra-osseous defect is more likely to occur. (Figure 7.5)

- The buccal bone is usually thinner than the corresponding palatal or lingual bone according to the biotype. Root prominence, such as in the case of canines or the mesio-buccal root of the first maxillary molars, may determine a further reduction of the bone thickness predisposing to buccal bone dehiscences and fenestrations. Eliot and Bowers (1963), studying human skulls, reported an incidence of bone defects of about 20%. Fenestrations were more frequent in the maxilla, whereas dehiscences occurred at a higher rate in the mandible. The occurrence of one of these defects during periodontal surgery may complicate the osseous recontouring or may determine a significant change in the treatment goals. (Figure 7.6)

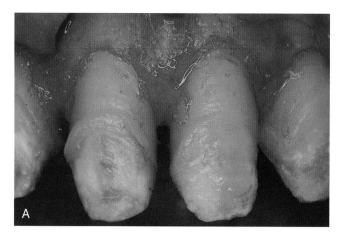 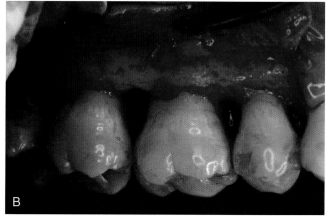

Figure 7.2. A, Surgical exposure of the alveolar crest around maxillary incisors during a crown lengthening procedure. Note how the bone architecture follows the CEJ outline, creating a scalloped morphology. B, A full-thickness flap of a maxillary posterior sextant for pocket elimination. The alveolar crest at the molar area runs with minimal scalloping according to the CEJ morphology.

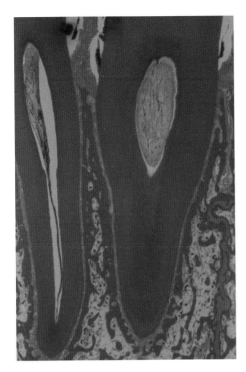

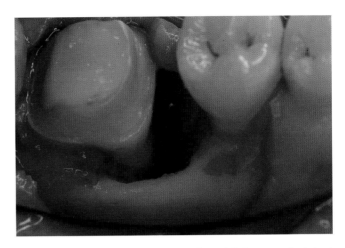

Figure 7.5. A large semi-circumferential three-wall defect around the mesio-lingual aspect of a mandibular first molar is exposed during surgery. The thickness of the lingual cortex and the inter-radicular distance account for the defect morphology.

Figure 7.3. Histologic specimen from a monkey (*Macaca fascicularis*) showing the interproximal bone septum between the canine and incisor. The coronal part of the crest consists of only cortical bone, while cancellous bone becomes evident toward the middle third of the septum. Courtesy of Dr. Morris Ruben, Boston, MA, USA.

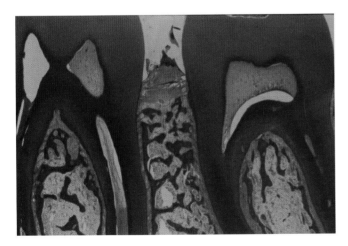

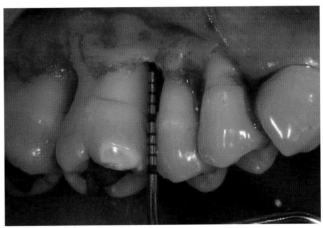

Figure 7.6. After flap elevation for pocket elimination, a dehiscence at the disto-buccal roots of the first molar has occurred. This finding greatly affects treatment strategy and approach. Courtesy of Dr. Alessandro Crea, Viterbo, Italy.

Figure 7.4. Histologic view of a block section taken from a non-human primate at the molar area. The interproximal distance is greater than 3 mm and cortical and cancellous bone are well represented. Courtesy of Dr. Morris Ruben, Boston, MA, USA.

PRINCIPLES

The principles of osseous resective surgery, as it is conceived today, date back to Schluger (1949) and Friedman (1955). Those authors reported the need for eliminating osseous defects so that a consistency between osseous topography and gingival tissue could be re-established, but at a more apical level. According to the *Glossary of Periodontal Terms*, osseous resective surgery includes two different steps: (1) osteoplasty, the reshaping of the alveolar process to achieve a more physiologic form without removing supporting bone, and (2) ostectomy, the excision of bone or portion of a bone that is part of a periodontal defect and includes removal of supporting bone.

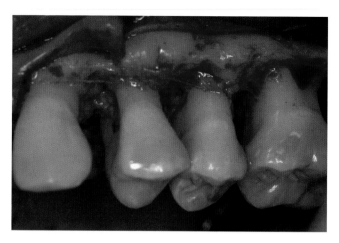

Figure 7.7. A thick buccal bony ledge can be observed after a full-thickness flap is raised. Bony ledges are often accompanied by infra-osseous defects and craters. Their elimination includes a generous osteoplasty to achieve a physiologic osseous anatomy.

Table 7.1 Indications and contraindications to the surgical therapy in the case of anterior areas with no prosthetic involvement.

Therapy	Indications	Notes
Non-surgical Therapy (SRP)	√ PPD > 4 mm √ Horizontal defects	Attention to thin biotypes for recessions
Access Surgery 1. Labial curtain 2. Papilla preservation	√ PPD > 6 mm √ Vertical defects √ Palatal defects	Attention to the high smile
Osseous resective surgery	√ Rarely √ Low lip line √ Low esthetic expectation	Attention to the post-op teeth sensitivity

Table 7.2 Indications and contraindications to the surgical therapy in the case of anterior areas with prosthetic involvement.

Therapy	Indications	Notes
Non-surgical Therapy (SRP)	√ PPD 4–5 mm √ Horizontal defects	Attention to thin biotypes for recessions
Access Surgery 1. Labial curtain 2. Papilla preservation	√ Palatal defects √ Severe buccal recessions and extremely long crowns	No if infrabony defect > 4 mm Attention to the high smile
Osseous resective surgery	√ PPD > 4 mm √ Medium and shallow intrabony defects	Att.: Crown-to-root ratio Att: Clinical crown length

According to Friedman (1955) osteoplasty, is indicated in the case of buccal and/or interpoximal thick bony ledges (Figure 7.7), whereas ostectomy should be used to correct shallow interproximal defects such as craters and hemisepti. This resective approach has several limitations and side effects, and often the application of these principles may determine extraction of involved teeth or an unacceptable esthetic result for the patient. Those limitations have been discussed by Siebert (1976), who reported that the main side effect was the loss of attachment induced by the surgery. He also listed a series of factors that should be taken into account before selecting ostectomy as the surgical treatment modality. Those factors include the length and shape of the roots, location and dimension of the defect, width of investing bone, root prominence, and relationship between the intrabony defects and the adjacent teeth or anatomic structures (maxillary sinus, alveolar nerve, etc). For these reasons, osseous resection underwent a series of modifications through the years, aiming to reduce the amount of bone removal during surgery and thus decreasing the resulting attachment loss.

It should be stressed that osseous resective surgery must be used cautiously whenever an area with esthetic concern is involved in the surgical plan. To simplify the surgical approach to esthetic areas, the key to deciding whether or not to use resective surgery is related to the presence of or a need for a prosthetic involvement. In those cases, osseous resection may be ideal. When there is no prosthetic commitment, only limited and selected cases, including patients with a low smile line and with low esthetic expectations, may be appropriate for this technique (Figure 7.8, Tables 7.1, 7.2).

TECHNIQUE

If osseous resective surgery is selected as a treatment option, several steps should be followed to correctly apply the technique.

Flap Design

Osseous resective surgery is usually coupled with an apical position of the flap. A para-marginal or sub-marginal incision using a 15 or 15C blade is carried out according to the soft tissue characteristics. A split or combined full-split flap may be used to expose the underlying alveolar bone. Releasing incisions may be necessary to gain better surgical visibility or to easily position the flap at the end of the surgery. Vertical incisions should always be carried out beyond the muco-

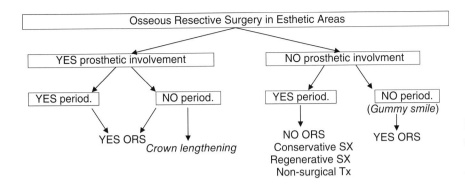

Osseous Resective Surgery in Esthetic Areas

YES prosthetic involvment

YES period.   NO period.

YES ORS
          Crown lengthening

NO prosthetic involvment

YES period.   NO period.
                    (*Gummy smile*)

NO ORS
Conservative SX   YES ORS
Regenerative SX
Non-surgical Tx

Figure 7.8. Strategic use of resective surgery according to the presence of prosthetic involvement and the diagnosis of periodontal disease.

gingival line buccally and lingually, while the palatal aspect should be extended far enough to allow flap mobilization. The main concern in designing the flap is to provide an adequate vascular supply to the margin of the mobilized flap. Therefore, the apical portion of the flap must be wider than the coronal one and should include the major vessel of the area. For this reason vertical releasing incisions should go by the following general principles: (a) must be bevelled, (b) must be divergent toward the apex, (c) should be placed at the mesial and/or distal line angle of the last tooth included in the surgical area, and (d) radicular and interpoximal areas must be avoided due to the major blood supply.

Degranulation and Root Debridement

Once the flap is reflected, degranulation of the soft tissue must be done with surgical curettes (Goldman-Fox n.2, n.3; Barnhardt n. 1/2, etc.) and with sonic/ultrasonic and hand scalers. Once the degranulation is completed and the defect can be identified thoroughly, the root surfaces should be cleaned and planed. Root preparation must be carried out with great care because it greatly influences the type of healing that will take place at the end of the surgical procedures. Polson and Caton described the factors influencing periodontal repair in a primate model (Polson and Caton, 1982). They showed that root surface alterations and contamination inhibit new connective tissue attachment and they stressed the importance of a complete root surface debridement for periodontal healing.

Identification and Measurement of the Defect

Once the surgical field is cleaned, the defect is measured and identified. This is critical in determining the amount of ostectomy and osteoplasty that is indicated. In addition, location of the furcation entrance, root trunk length, or anatomical characteristics of the surgical area must be identified.

Osteoplasty/Ostectomy

The first step is reducing the interpoximal bone thickness. This procedure, called grooving, determines the amount of

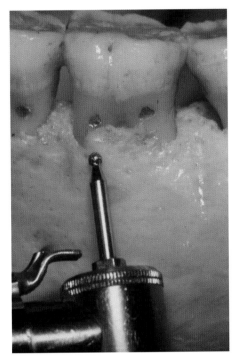

Figure 7.9. A diamond coarse round bur (Brassler, USA) can be used to perform osteoplasty. Due to its moderate cutting ability, compared to the carbide bur, it may be indicated whenever minimal osteoplasty must be done.

osteoplasty that is needed at the radicular bone. In the case of a very thin buccal or palatal/lingual bone, a minimal or no osteoplasty is required. In other instances, a thick bony ledge may be present, requiring aggressive bone re-contouring. This is usually done with diamond coarse or carbide round burs mounted on a hand piece or a high speed hand piece under abundant water cooling irrigation (Figure 7.9). In the case of a bony ledge, a thin cortical layer may be encountered and if care is not taken during the osteoplasty a deep groove into the ledge may be produced as the bur drops into the cancellous bone once the resistance offered by the cortical bone is gone.

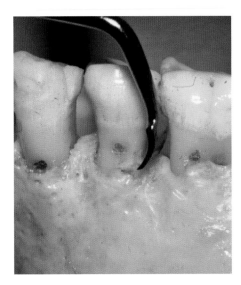

Figure 7.10. A back action (Rhodes 36–37 Hu-friedy, USA) is used in a dry mandible to demonstrate how to perform fine ostectomy. The blade of the instrument is placed on the radicular bone and moved backwards toward the root to eliminate the supporting bone involved in the defect.

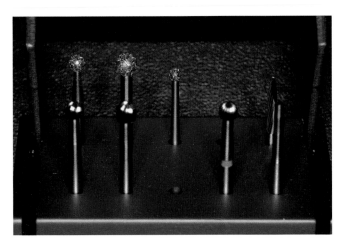

Figure 7.11. An osseous resective surgery bur kit (Brassler, USA), including different sized round burs made of diamond coarse and carbide. The end-cutting bur 957c-H207C is used to remove supporting bone around the tooth without damaging the root surface.

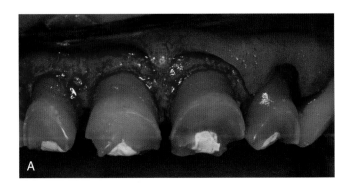
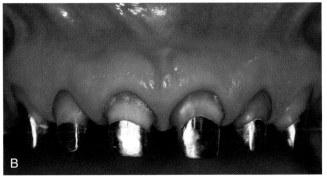

Figure 7.12. A, It may be useful to create a bone ledge in the esthetic area. In this case a crown lengthening has been done and a certain degree of crestal thickness has been intentionally achieved. B, Six months after surgery and before final prosthetic delivery. It is observable that the thickness of crest contributed to the creation of a thick and firm gingival unit.

As soon as the grooving is accomplished, a radicular blending must be done to produce a smooth and blended surface (also known as a sluice-way profile) to enhance flap adaptation. During this step a careful evaluation of root position and anatomy will reduce the risk of causing any fenestration or dehiscence. At this point ostectomy comes into play. One wall, craters, or other defects should be removed and interpoximal and radicular bone designed to achieve a positive architecture. Radicular bone removal is usually carried out with hand instruments. The Ochsenbain chisel (n.1 and 2) and back baction chisel (Rhodes 36–37) (Figure 7.10) are the most popular instruments used for this purpose. Rotary instruments also may be used, but great care must be taken so as to not damage the root while carrying out the ostec-

tomy. Special burs with only an end-cutting head have been designed for this purpose and may be very useful in the interpoximal areas (Figure 7.11).

The more bone that is removed from the radicular or interpoximal areas, the thicker the alveolar margin; this phenomenon is known as ledging. The desired newly established alveolar bone morphology should have a knife-edged profile to allow better flap adaptation and reduce the chance of pocket re-formation. However, there are instances, such as during crown lengthening, in which a certain degree of margin thickness (ledge) is desirable to support soft tissue stability (Figure 7.12).

The last surgical step is the correction of the interdental area. The presence of a crater or a one-wall defect may be managed according to the location and anatomy of the tooth, either by a complete flattening of the crest or by a palatal/lingual approach. This can be done initially with a round bur and completed with bone files (Sugerman file, Kramer and Nevins, etc.). In addition, the removal of the so-called widow's peak is critical. These peaks consist of residual bone left at the facial and palatal/lingual line angles of the teeth. During the healing process, the persistence of these formations may lead to a soft tissue bridging with a re-pocketing of the area. Their elimination is achieved with hand chisels (Wiedelstadt n.1 and n.2) that are run into the interdental area against the radicular surfaces.

Another important factor that influences the ability to achieve a positive architecture is the amount of the residual attachment apparatus. Performing osseous resection to eliminate pockets and defects should not jeopardize tooth stability. The length and anatomy of the roots and evaluation of the residual periodontal support help determine whether osseous resection may be the treatment of choice. The amount of bone that is removed during osseous surgery may vary according to the defect characteristics, the bone architecture, and the teeth morphology. Selipsky (1976) showed that an average of 0.6 mm of support per tooth may be removed with osseous resective surgery. He concluded that although a significant amount of the total bone had to be removed, only a minimal amount of the removed portion would be the supporting apparatus. The increase of mobility following the surgical therapy is transitory and returns to the pre-operative level in about 12 months.

Suturing

Once the osseous re-contour is completed the flap is placed apical to the pre-operative margin. Its position may be apical to or at the osseous crest. In the first case, a small portion of exposed bone, with or without its periosteum, is left exposed. A vertical or horizontal periosteal mattress suture may be used to hold the flap in position; the sutures may be interrupted or continuous. The use of sling sutures is also recommended any time the lingual/palatal or buccal flap must be placed at a different level. A periodontal dressing may or may not be used according to the operator's preference. In the authors' experience it seems that periodontal eugenol-free dressing (Coe-pack) may be indicated any time the flap is positioned apical to the osseous crest to improve patient comfort during healing and reduce the risk for flap displacement during healing. However, it is important to remember that the use of a periodontal dressing may delay the healing process and therefore routine use is no longer justified.

MODIFICATIONS TO THE ORIGINAL SURGICAL APPROACH

Palatal Approach

Ochsenbein and Bohannan (1963) were the first to introduce a modification of the original protocols, by describing the palatal approach. This approach was based on the observation that, due to teeth location and alveolar bone anatomy, infraosseous defects in the maxillary arch were located mainly interproximally and palatally. The palatal approach has several advantages: (a) the presence of an abundant amount of keratinized tissue on the palatal side, (b) an increased thickness of the alveolar bone compared to the buccal aspect, (c) a wider embrasure area between the molars, facilitating the surgical access, and (d) the cleansing effect of the tongue in the post-operative period.

By using this approach a palatally inclined ramp is created with minimal ostectomy. The majority of the osteoplasty and ostectomy are carried out from the palatal aspect and only minimal osseous contour is done buccally, preserving furcation entrance integrity in the molars and reducing the amount of root exposure in esthetically sensitive areas. In 1964, the same authors classified the interproximal defects (craters) in four different entities. Class I defect was characterized by a 2-mm to 3-mm deep component with thick facial and palatal walls; Class II was 4 mm to 5 mm deep with thin facial and palatal walls; Class III more than 6 mm deep with a sharp drop from the walls to a flat base, and Class IV, the least common situation, was characterized by a crater with a variable depth but extremely thin buccal and palatal walls. The authors associated a treatment option with each defect so that Class I could be managed only with palatal ramping, while Class II and III should be approached with both buccal and palatal ramping, and treatment of Class IV, although very unfavorable, included the elimination of buccal and palatal walls.

Lingual Approach

The same concept used in the maxilla was later introduced for the mandible. Tibbets et al. (1976) reported on how the mandibular molars and premolars should be approached from the lingual aspect. The rationale for this lies in the observation that molars and premolars have a lingual inclination (Wilson's curve around 29 degrees for the molars and 9 degrees for the premolars) so that the entrance of the lingual furcation is located at a more apical position compared to the buccal one. Furthermore, the lingual bone is thicker compared to the buccal (Figure 7.13) and there is always an adequate amount of keratinized tissue on this side. As for the palatal approach, this technique should be used to minimize the amount of ostectomy carried out in the buccal area, preserving the furcation integrity and reducing the total amount of attachment loss (Figure 7.14 a-b).

Fiber Retention Osseous Resective Surgery

Another and more recent modification of the osseous resective surgical technique has been presented by Carnevale (2007). This technique is based on the concept that supracrestal fibers inserted into the root cementum are always present coronal to the alveolar crest, both in diseased and healthy situations (Gargiulo et al., 1961; Carnevale et al., 1985). Therefore, it seems reasonable from a biological and clinical standpoint that preservation of those fibers during surgery may have two effects: (a) relocating the deepest portion of the defect at a more coronal position, and (b) reducing the amount of ostectomy required to eliminate the defect. In other words, the presence of a connective tissue attachment coronal to the crest determines a coronal shift of the apical component of the osseous defect.

The technique includes a split thinned flap and the careful removal of the soft tissue using a blade or an interproximal knife (Goldman-Fox n.11, Orban 5/6, Buck 1/2). This sharp dissection is followed by the identification of the residual attachment apparatus within the bone defect using a periodontal probe. The non-attached soft tissue is then removed and resection of the osseous crest is carried out. At the end of the alveolar bone re-contouring, only bone with attached fibers should be left around the tooth. This technique has been proven to be effective in reducing and maintaining probing depth within the normal range. Carnevale et al. (1991) reported on 304 periodontally compromised patients treated with the fiber retention osseous resective surgery who were followed for three to 17 years. The majority of the patients (86%) belonged to ADA case types 3 and 4. Patients were further divided into three groups according to the length of the follow-up period. Ninety-two patients were followed for 11.3 years. At the end of the study only 147 out of 8,572 sites were deeper than 4 mm (1.72% of the total sites), demonstrating a remarkable long-term stability of the results achieved at the completion of active therapy.

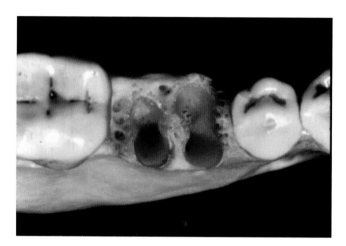

Figure 7.13. Photograph of a dry human mandible showing the alveolar crest after removal of a first molar. The buccal bone is a very thin lamina compared to the lingual crest. Removal of lingual bone to correct a periodontal defect is preferred to prevent furcation exposure and severe buccal dehiscence.

Data on teeth extraction also have been reported by the authors. It is significant that the majority of the teeth (576, that is, 7.5% of the total sample) were extracted during active treatment. Most of these teeth (63.7%) belonged to patients falling in the ADA case type 4 category, and the main reason for their loss was advance periodontal breakdown. During supportive therapy, however, the incidence of teeth extraction was dramatically reduced (67 teeth; 0.9% of the total sample) and limited to a subgroup of 50 patients. These results confirmed the effectiveness of this technique in treating and controlling advanced periodontal disease.

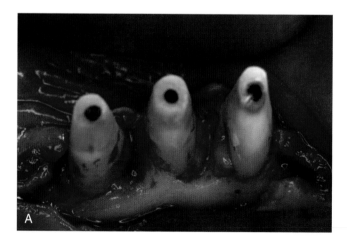
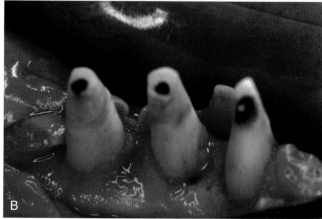

Figure 7.14. A, Craters and combined infrabony defect less than 3 mm deep lingually to prosthetic abutments. Lingual osteoplasty and minimal ostectomy are indicated to manage this defect. B, The result after osseous re-contouring and tooth preparation. No defects remain.

Furthermore, this technique should be considered a very reliable option in the case of complex perio-prosthetic case involvement.

SOFT TISSUE MANAGEMENT

The soft tissue component must be managed during the osseous surgery. Positioning the gingival margin apical to the pre-operative level is recommended any time elimination of the defect is indicated. This can be done in several ways according to the soft tissue biotype and osseous determinants.

Buccal/Facial Flap

Whenever an adequate band of keratinized tissue is present a sub-marginal scalloped incision may be outlined about 1 mm to 2 mm apical to the gingival margin or as deep as the required probing depth (Figure 7.15). A full-thickness thinned flap up the mucogingival line followed by a partial dissection or a complete partial-thickness flap may be elevated to gain access to the underlying bone. In the case of inadequate or minimal keratinized gingiva an intra-sulcular incision is preferred to preserve as much attached gingiva as possible. In the case of a very thin biotype a mucoperiosteal flap is preferred because the chance of flap perforation and necrosis may increase (Wood et al., 1972). Once the flap is elevated and osseous recontouring is performed, the mobility of the flap should be tested so that a passive positioning is obtained at or apical to the newly recontoured alveolar crest. As previously described, if vertical releasing incisions are indicated to freely move the flap, these should be extended into the alveolar mucosa.

Palatal Flap

A different approach is required on the palatal side because the gingiva in this area is completely keratinized and cannot be moved in an apico-coronal position. This approach, best known as palatal thinned flap, is used any time pocket reduction or elimination is required. The primary scalloped incision should be outlined according to the probing depth and following the anatomy of the teeth involved in the surgical area. For instance, the primary incision around a second premolar is more concave compared to that around a first molar. Another factor that influences flap design is root anatomy and morphology. As the defect moves apically, the size of the roots narrows. So in the case of a deep probing around the palatal root of a maxillary first molar, the scalloping should be calibrated to the root morphology rather than the mesio-distal dimension of the clinical crown. It is therefore root morphology that dictates the incision outline, rather than clinical crown anatomy. In addition, tooth position and consequently root direction must be considered in the surgical planning. Most of the time palatal roots of maxillary first and second molars have a disto-palatal direction. This must be considered in the flap design.

The palatal vault is another important anatomic issue for the thinned palatal flap. In the case of a high vault palate the incision may correspond to the probing depth, while in the case of a flat vault it should be outlined close to the gingival margin. This is mainly due to the presence of the greater palatal artery that runs into the soft tissue at a distance from the CEJ of the molars that varies according to the vault extension (Reiser et al., 1996).

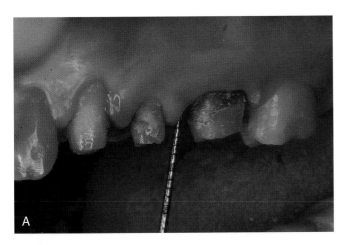
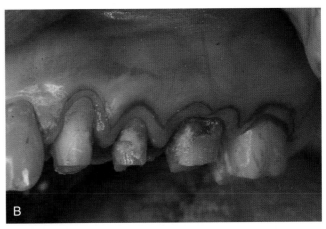

Figure 7.15. A, Pre-surgical probing for crown lengthening. Surgical incisions are planned according to probing depth, toothy and root anatomy, and amount of keratinized tissue. B, In this case the abundance of keratinized tissue allows the outline of a submarginal scalloped full-thickness flap. Surgical papillae are created interproximally and facial to the furcation entrance to protect this area during healing.

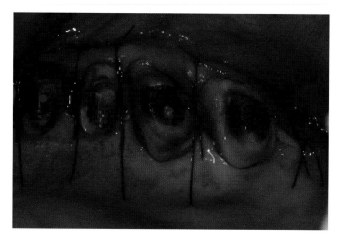

Figure 7.16. If properly outlined, a palatal thinned flap will drop on the re-contoured alveolar crest following the root anatomy. Minimal or no trimming should be required if proper tissue incisions are made. The picture shows a passive adaptation of a thinned flap. Note how the primary incisions have been designed according to the root position and anatomy.

A thinned flap is indicated to reduce the soft tissue component and achieve a pocket reduction with a better flap adaptation. The final crest morphology should be estimated during flap incisions so that minimal trimming of the flap is needed at the end of the surgery (Figure 7.16). A bone sounding under anaesthesia is required to determine the pre-operative bone contour. The periodontal probe is run into the palatal tissue until it stops, so that the thickness of the gingiva may be estimated.

The presence of an exostosis or osseous defect also may be recorded. This information will help the operator to create an evenly thinned flap along its entire extension. An interproximal thickening of the flap may determine poor tissue adaptation at the radicular aspect of the bone, thus creating an anatomical dead space that may result in a sloughing of the marginal tissue.

Remember that flap design and osseous anatomy are by far more crucial than the suturing technique in achieving passive flap adaptation. However, care must be taken during suturing to hold the flap in the proper position.

EFFECT OF SURGERY ON THE ALVEOLAR BONE

Flap elevation with or without bone reshaping determines a certain degree of crestal bone remodelling, leading to a loss of bone ranging from 0mm to 0.8mm (Donnenfeld et al., 1964). Studying the amount of post-surgical bone remodelling in a human model, Moghaddas and Stahl (1980) reported that the net bone loss at six months after osseous surgery combined with a full-thickness flap varied according to the location. Crestal bone loss averaged 0.23mm in the interproximal space, 0.55mm at the radicular aspect, and 0.88mm in the furcation region of a molar. In their study the three months' data did not reach any statistically significant difference from the six months' data.

Another interesting finding of this work was that no correlation could be made between the amount of resection and the degree of remodelling. During a re-entry procedure, Donnenfeld and co-workers (1970) measured the amount of bone remodelling that took place in three patients undergoing osseous resective procedures both immediately after surgery and at six months. They reported an average of 0.6mm of bone loss interproximally and 1mm at the radicular location. Another study (Smith et al., 1980) described the bone loss after osseous resective surgery only through a bone sounding procedure at six months. They found 0.2mm of radicular bone loss and 0.3mm of interproximal bone loss. Pennell and co-workers (1967) described in a landmark paper the pattern of wound healing obtained from 34 teeth from 20 patients treated with a full-thickness flap followed by osteoplasty on 5mm of marginal bone and ostectomy at the first mm of crestal bone. The post surgical observation period ranged from 14 to 545 days and they reported an average bone crest resorption of 0.54mm. The majority of the teeth (82%) showed less than 1mm of resorption, while severe bone loss (more than 3mm) was recorded in only two cases.

Histologic Effect of Osseous Surgery

The best histologic evidence on the effect of resective procedures on the alveolar crest are reported by Wilderman et al. (1970). The sample included 23 block sections of teeth that underwent a mucoperiosteal flap followed by osteoplasty in the first 5mm of alveolar bone and 1mm of crestal bone reduction. The effect of bone surgery varies according to the nature of the alveolar bone. Superficial bone necrosis with intense osteoclastic activity was a common finding. In the case of a thin alveolar bone, resorption took place at the periodontal ligament side, while when a thick bone was found, the osteoclastic activity started within the marrow spaces toward the periosteal side. Osteoblastic activity reached its peak after 21 days, and after six months very little additional bone remodelling could be detected.

Interestingly, the mean loss of bone was 0.8mm in the case of a thick alveolar crest, while it reached 3.1mm in the case of a thin crest. This may be due to the different intrinsic healing potential of different bone anatomy. Thick cancellous bone holds better healing potential compared to thin cortical bone. Therefore, great attention must be paid to the quality of the bone during osseous surgery because the knowledge of these characteristics may be of great importance in determining the final surgical result.

EVIDENCE-BASED OUTCOMES

In the past 50 years a number of studies comparing different treatment approaches to periodontal pockets have been published. It is worth noticing that different conclusions may be drawn from the results presented with a certain degree of discrepancy. Evidence-based dentistry, as it is established today, is a very important tool for gaining a better understanding of the limitations and benefits of different treatment options. However, ideal studies fulfilling all of the requisites for the highest scientific evidence have yet to be performed. This chapter attempts to summarize the results of some of the most representative studies to give the reader some indications that may be useful in a clinical setting. A more in-depth and precise examination of the literature on this topic is suggested to gain a broader understanding of each of the studies quoted.

Osseous resective surgery has been studied alone and compared with other surgical and nonsurgical techniques in several longitudinal studies. Most of the studies reported on short-term results, while only a few extended to a five-year follow-up. Here we discuss only those studies with at least five years of follow-up. Although there are some differences, the layout of these studies is somewhat similar as different modalities of treatment have been tested in a split mouth design. The treatments rendered were osseous resective surgery with apical positioning of the flap, modified Widman flap surgery, and scaling and root planing. The results have been analyzed according to the initial probing depth. Three depth categories have been identified: 1 mm to 3 mm, 4 mm to 6 mm, and greater than 7 mm.

Knowles and co-workers (1979) treated 72 patients and found that while in a 1-mm to 3-mm depth there was a slight loss of attachment with all of the treatment modalities (thus demonstrating that there is no indication for any kind of treatment in a shallow pocket), for the 4 mm to 6 mm category osseous resective surgery achieved greater pocket depth reduction compared to scaling and root planing but similar results compared to Widman flap surgery. Interestingly, in this depth category all three modalities determined the same amount of attachment level gain. For the greater than 7 mm pockets, all of the treatments reduced the probing depth, but the Widman flap achieved a more significant reduction and a greater gain of attachment compared to the other two.

Ramfjord et al., in 1987, published a second study with a five-year follow-up. The general conclusions were similar to those previously reported except for the greater than 7 mm pockets. In this category the probing depth reduction, although greater compared to the other probing categories, did not show any significant difference in any of the three therapies (ORS 3.53 mm, MWF 3.13 mm, SRP 2.92 mm). This finding was also true for the attachment level gain; none

of the treatments was superior to the others. Comparing the results of the one year of maintenance with the final examination at five years, it is notable that some periodontal deterioration took place in most of the patients. Although no statistically significant differences could be reported between the treatments in terms of probing depth reduction and gain of attachment, the incidence of loosing sites was twice in the Widman flap and scaling-treated quadrants compared to the resective surgery quadrants. It is also noteworthy that no molar furcations were included in this study.

In a similar study, Kaldahl and co-workers (1996) reported on 72 patients who were followed for more than five years. Osseous resective surgery was able to produce a greater probing depth reduction compared to Widman flap surgery and scaling and root planing during the entire study in the 5 mm to 6 mm pocket category (−1.85 mm for ORS, −1.48 for MWF, −1.52 for SRP). In terms of attachment level gain, osseous resective surgery had the least gain, 0.44 mm, while modified Widman flap surgery (0.60 mm) and scaling and root planing (0.90 mm) showed the greatest performance. In the greater than 7 mm pocket category, osseous resection was the most efficacious treatment in probing reduction (3.38 mm) compared to the other two (MWF 3.09 mm, SRP 2.88 mm). No statistically significant difference could be found in terms of clinical attachment gain between the three therapies at five years (ORS 1.83 mm, MWF 2.07 mm, SRP 1.88 mm).

Several considerations should be made before drawing a definitive conclusion from these studies. Probing depth alone does not reflect the anatomy and morphology of the underlying bony defect, so a deeper or shallower intrabony defect associated with the same probing depth may respond differently to the same treatment modality. The split mouth design may carry an innate bias related to the effect that one treatment may have on the others over the long term. Also, clear endpoints in the performance of osseous surgery have not been stated in any of the studies except those from the Nebraska group (Kaldahl et al., 1996). In this study the achievement of a positive architecture led to the extraction of several teeth and roots during surgery. This is clearly in contrast to other studies in which no mention of root resection or extraction was reported (Knowles et al., 1979; Ramfjord et al., 1987). This may be considered a major limitation in defining the effect of a specific treatment modality.

Another interesting point is the fact that attachment loosing sites appeared to have a higher incidence in those quadrants not treated with osseous resection. Usually the statistical comparison between treatments that has been reported has been based on the mean changes. Now if the number of attachment loosing sites is relatively small, it may be overshadowed by the majority of the stable sites. However, a site analysis may bring up differences that may be significant in the clinical setting. Therefore, the fact that patients treated with osseous resective procedures have a low incidence of attachment loosing sites (Kalkwarf et al., 1988; Kaldhal et al., 1996; Carnevale et al., 2007) may be very important in the case of perio-prosthetic rehabilitation in which disease recurrence may determine prosthetic failure.

A possible explanation for this stability of the apical positioning of the flap has been reported as a major contributor. Several studies (Mombelli et al., 1995; Levy et al., 2002) have shown that the apical displacement of the gingival margin exposing the previously contaminated root determines the formation of a new dento-gingival unit apical to the diseased cementum. This may also determine a positive shift of the microflora by modifying the existing habitat (Levy et al., 2002) and reduce the chance for micro-organisms (that have been dormant in the dentinal tubuli) to inhabit the newly formed shallow sulcus (Adriaens et al., 1988).

Treatment of Furcated Molars with Resective Techniques

Furcation lesions traditionally have been seen as a major challenge for periodontists and restorative dentists. Complicated root anatomy combined with limited access to the area due to teeth location have been cited for the poor prognosis of those areas. Furcation anatomy presents several characteristics that must be known before continuing with their treatment. Furcation entrance size, root trunk length, root concavities, and dome morphology all contributes to make treatment of furcation involvement a difficult task.

Classification of Furcation Involvement

Once a furcation is periodontally involved different treatment options may be contemplated in relation to the degree of involvement. A furcation lesion may be detected using a dedicated curved probe (Nabers probe) with color marking every 3 mm. Hamp et al. (1975) categorized furcation defects according to the degree of horizontal probing. Three different classes of severity were identified: Class I, when the probing was in the 3 mm range; Class II, if the probing was greater than 3 mm but not passing through the furcation; and Class III, if a through and through lesion was detectable. Tarnow and Fletcher (1984) added to the Hamp classification the evaluation of the vertical probing, identifying three different categories: Subclass A, 1 mm to 3 mm; Subclass B, 4 mm to 6 mm; and Subclass C, greater than 6 mm. According to the authors, this may help clinicians to improve treatment choices and predictability.

Ability to Remove Calculus

Furcation is a critical area for cleaning. Caffesse and co-workers (1986) showed that even with an open approach it was very difficult to achieve complete removal of the calculus from an involved furcation area. Matia et al. (1987), using a surgical approach, was able to remove calculus from only seven out of the 26 treated furcation surfaces. These difficulties in achieving a satisfactory result are determined mainly by the complicated anatomy of the area.

Molar Root Anatomy

Bower (1979) and Gher and Vernino (1980), analyzing extracted maxillary and mandibular molars, reported that the furcation aspect of mandibular molars presents a concavity up to 1 mm deep 100% of the time for the mesial root and 99% of the time for the distal root. In the maxillary molars 100% of the mesio-buccal roots have a 1 mm deep concavity while the distal has this concavity 97% of the time and the palatal has this 17% of the time. Furthermore, 75% of the time the furcation entrance is less than 1 mm, limiting the accessibility to scalers and sonic devices. For these reasons new designs and miniaturized hand and sonic instruments have been introduced in the market and have become very popular. In spite of these technological advancements, each clinician should bear in mind that the result in treating a furcation depends on the strategic value of the tooth.

Enamel Pearl Projections

Other anatomical determinants may complicate the furcation area. Enamel pearl projections have been reported in the literature as co-factors for furcation lesion formation. Masters and Hoskins (1964) found that cervical enamel projections were present at 29% of the buccal surfaces of mandibular molars, while only 17% of the observed maxillary molars had the same anatomical feature. Moskow and Canut (1990) found a lower incidence of the enamel pearl projections, with a range from 1.1% to 9.7%. The teeth with the highest frequency were the maxillary third and second molars. Two different papers (Bissada and Abdelmalek, 1973; Swan and Hurt, 1976) reported a 50% correlation between furcation involvement and enamel pearl projections. In 1987 Hou and Tsai were able to correlate furcation involvement with the presence of cervical enamel projections based on a study of 87 furcated molars that showed cervical enamel projections in 63% of the cases.

Intermediate Bifurcational Ridge

These formations can be found on the mandibular molars; they consist of cementum formation originating from the mesial surface of the distal root, extending to the mesial root. Everett et al. (1958) found that 73% of the observed extracted mandibular molars were affected by these anatomical aberrations.

Accessory Pulp Canals

Since Bender and Seltzer (1972) reported on the presence of a great number of accessory pulp canals in the furcation area of molars, many other authors have investigated the incidence of these canals and their role in the establishment of periodontal lesions. While there is enough evidence to support the fact that accessory pulp canals open in the furcation area with a great deal of frequency (with a range of 27.4% to 76%) (Lowman et al., 1973; Vertucci and Williams, 1974; Burch and Hulen, 1974; Gutman, 1978), there is still some controversy regarding their role in the pathogenesis of a periodontal lesion.

Resective Options

According to the 1992 *Glossary of Periodontal Terms* we can define the following treatment modalities:

Root amputation: The surgical removal of a root without the related crown portion (this can be done before or after the endodontic treatment).

Root resection: The removal of a root and the related crown portion from a multi-rooted tooth.

Root separation: The surgical sectioning of the root complex and the maintenance of all roots.

Hemisection: The surgical separation of a multi-rooted tooth with the extraction of one root with the overhanging crown. Usually refers to mandibular molars.

Tunnelization: Conservative treatment by creating a space between the roots that can be cleaned by the patient. (Usually refers to mandibular molars.)

The modalities are described in detail below.

Root Amputation

This treatment may be considered a conservative treatment modality; it may not include the prosthetic restoration of the involved tooth. This may be indicated whenever one of the roots is involved periodontally or endodontically and the overhanging crown is sound (Figure 7.17 a,b). In this case, after a flap is raised the root is cut right at its emergence from the root trunk. A fissure bur is used to bevel the amputation. A minimal ostectomy should be performed on the buccal aspect of the root (or palatal aspect in the case of a palatal

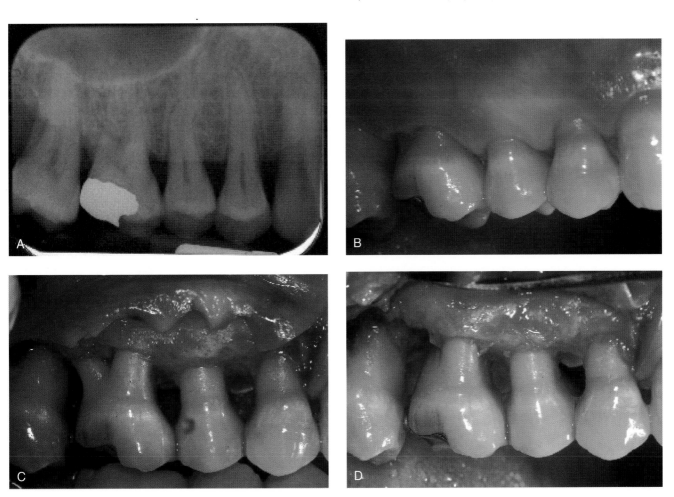

Figure 7.17. A, Radiograph of a maxillary first molar with a root proximity and a Class II defect of the buccal furcation. B, Clinical view, pre-operative. C, After mucoperiosteal flap elevation, the buccal furcation is clearly visible. D, The root amputation is performed by cutting the base of the disto-buccal root with a fissure bur to create a sluiceway to allow proper cleaning.

maxillary molar) to allow the extraction of the root without the risk of buccal bony plate fracture (Figure 7.17 c,d). Once the root is extracted the orifice on the crown should be filled and the flap sutured back. Smukler and Tagger (1976) showed in a clinical and histological study that this procedure may be carried out as an emergency procedure before endodontic treatment has been performed. The pulp of the amputated molars remains vital for up to two weeks without symptoms. However, all efforts should be made to treat the tooth endodontically before the amputation is performed.

Evidence: There is scarce evidence regarding the long-term effect of this modality of treatment.

Root Resection/Separation/Hemisection

In the case of Class II and III furcation involvement, a root resection or separation may be considered. Several factors should be evaluated before considering this option: root anatomy, root length, amount of attachment loss and attachment apparatus left on the residual roots, tooth mobility before resection, restorability of the crown, strategic importance, and alternative treatment. This treatment includes endodontic therapy, tooth reconstruction, and prosthetic coverage. All of the operators involved in the treatment must be acquainted with the objectives of the treatment so that appropriate minimally invasive root canal shaping and conservative root preparation is done.

Once the tooth has been judged appropriate for this treatment, it must undergo endodontic therapy first and then must be prepared for a complete crown coverage (Figure 7.18). After raising a flap, the furcation entrance must be clearly identified and the anatomy of the root selected for resection carefully evaluated (Figure 7.19). Using a carbide or diamond fissure bur, a trough will be outlined connecting the entrances of the two furcations. The extraction can be done once the root and the related portion of the crown are isolated (Figure 7.20). Some crestal bone may be removed to facilitate root mobilization and minimize the chance of fracture of the buccal bony plate during root extraction. At this point the residual tooth should be checked for any further furcation involvement; if this is the case a separation of the residual roots may be considered.

It is very important in this procedure to consider each separated root as an individual unit and the furcation space as an interdental area. Osseous surgery around each of the resected roots should therefore follow the same basic principles of creating a positive architecture. The amount of the attachment apparatus left on each root combined with root morphology and length determines the degree of stability of the root. It should be remembered that the majority of the attachment apparatus of a maxillary molar is in the root trunk area and that the mesio-buccal root has a greater attachment area followed by the palatal and disto-buccal roots. A maxillary molar with a short root trunk will be affected by a furcation lesion earlier, but may have a better prognosis if resective procedures are used as most of the attachment is still present. On the contrary, a long root trunk, once involved, has a lesser chance to be treated with resective means because the amount of residual attachment on the remaining root is reduced. Therefore, the root to be resected should be carefully selected both pre- and intra-operatively, particularly when mesio-buccal or palatal roots are indicated for extraction.

After root extraction and/or separation, the tooth must be reshaped and prepared to ensure physiologic soft tissue adaptation and allow patient cleansing maneuvers.

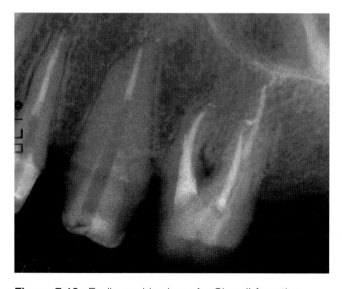

Figure 7.18. Radiographic view of a Class II furcation.

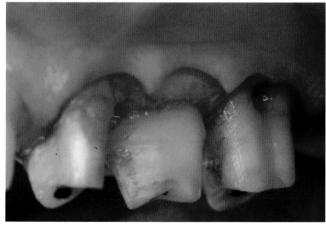

Figure 7.19. The furcation is identified and measured at flap elevation.

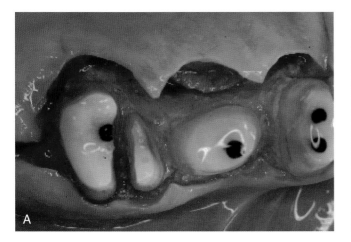

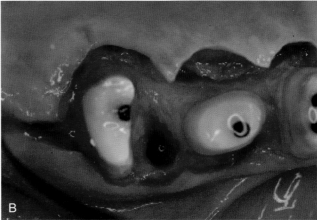

Figure 7.20. The mesio-buccal root is isolated (A) and extracted (B).

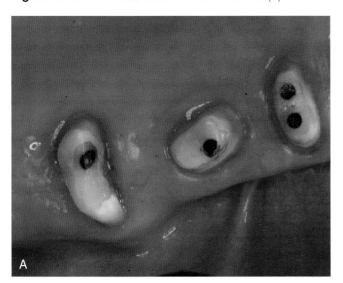

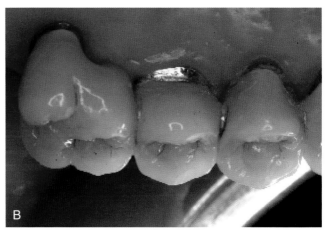

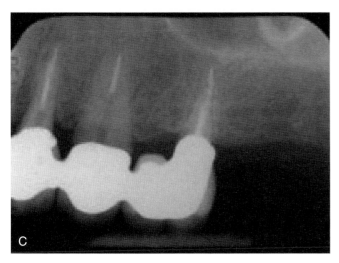

Figure 7.21. A, Two months healing demonstrates good tissue quality and adequate plaque control by the patient. B, Clinical view two years after crown delivery. C, Two-year radiographic control. Courtesy of prosthodontist Dr. Paolo Manicone, Rome, Italy.

Osteoplasty of the residual alveolus also may be indicated to allow better flap adaptation.

Temporary restorations play a significant role in this treatment technique because they ensure stability and protection of the residual tooth during the healing period. At the end of the surgery the temporary restorations should be relined and adapted, leaving the margin at least 3 mm away from the osseous crest to allow tissue maturation and establishment of physiologic supra-crestal gingival tissue (Figure 7.21). Kon and Majzoub (1992) reported that the distance between the pulp floor and the furcation entrance in maxillary resected first molars was, on average, less than 3 mm (Figure 7.22). The significance of this finding may have a major restorative impact because it may imply that all of the restorations in those areas may violate the supra-crestal gingival tissue dimension.

Root resection for mandibular molars deserves some additional considerations. Mesial root anatomy is far more complex compared to the distal root anatomy because it contains two canals and in 100% of the cases has a curvature and a deep concavity on the furcation aspect (Bower, 1979). Removal of the mesial root is therefore preferable because the distal root may be easier to restore and manage periodontally. Fracture of the resected mandibular molar is more frequent when the mesial root is retained (Langer et al., 1981). In the author's experience resection of the mandibular molar may be indicated when the adjacent teeth are involved in the prosthetic plan (Figure 7.23).

The restoration of a resected mandibular molar with an individual crown is the least advantageous because a mesial or distal cantilever is created, along with a great chance of fracture. On the contrary, once the resected molar is involved in a more extended bridgework, the mechanical loading is

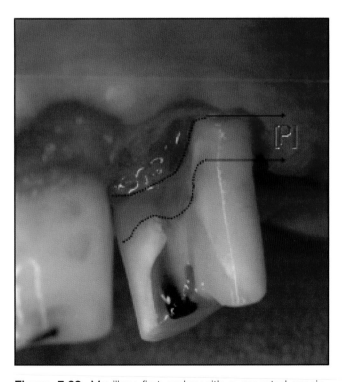

Figure 7.22. Maxillary first molar with a resected mesio-buccal root. The distance between the pulp chamber and the furcation entrance (P) is on average less than 3 mm, as in this case.

distributed along the entire bridge span, reducing the risk for fracture. Prosthetic management of resected teeth is beyond the scope of this chapter, but usually requires conservative preparations to spare as much tooth structure as possible to avoid weakening the abutments.

Mandibular furcated molars, and to a lesser extent maxillary molars, may also be treated by root separation, better known as hemisection. In this instance the roots are separated and maintained. This procedure may be indicated whenever each of the roots has an adequate periodontal apparatus and is judged to be able to be maintained from a prosthetic and endodontic standpoint. The surgical principles are the same as for root resection; however, prosthetic management may differ because a tunnelled molar crown must be fabricated to ensure good access for home care (Figure 7.24). The interproximal distance between the roots must be adequate to allow space for the crown margin (that should only be made of metal) and for interproximal space. Therefore, molars with a narrow inter-radicular space or with roots that connect or converge toward the apex may not be candidates for this treatment modality. The use of an orthodontic device to increase the inter-radicular space has also been advocated, even though it may increase the complexity and length of the therapy.

Evidence: Gathering a general consensus on the effectiveness of root resection therapy on a long-term basis may not be so easy. Conflicting data can be found in the scientific literature regarding this subject. Poor treatment outcomes on a long-term basis have been reported by Langer et al. (1981), who in a 10-year study found that 38 of 100 resected molars had to be extracted. The main reasons for failure were root fracture (18%), periodontal breakdown (10%), and endodontic lesion (7%). Only three teeth failed because of cemental leakage and recurrent decay. Buhler (1988) reported a 32% failure rate at 10 years on 34 resected molars. Again, the main causes of failure were endodontic pathology and root fracture, while only one tooth was extracted due to periodontal breakdown. The same failure rate was found by Blomlof et al. (1997) in a follow-up three to 10 years later. The results of this study should be interpreted with caution because the authors compared the survival of 146 root-resected molars with 100 endodontically treated single-rooted teeth. Interestingly, at five years the survival rate between the two groups did not differ significantly (82% vs. 83%), while at 10 years the survival rate for multi-rooted teeth dropped to 68% compared to 77% of single-rooted teeth. These differences, however, did not provide statistical significance. In this study the primary reason for failure was recurrence of periodontitis, and smoking was identified as a strong risk factor in this group of patients.

On the other hand, several studies report favorable results with the use of root resection. Taken together, the failure rate

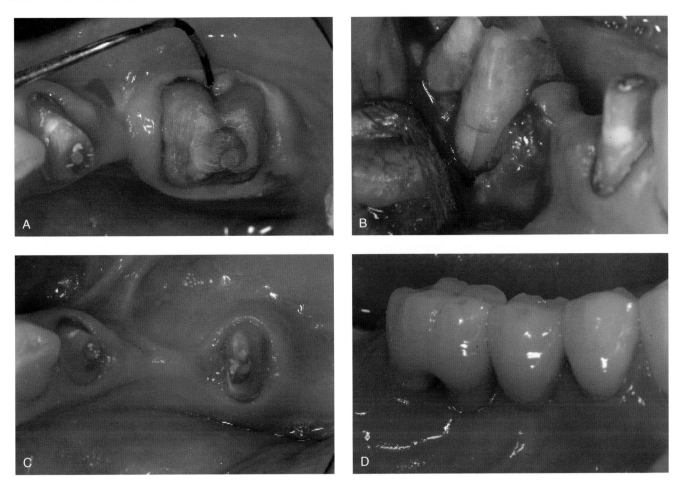

Figure 7.23. A, Lower right first molar with a Class I furcation. B, A vertical fracture of the mesial root is found and the tooth is resected with the extraction of the mesial root. C, Three months after the extraction the distal root is checked for stability and a final fixed partial denture is delivered. D, The pontic design should be adequate to allow good home care. Courtesy of prosthodontist Dr. Paolo Manicone, Rome, Italy.

described in those studies ranged from zero to 8%, at two to 23 years of follow-up. Hamp et al. (1975) reported on the effect of various treatment modalities in the case of furcation involvement of 310 molars. Eighty-seven of these teeth received root resection. After five years no teeth were lost and periodontal conditions were stable; only two teeth had a probing depth greater than 6 mm. This would indicate that a change in the supra- and sub-gingival environment, allowing good self-performed home care, may be critical for periodontal stability. The same periodontal success has been reported by Erpenstein (1983), treating 34 molars with root resection. During the average follow-up time of 2.9 years (range one to seven years) only four teeth were lost, three of which had endodontic failure.

The main study dealing with root resection therapy is the one from Carnevale and co-workers (1998), who treated 194 patients for a total of 488 resected molars. All of the teeth were prosthetically restored. The follow-up time ranged from three to 11 years. At the end of the study all of the patients were included in a strict regimen of supportive therapy. The success rate was 94% (28 teeth failed) and the reasons for failure included endodontic recurrence (four teeth), caries (nine teeth), abutment fracture (three teeth), and root fracture (nine teeth). Three teeth with a probing depth of greater than 5 mm were also included as failures. The conclusion of this study was that resective therapy may be considered to be a viable option in the treatment of advanced periodontal disease on a long-term basis.

Comments: Root resection therapy is a highly demanding procedure that can still be considered an option in the armamentarium of a periodontist. The introduction of implant therapy has greatly affected the application of this technique in the daily practice. Nevertheless, any time the decision whether to treat and maintain a multi-rooted tooth or extract and replace it with an implant has to be made, there are several considerations. These considerations must be made

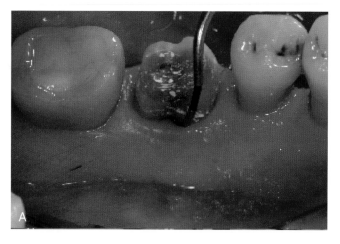

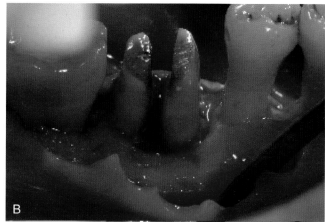

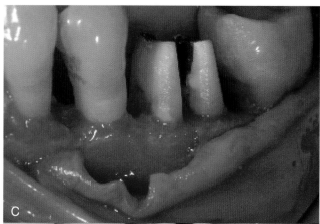

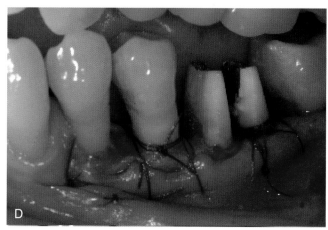

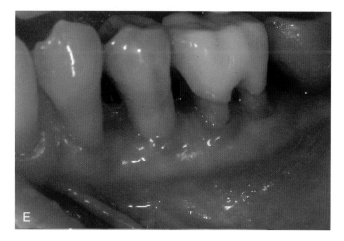

Figure 7.24. A, A Class II lingual furcation is detected at the lower left first molar. B, A root resection is performed and an osteoplasty is also carried out to reduce the infrabony defect around the roots on the lingual side. C, A buccally minimal ostectomy is necessary. D, The buccal flap is apically repositioned using continuous sling vertical mattress sutures. E, Three weeks' healing after surgery. Courtesy of prosthodontist Dr. Antonello Pavone, Rome, Italy.

by every single member of the restorative team because a team effort is required to achieve a predictable result:

- The endodontist should perform the least invasive therapy possible, sparing as much root structure as possible.

- A fiber post or post and core reconstruction with a temporary crown should be done before resective surgery is initiated.

- A positive architecture must be achieved during surgery and the tooth profile must be reshaped to ensure good access for maintenance and easy prosthetic finalization.

- The precision of the final crown is a critical step and the lab technician should be instructed to create space for cleaning.

- A strict periodontal support program is critical to achieve long-term success, as has been widely demonstrated by several authors (Axelsson et al., 1981).

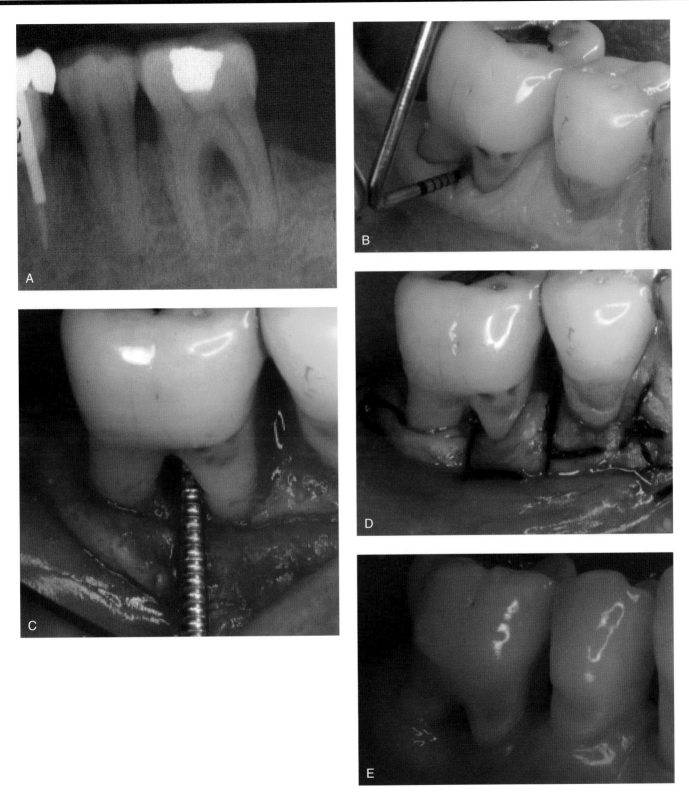

Figure 7.25. A, A Class III furcation defect is documented radiographically, and B, clinically. C, Tunnelization is performed, and using a Sugerman bone file, the interradicular space is widened and the bone crest flattened. D, Silk sutures provide apical displacement of the tissue. E, Six months' healing shows an adequate opening of the furcation area for cleaning. F, Radiograph at one year, suggesting corticalization of the inter-radicular bone crest at the first molar with no sign of further loss of support.

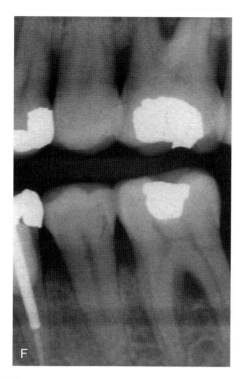

Figure 7.25. continued

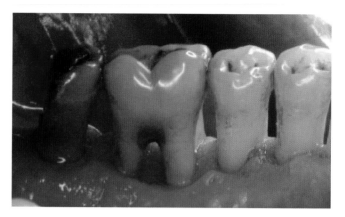

Figure 7.26. Caries at the furcation of a tunnelized lower left first molar. The unrestored mesial root of a resected second molar is also present. The lack of an adequate prosthetic plan may well be considered a major drawback in this case.

Although all of these steps may seem overwhelming, the extraction of a periodontally compromised maxillary molar and its replacement with an implant may not be as hard as it seems. One should note that most of the time the sinus in that area is highly pneumatized and drops into the inter-radicular space. Once the tooth is extracted, an alveolar bone remodelling takes place, further reducing the amount of remaining crestal bone. Furthermore, posterior maxillary sextants are physiologically associated with poor bone quality, which is directly correlated with a higher implant failure rate (Jaffin and Berman, 1991). Therefore, the alternative to root resection therapy may be tooth extraction followed by sinus elevation surgery and implant placement. Although this procedure is now considered to be routine, with good results (Del Fabbro et al., 2004), the data are rarely higher than those reported by Carnevale et al. (1998). A careful evaluation of each individual case, considering patient risk profile, local determinants, and possible alternatives, is always recommended.

Tunnelization

This conservative technique has been employed in the treatment of advanced furcation lesions that mainly affect mandibular molars. The primary indication for this approach is the case of an existing Class III furcation with no or a minimal vertical component (Figure 7.25). The anatomy of the affected molar is critical to determining the possibility of performing this procedure. Usually a short or medium root trunk with divergent and long roots may be considered as an ideal candidate for this treatment. The technique includes a certain degree of osteoplasty/ostectomy to widen the furcation entrance and achieve a flat bone crest anatomy.

Some odontoplasty has also been proposed to obtain better access to the furcation area. This should be done with great care because it may cause tooth hypersensitivity. Therefore, it is suggested that odontoplasty of the furcation entrance only be performed in the case of an endodontic-treated tooth or when the distance between the dome of the furcation and the floor of the pulp chamber is adequate. Once the osseous resection is accomplished the flap is apically positioned and a mattress suture is passed through the furcation to hold down the flap. As soon as the sutures are removed the patient must be instructed to use an interproximal brush or a superfloss to ensure good cleaning of the area.

Evidence: No large studies reporting on this technique have been published in the literature. Relative periodontal stability has been reported using this technique (Little et al., 1995; Muller et al., 1995). According to several authors, the major complication is related to the development of caries in the furcation area (Figure 7.26), with an incidence that ranged from 10% to 57% up to five years. (Hamp et al., 1975; Hellden et al., 1989; Ravald and Hamp, 1981). Other authors were unable to report the same cario-susceptibility and described more favorable long-term results. A recent publication by Feres and co-workers (2006) reported on 30 tunnelized teeth in 18 subjects who were followed for a mean period of 3.6 years. Four teeth (13.4%) showed active caries, while there was no difference in the carious lesion between the inner and outer furcation area. Probing depth was, however, higher inside of the furcation compared to the radicular and interproximal sites.

AUTHOR'S VIEWS/COMMENTS

This treatment should be reserved for those cases in which a compromised treatment option is selected for strategic or financial reasons. In addition, careful analysis of the tooth anatomy and morphology (root length, interradicular space, root curvatures, etc.) must be reviewed before performing the procedure.

REFERENCES

Adriaens PA, DeBoever JA, Loesche WJ. 1988. Bacterial invasion in root cementum and radicular dentin of periodontally diseased teeth in humans—A reservoir of periodontopathic bacteria. *J. Periodontol.*, 59, 222–230.

Axelsson P and Lindhe J. 1981. Effect of controlled oral hygiene procedures on caries and periodontal disease in adults. *J Clin Periodontol.* 8(3), 239–248.

Barrington, E.P. 1981. An overview of periodontal surgical procedures. *J. Periodontol.*, 52, 518–528.

Becker W, et al. 1997. Alveolar bone anatomic profiles as measured from dry skulls. Clinical ramification. *J. Clin. Perio.*, 24, 727–780.

Bender IB, Seltzer S. 1972. The effect of periodontal disease on the pulp. *Oral Surg. Oral Med. Oral Pathol.*, 33, 458–474.

Bissada NF, Abdelmalek RG. 1973. Incidence of cervical enamel projections and its relationship to furcation involvement in Egyptian skulls. *J. Periodontol.*, 44, 583–585.

Blomlof L, Jansson L, Applegren R, Enhevid H, Lidskog S. 1997. Prognosis and mortality of root resected molars. *Int. J. Period. Rest. Dent.*, 17, 191–201.

Bower RC. 1979. Furcation morphology relative to periodontal treatment—furcation entrance architecture. *J. Periodontol.*, 50, 23.

Bower RC. 1979. Furcation morphology relative to periodontal treatment—furcation root surface anatomy. *J. Periodontol.*, 50, 366.

Buhler H. 1988. Evaluation of root-resected teeth. *J. Peridontol.*, 59, 805–810.

Burch JC, Hulen S. 1974. A study of the presence of accessory foramina and the topography of lower molar furcations. *Oral Surg. Oral Med. Oral Pathol.*, 38, 451–454.

Caffesse R, et al. 1986. Scaling and root planing with and without periodontal flap surgery. *J. Clin. Periodontol.*, 13, 205.

Carnevale G, Cordioli G, Mazzocco C, Brugnolo C. 1985. La tecnica della conservazione delle fibre gengivali. *Dental Cadmos*, 19, 15–40.

Carnevale G. 2007. Fibre retention osseous resective surgery: a novel conservative approach for pocket elimination. *J. Clin. Periodontol.*, 34, 182–187.

Carnevale G, Pontoriero R, Di Febo G. 1998. Long term effects of root resective therapy in furcation involved molars. *J. Clin. Periodontol.*, 25, 209–214.

Carnevale G, Di Febo G, Tonelli MP, Marin C, Fuzzi M. 1991. A retrospective analysis of the periodontal-prosthetic treatment of molars with interradicular lesions. *Int. J. Perio. Rest. Dent.*, 11(3), 189–204.

Del Fabbro M, Testori T, Francetti L, Weinstein R. 2004. Systematic review of survival rates for implants placed in the grafted maxillary sinus. *Int. J. Period. Rest. Dent.*, 24, 565–577.

Donnenfeld O, Hoag PM, Weissman DP. 1970. A clinical study on the effects of osteoplasty. *J. Periodontol.*, 41, 131–141.

Donnenfeld OW, Marks RM, Glickman I. 1964. The apically repositioned flap: A clinical study. *J. Periodontol.*, 35, 381–387.

Elliott GM, Bowers GM. 1963. Alveolar dehiscences and fenestrations. *Periodontics*, 1, 245–248.

Erpenstein H. 1983. A three-year study of hemisected molars. *J. Clin. Periodontol.*, 10, 1–10.

Everett FG, Jump EB, Holder TD, Williams GC. 1958. The intermediate bifurcational ridge: a study of the morphology of the bifurcation of the lower first molar. *J. Dent. Res.*, 17, 62.

Feres M, Araujo MW, Figueiredo LC, Opperman RV. 2006. Clinical evaluation of tunneled molars: a retrospective study. *J. Int. Acad. Periodontol.*, 8, 96–103.

Friedman N. 1955. Periodontal osseous surgery: Osteoplasty and ostectomy. *J. Periodontol.*, 26, 257–269.

Gargiulo A, Wantz F, Orban B. 1961. Dimensions of the dentogingival junction in humans. *J. Periodontol.*, 32, 261.

Gher ME, Vernino AR. 1980. Root morphology—Clinical significance in pathogenesis and treatment of periodontal disease. *J. Am. Dent. Assoc.*, 101, 627–633.

Gutman JL. 1978. Prevalence, location and patency of accessory canals in the furcation region of permanent molars. *J. Periodontol.*, 49, 21–26.

Hamp SE, Nyman S, Lindhe J. 1975. Periodontal treatment of multirooted teeth. Results after 5 years. *J. Clin. Periodontol.*, 2, 126–132.

Hellden LB, Elliot A, Steffensen B, Steffensen, J. 1989. The prognosis of tunnel preparations in treatment of class III furcations. A follow-up study. *J. Periodontol.* 60, 182.

Ingber JS, Rose LF, Coslet JG. 1977. The biologic width: A concept in periodontics and restorative dentistry. *Alpha Omegan.* 10, 62–65.

Jaffin CL, Berman BA. 1991. The excessive loss of Branemark fixtures in type IV bone. A 5-year study. *J. Periodontol.*, 6, 2–5.

Kaldahl W, Kalkwarf K, Patil KI, et al. 1996. Long-term evaluation of periodontal therapy: I. Response to 4 therapeutic modalities. *J. Periodontol.*, 67, 93–102.

Kalkwarf KL, et al. 1988. Evaluation of furcation region response to periodontal therapy. *J. Periodontol.*, 59(12), 794–804.

Knowles J, et al. 1979. Results of periodontal treatment related to pocket depth and attachment level—Eight years. *J. Periodontol.*, 50, 225.

Langer B, Stein SD, Wagenberg B. 1981. An evaluation of root resections. A ten-year study. *J. Periodontol.*, 52(12), 719.

Levy RM, Giannobile WV, Magda F, Haffajee AD, Smith C, Socransky SS. 2002. The effect of apically positioned flap surgery on the clinical parameters and the composition of subgingival microbiota. A 12-month study. *Int. J. Period. Rest. Dent.*, 22, 209–219.

Little L, Beck B, Bagci B, Horton J. 1995. Lack of furcal bone loss following the tunneling procedure. *J. Clin. Periodontol.*, 22, 637–641.

Lowman JV, Burke RS, Pelleu GB. 1973. Patent accessory canals: incidence in the molar furcation region. *Oral Surg. Oral Med. Oral Pathol.*, 36, 580–584.

Majzoub Z, Kon S. 1992. Root Resection of Maxillary First Molars. *J. Periodontol.*, 63, 290–296.

Masters DH, Hoskins SW. 1964. Projections of cervical enamel in molar furcations. *J. Periodontol.*, 35, 49–53.

Matherson DG. 1988. An evaluation of healing following periodontal osseous surgery in monkeys. *Int. J. Period. Rest. Dent.*, 8, 9–39.

Matia J, et al. 1987. Efficiency of scaling of the molar furcation area with and without surgical access. *Int. J. Perio. Rest. Dent.*, 6, 25.

Moghaddas H, Stahl SS. 1980. Alveolar bone remodeling following osseous surgery. A clinical study. *J. Periodontol.*, Jul;51(7), 376–381.

Mombelli A, Nyman S, Bragger U, Wennstrom J, Lang NP. 1995. Clinical and microbiological changes associated with an altered subgingival environment induced by periodontal pocket reduction. *J. Clin. Periodontol.*, 22, 780–787.

Moskow BS, Canut PM. 1990. Studies on root enamel (II) Enamel pearls. A review of their morphology, localization, nomenclature, occurrence, classification, histogenesis and incidence. *J. Clin. Periodontol.*, 17, 275–281.

Muller HP, Eger T, Lange DE. 1995. Management of furcation-involved teeth. A retrospective analysis. *J. Clin. Periodontol.*, 22, 911–917.

Ochsenbein C. 1986. A primer for osseous surgery. *Int. J. Perio. Rest. Dent.*, 6(1), 8–47.

Ochsenbein C, Bohannan HM. 1963. The palatal approach to osseous surgery. I. Rationale. *J. Periodontol.*, 34, 60–68.

Pennell B, King KO, Wilderman MN, Barron JM. 1967. Repair of the alveolar process following osseous surgery. *J. Periodontol.*, 38, 426–431.

Polson AM and Catou J. 1982. Factors influencing periodontal repair and regenerization. *J Periodontol.* 53(7), 420–424.

Ramfjord S, et al. 1987. Four modalities of periodontal treatment compared over five years. *J. Clin. Periodontol.*, 14, 445.

Ravald N, Hamp SE. 1981. Prediction of root surface caries in patients treated for advance periodontal disease. *J. Clin. Periodontol.*, 8, 400–414.

Reiser GM, Bruno JF, Mahan PE, Larkin PE. 1996. The subepithelial connective tissue graft palatal donor site: anatomic considerations for surgeons. *Int. J. Perio. Rest. Dent.*, 16, 130–137.

Schluger S. 1949. Osseous resection—A basic principle in periodontal surgery. *Oral Surg.*, 2, 316–325.

Selipsky H. 1976. Osseous surgery. How much need we compromise? *Dent. Clin. North Am.*, 20, 79–106.

Siebert J. 1976. Treatment of infrabony lesions by surgical resection procedures: In: Stahl SS, ed. *Periodontal Surgery: Biologic Basis and Technique.* Springfield, IL: Charles C. Thomas.

Smith DH, Ammons WF, Van Belle G. 1980. A longitudinal study of periodontal status comparing osseous recontouring with flap curettage. I. Results after 6 months. *J. Periodontol.*, 51, 367.

Smukler H, Tagger M. 1976. Vital root amputation: A clinical and histological study. *J. Periodontol.*, 47, 324–330.

Swan RH, Hurt WC. 1976. Cervical enamel projections as an etiologic factor in furcation involvement. *J. Am. Dent. Assoc.*, 93, 342–345.

Tal H. 1984. Relationship between the interproximal distance of roots and the prevalence of intrabony pockets. *J. Periodontol.*, 55, 604–607.

Tarnow D, Fletcher, P. 1984. Classification of the vertical component of furcation involvement. *J. Periodontol.*, 55, 283–284.

Tibbets L, Ochsenbein C, Loughlin DM. 1976. Rationale for the lingual approach to mandibular osseous surgery. *Dent. Clin. North Am.*, 20, 61–78.

Vertucci FJ, Williams RG. 1974. Furcation canals in the human mandibular first molar. *Oral Surg. Oral Med. Oral Pathol.*, 38, 308–314.

Wilderman MN, Pennell B, King KO, Barron JM. 1970. Histogenesis of repair following osseous surgery. *J. Periodontol.*, 41, 551–565.

Wood DL, Hoag PM, Donnenfeld O, Rosenfeld LD. 1972. Alveolar crest reduction following full and partial thickness flaps. *J. Periodontol.*, 43, 141–144.

Chapter 8 Regenerative Periodontal Therapy

INTRODUCTION

The aim of periodontal regeneration is complete restoration of the attachment apparatus. Specific components such as periodontal ligament, cementum, and alveolar bone must contribute to this biological process for regeneration to occur. Periodontal ligament cells, osteoblasts, and cementoblasts must be in the regenerative site to achieve a clinically acceptable result. Regeneration, in contrast to conventional periodontal resective surgery, achieves pocket elimination/reduction and attachment gain by a biological process and not repair. Furthermore, pocket elimination procedures result in attachment loss that may cause root caries, sensitivity, and an esthetically compromised dentition. Meanwhile, regenerative surgical procedures alter factors during the wound healing process that shift repair to restoration of architecture. Ideally, a patient who suffered from periodontitis should have a periodontium comparable to a periodontally healthy individual following a regenerative treatment.

Regenerative periodontal procedures require biomaterials that lead to regeneration of the periodontal ligament (PDL) and new attachment. Earlier periodontal procedures for regeneration included bone and/or bone substitutes alone. A variety of barrier membranes to contain the graft material were later added to the procedure. In addition, graft materials or carrier materials (scaffold) are necessary depending on the purpose, e.g., space to be maintained at the site, and/or delivery of growth/regeneration factors. An ideal grafting material should deliver the regenerative signals in an optimal manner to stimulate a cellular response.

The specific predictability of periodontal regenerative procedures has focused on its indications. In general, the morphology of the bone defect limits the outcome. The procedures aim first to eliminate or reduce periodontal pockets, second to restore the lost alveolar process with regeneration of PDL and bone, and last to regenerate a functional attachment apparatus, ideally to periodontally healthy levels (Schallhorn, 1977). In general, indications for a regenerative procedure are deep intraosseous defects or cases in which osseous resective surgery is contraindicated because a substantial amount of supporting bone has been lost. In localized aggressive periodontitis, a regenerative approach should be considered first because osseous resective therapy can cause more harm. Regeneration minimizes post surgical clinical attachment loss.

Periodontal regeneration can be achieved by various techniques. These methods can be generally classified into grafting alone, guided tissue regeneration (graft and membrane), and growth factor stimulated regeneration. Grafting procedures alone can involve several material types including autogenous, allograft, xenograft, and alloplasts (Box 8.1). A variety of materials have the potential for periodontal stimulation for bone grafts. Materials commonly used for that purpose are osteogenic (bone graft material that has viable cells that can produce bone), osteoinductive (bone graft material that contains factors that may stimulate new bone growth), and osteoconductive (bone graft material that does not have any bone stimulatory factors in it but rather acts as a scaffold for bone growth).

Regeneration associated with grafting may result in long junctional epithelium because new PDL, cementum, and connective tissue (CT) attachment may not be established. However, acceptable clinical healing, including pocket reduction and attachment gain, may occur. Initial efforts to achieve guided tissue regeneration (GTR) aim to regenerate PDL and the rest of the periodontium by isolating the defect with barrier membranes and/or grafting to maintain space so that the regeneration can take place. Guided tissue regeneration is based on the exclusion of connective tissue and epithelium in favor of PDL regeneration, and following establishment of a new attachment. Thus, GTR is the purposeful selection of cell types that repopulate at the wound with the intention of directing the healing tissue composition. Barrier materials include natural absorbable polymers such as collagen (Types I, II, III, IV) and collagen and glucoseaminoglycan (GAG) copolymer; synthetic absorbable polymers such as polylactic acid and polyglycolic acid; fibrin; synthetic non-resorbable polymer polytetraflouroethylene (PTFE); synthetic ceramics such as calcium phosphate; and natural bone mineral.

Recently, the stimulation of periodontal regeneration with growth factors has become an effective and predictable technique. Based on biological enhancement of wound healing, these molecules produce a true histological regeneration. Growth/regeneration factors and differentiation factors such as enamel matrix proteins (amelogenin), polypeptide mitogens such as bone morphogenic protein-2(BMP-2), growth factors such as platelet derived growth factor (PDGF), and a combination of growth factors such as platelet rich plasma (PRP) are being used to stimulate regeneration. These molecules augment and/or stimulate the

BOX 8.1. Graft Material Types

Autogenous graft: Bone graft obtained from the same person either from intraoral or extraoral donor sites.

Allograft: Bone graft obtained from the same species as the recipient. A human bone graft is obtained from a donor (cadaver) and processed to decontaminate the graft material and make the particulate size adequate to use intraorally. Demineralized freeze-dried bone allograft (DFDBA) is the classical bone graft material used for GTR purposes.

Xenograft: Bone graft obtained from a different species than the recipient. An animal (typically cow) bone graft is obtained and processed to decontaminate the graft material and make the particulate size adequate to use intraorally.

Alloplasts: Synthetic or natural materials that can act as scaffold during bone regeneration. These materials must be bioinert and resorbable in the recipient site.

natural healing response and include stimulatory effects on angiogenesis, cellular differentiation, cellular proliferation, cellular ingrowth, and extracellular matrix biosynthesis, respectively. The stimulation by signaling molecules (growth factors) has improved the predictability in periodontal defects.

PERIODONTAL REGENERATIVE TECHNIQUES

The contemporary periodontal approach should eliminate the etiology and correct the defects by returning the periodontium to healthier levels. Periodontal regenerative procedures are necessary to achieve this goal (Figure 8.1). The advantage to periodontal regeneration not only includes attachment gain, but also provides benefits in areas with local or dental anatomical factors such as root concavities or where deep interproximal periodontal breakdown occurs. In addition, esthetics may be enhanced.

Guided Tissue Regeneration

Guided tissue regeneration is based on several key concepts such as new attachment, reattachment, regeneration, and repair. The term guided tissue regeneration was first used when a new connective tissue attachment was demonstrated with human histology by using a ePTFE membrane (nonresorbable) (Gottlow et al., 1986). Additional terminology includes new attachment (union of connective tissue or epithelium with root surface that has been deprived of its original attachment), reattachment (reunion of epithelium or connective tissue with root surfaces and bone such as occurs after incision or injury), regeneration (a histological term describing

the reconstruction of an injured part), and repair (healing of a wound that is not fully restored to its original form and function).

Exclusion of epithelium is a critical component of barrier membrane regeneration. Epithelial cells migrate three to five times faster than PDL cells. As a result, the invasion by the epithelium does not allow PDL to regenerate. The first study showing that histological new attachment was possible used a Millipore filter to exclude epithelium (Nyman et al., 1982a,b), which showed that space creation by a membrane and/or graft is effective in periodontal regeneration. Cellular response investigations indicate that wound healing originates from the PDL (Aukhil et al., 1986). The peak mitotic activity of PDL occurs at approximately three weeks (Nyman, 1982). The importance of the PDL cell response in GTR is also critical to cementum formation, which allows PDL fibers to attach. Therefore, cementum formation is considered the rate-limiting step in periodontal regeneration (Caton et al., 1987).

Several factors are important in the outcome of guided tissue regeneration, including periodontal defect morphology, remaining periodontium, and practitioner skill. Guided tissue regeneration is technique-sensitive because the surgical area is narrow and soft tissue management is difficult. Meanwhile, flap design must consider primary closure of the surgical site to achieve full coverage of the regenerative membrane. An optimal amount of tissue must be retained in the flap design; typically, intrasulcular incisions are preferred. Releasing incisions also may be used as necessary (anatomy permitting) because access for thorough debridement of the surgical site from granulation tissue is important for success. Vertical incisions may also facilitate proper flap coverage of the membrane and graft material placement.

Following adequate flap elevation, the root surface must be debrided and deposits removed for new attachment. The consensus is that root conditioning with chemical agents is not recommended because no clear benefits have been established (Mariotti, 2003). Root surface mechanical preparation is essential in conjunction with hand instrumentation (curettes) or sonic or ultrasonic hand pieces.

Membrane adaptation around the tooth and onto the defect must be optimal to favor PDL growth without any significant epithelial downgrowth. Any significant irregularity of the bone that may affect the position of the membrane should be eliminated with conservative osteoplasty. As necessary, the membrane must be trimmed accordingly, adapted, and sutured around the tooth. Flap adaptation should be maximized around the tooth and onto the membrane for proper coverage. In addition, the flap should be passive onto the surgical site to prevent any dehiscence during the healing period. Suture material such as ePTFE or polyglycolic acid material should be chosen to close the site because these

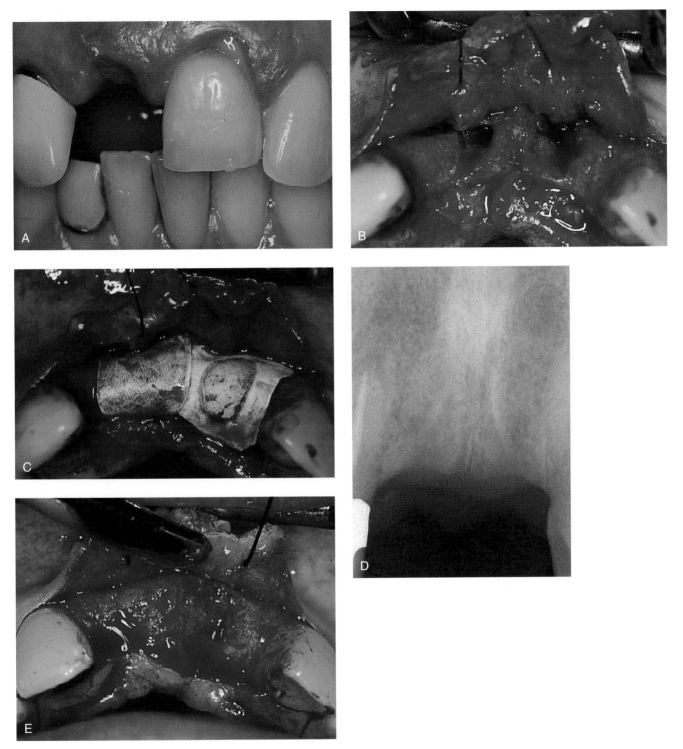

Figure 8.1. Extraction and ridge augmentation in the anterior maxilla with bone graft and resorbable membrane by guided tissue regeneration principles, implant placement, and final restoration. A, Fractured upper left central incisor (pus is noticeable on the gingival margin) and missing upper right central incisor. B, Upon flap reflection, extraction and degranulation were completed. Buccal plates for both sockets were entirely resorbed. C, Bone graft and resorbable membranes are in place. The membranes are critical for epithelial exclusion in favor of proper bone regrowth in the area. D, Radiographic evaluation prior to implant placement, approximately four months after bone grafting, reveals uniform bone formation. E, Complete clinical bone regeneration achieved approximately four months later. F, Implant placement at bone regenerated site to replace upper right central incisor and upper left central incisor. G, Final implant-supported fixed restorations for upper right central incisor and upper left central incisor with a desirable esthetic result.

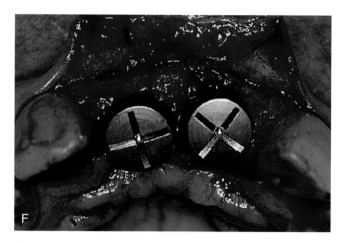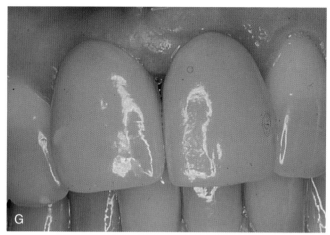

Figure 8.1. *Continued*

retain the least amount of plaque. Finally, a periodontal dressing may be used to secure the surgical area, especially from food impaction or trauma. Postoperative care is important and patients are typically prescribed an antibiotic, anti-inflammatory, and antibacterial rinse during the initial healing period.

Pontoriero et al. (1987, 1995) demonstrated in a series of studies that GTR is a predictable procedure for Class II furcations (Hamp classification) compared to open flap debridement. However, that predictability decreased significantly for Class III furcation-involved molars. For maxillary molars, buccal furcations are more predictable than the interproximal area. Meanwhile, a six month re-entry study showed that results were enhanced with GTR with a non-resorbable membrane and DFDBA, compared to GTR alone. The GTR and DFDBA combination produced more defect fill and pocket depth reduction and a greater gain in the clinical attachment level (Anderegg et al., 1991).

Depending on the number of bone wall defects, GTR showed 95% fill of three-wall, 82% fill of two-wall, and 39% fill of one-wall. Overall, a 73% defect fill was achieved (Cortellini et al., 1993a, b). In terms of defect fill, the areas of deepest probing depth demonstrated the greatest pocket depth (PD) reduction and clinical attachment level (CAL) gain (Selvig et al., 1993). Long-term results indicate that CAL gains were maintained four to five years following GTR (Gottlow et al., 1992). Good oral hygiene and patient compliance were found to be critical in long-term stability of GTR procedures (Cortellini et al., 1994).

Signaling Molecules in Periodontal Tissue Regeneration

There has been mounting evidence that the choice of graft material may play a significant role in altering the wound healing, from repair to regeneration. The analysis of autograft

or allograft has found that signaling molecules contained in the material may stimulate regeneration. The molecular bases of these factors have been identified, characterized, and produced in large quantities. Several signaling molecules are currently being investigated with preclinical and clinical studies.

Enamel Matrix Proteins

Enamel matrix protein (EMP) or enamel matrix derivative (EMD) is a commercially available regenerative material. Amelogenin is the main constituent (95%) of this group of proteins; the remaining approximate 5% are other less characterized proteins. These proteins, especially amelogenin, are thought to be involved in acellular cementum, PDL, and alveolar bone development. The EMD that is currently available is isolated from porcine tooth buds (Hammarström, 1997). These porcine-derived proteins are very similar to proteins expressed during human enamelogenesis, but there are small genetic differences (Gestrelius et al., 1997a,b). In vitro studies with enamel proteins suggested that periodontal ligament cells' RNA expression is stimulated. Enamel proteins improved PDL cell function, particularly their effects on cell metabolism (Barkana et al., 2007). In addition, enamel proteins contributed to new blood vessel formation (Schlueter et al., 2007).

Osteoblast growth and differentiation, another critical component for periodontal regeneration, has been shown to be enhanced by EMD. In vitro studies indicate that EMD contributes to osteoblastic activity on human osteoblasts. In addition, it limits bone resorptive/osteoclastic activity. Moreover, important osteoblastic activity markers were enhanced at two and three weeks, an indication of continued biological activity (Galli et al., 2006).

Further evaluation of enamel matrix proteins for periodontal regeneration in a mouse model demonstrated that new cellular cementum-like tissue formed along EMP-treated root slices (Song et al., 2007). Meanwhile, in order to understand the effects on soft tissues, human gingival fibroblast cells were treated with EMD and the cell cycle was assessed. The results suggested that EMD induced mitogenic activity for gingival fibroblasts, which may explain better soft tissue healing clinically (Zeldich et al., 2007).

Clinical investigations have demonstrated multiple benefits of the regeneration of periodontal support with EMD. The use of EMD in patients with lower molar Class II buccal furcation defects resulted in reduced horizontal probing at 14 months post-surgery as compared to those treated with traditional GTR (Hoffmann et al., 2006). Another trial evaluating contra-lateral randomized infrabony defects using EMD vs. GTR with resorbable membrane demonstrated similar improvements. These improvements in periodontal parameters were main-tained up to eight years (Sculean et al., 2006). In addition numerous clinical case series have indicated positive results with EMD (Cortellini and Tonetti, 2007). A localized bone defect associated with a palatal groove was successfully treated with EMD. This particular treatment is limited to a case report with 8 mm clinical attachment gain and 2 mm of residual probing depth one year post surgically. However, it is viable evidence of the success for regenerative treatment in such complex lesions with EMD (Zuchelli et al., 2006).

Recombinant Human Platelet-derived Growth Factor

Recombinant human platelet-derived growth factor (rhPDGF) is a polypeptide growth factor which has been shown to stimulate periodontal regeneration. rhPDGF has specific effects on wound healing properties, including the regenera-tion of periodontium. rhPDGF is especially a strong mitogen for mesenchymal cells. Indeed, it has been shown that human osteoblastic cells produce PDGF. On a molecular basis, pdgf-a gene expression results in the PDGF protein. PDGF has PDGF-AA (acidic) and PDGF-BB (basic) variant forms. While human osteoblasts respond to PDGF-BB uni-formly, there is an inconsistent response to PDGF-AA (Zhang et al., 1991).

Originally platelet-derived growth factor (PDGF) and insulin-like growth factor-I (IGF-I) were found, in combination, to synergistically upregulate DNA and protein synthesis in osteoblasts. Additional in vivo findings indicated that this effect would be achieved on soft tissue. Early studies sug-gested and evaluated the synergistic effects of PDGF and IGF-1 in periodontal defects in canine and human models with naturally occurring periodontitis. In preclinical models, rhPDGF-BB and rhIGF-1 in a carrier gel were applied on the root surfaces of periodontitis-affected teeth in conjunction with an open flap debridement procedure. Histological analy-sis of control carrier gel specimens indicated the presence

of long junctional epithelium without any clear new attach-ment in two weeks. As expected, PDGF/IGF-1-treated sites demonstrated considerable new attachment as well as new bone highly populated with osteoblasts and new cementum. Significant osteoblast presence in PDGF-applied specimens was evidence of bone regeneration that perhaps would con-tinue beyond two weeks.

Similarly, a carrier gel, with or without radioactively labeled rhPDGF-BB and rhIGF-1, was applied during periodontal surgery on beagles with naturally occurring periodontal disease. This experimental design made it possible to show the clearance rate of rhPDGF-BB and rhIGF-1 protein. The results revealed that the half-life of the molecules at the site of application was three hours for IGF-I and up to 4.2 hours for PDGF-BB. Almost all of the radioactively labeled protein was cleared after 96 hours, and two weeks later no radioac-tivity was detected. However, twice as much radioactive material was bound at the surgical site in the experimental group, which indicated that PDGF and IGF-1 bind on the target cells, which would trigger biological activity during periodontal regeneration. Histomorphometric analyses on two- and five-week specimens demonstrated five- to ten-fold increases in new bone and cementum as compared to con-trols (Lynch et al., 1991).

Meanwhile, the mitogenic effect of natural platelet-derived growth factor (nPDGF) on periodontal ligament fibroblast-like cells was investigated by using radioactive isotope incor-poration in DNA. nPDGF stimulated approximately three times more DNA synthesis compared to the control and two times more compared to fibroblast growth factor (Blom et al., 1994). In vitro or laboratory findings are ultimately important for clinical practice to provide a proof of principle basis for biological activity. In that regard, in order for PDGF to optimally stimulate periodontal regeneration, the PDGF protein must bind its cellular receptor in periodontal tissues. Moreover, periodontal ligament cells may have the ability to differentiate into cementoblasts and/or osteoblasts with this stimulation.

Although PDGF-BB is well established as a key stimulator for periodontal regeneration in vitro and in vivo, further clinical studies were required to validate its effects on human peri-odontal defects. A split-mouth study was carried out with rhPDGF-BB and rhIGF-I in a carrier gel. Re-entry surgical procedures were performed to assess bone fill six to nine months following treatment. Results demonstrated that 2.08 mm of new vertical bone height gain and 42.3% osseous defect fill in rhPDGF-BB/rhIGF-1-treated defects occurred in comparison to 0.75 mm and 18.5% for the control sides (Howell et al., 1997).

In another study, purified recombinant human platelet-derived growth factor-BB alone (without IGF) with bone allograft as the carrier was tested on interproximal intrabony defects and molar Class II furcation defects. Patients with teeth with advanced periodontal disease and poor prognosis that required extraction participated in the study. After the surgical debridement and notch placement on the root surfaces, osseous defects were filled with demineralized freeze-dried bone allograft (DFDBA) with one of three concentrations of rhPDGF-BB (0.5 mg/ml, 1 mg/ml, or 5 mg/ml). Bloc sections were taken, including the hopeless teeth and surrounding bone nine months following surgeries. Histomorphometric analyses were done in reference to the notch placed on the root surface. In the rhPDGF and allograft-treated defects, the vertical probing depth reductions as well as clinical attachment level gain for interproximal defects were approximately 6 mm, while radiographic bone fill was approximately 2 mm. Furcation defects treated with rhPDGF/allograft demonstrated a horizontal and vertical pocket depth reduction with clinical attachment level gain approximately of 3 mm. Moreover, histological evaluation indicated regeneration of a complete periodontal attachment apparatus with new cementum, PDL, and bone. Overall, this study demonstrated that rhPDGF-BB alone stimulates periodontal regeneration in both Class II furcations and interproximal intrabony defects (Nevins et al., 2003).

Further evaluations on clinical and histological response to rhPDGF-BB on Class II furcation defects were done with a similar study design. rhPDGF-BB stimulated periodontal regeneration, resulting in significant gains in horizontal and vertical probing depths and attachment levels. Similar to the previous study by the same investigators, histological specimens demonstrated that periodontal regeneration with new bone, cementum, and periodontal ligament used rhPDGF-BB with a xenograft (Camelo et al., 2003). Therefore, preliminary studies showed periodontal regeneration by returning attachment apparatus to healthier levels.

Following these findings, a prospective randomized, clinical study to determine the safety and effectiveness of rhPDGF-BB was completed. rhPDGF-BB and β-tricalcium phosphate (β-TCP) were used to treat advanced periodontal osseous defects and for comparison with the control. In this multi-center study, patients who required surgical treatment for a 4-mm or greater intrabony periodontal defect participated and were evaluated after six months. Experimental groups consisted of beta-TCP and either 0.3 mg/ml rhPDGF-BB or 1.0 mg/ml rhPDGF-BB, while the control consisted of β-TCP alone. The results demonstrated that rhPDGF-BB was safe for clinical use, since no adverse effects were detected. The clinical parameters that were used assessed PDGF-BB effects including clinical attachment levels, gingival recession, and radiographic linear bone growth and percent bone fill. The clinical attachment level gain was 3.8 mm for 0.3 mg/ml rhPDGF and was significantly higher compared to β-TCP alone at three months following the surgical procedures.

However, at six months this difference was not statistically significant. The initial clinical attachment level gain acceleration with 0.3 mg/ml rhPDGF consequently caused a more significant clinical attachment level gain between baseline and six months compared to the control. Furthermore, at six months, rhPDGF-BB (0.3 mg/ml) treated sites also had significantly more linear bone gain (2.6 mm) and percent defect fill (57%) compared to 0.9 mm and 18% for the control group (Nevins et al., 2005).

The stability of the treatment during this clinical study was followed 18 or 24 months post surgically. All of the cases except one had their clinical attachment levels remaining intact. Moreover, linear bone gain and percent bone fill further improved compared to the six-month postsurgical results. The rhPDGF-BB-treated patients exhibited increased radiographic defect fill at 18 to 24 months post surgery compared to six months post surgery (McGuire et al., 2006).

In summary, this multi-center study demonstrated the safety of rhPDGF-BB for clinical treatment of periodontal defects. Treatment with rhPDGF-BB improved clinical attachment level gain at three months and maintained it up to 24 months. The results beyond six months showed further improvements in bone defect fill. the improvement of clinical attachment level is even more significant considering the multi-center nature of this study and the possible variability between both the operators and bone defects, despite standardization. Finally, expedited healing may be reflected in patient post surgical satisfaction and translate into easier patient management.

Predictable site development for dental implant placement and acceleration of healing at those sites are areas of interest to clinicians. In particular, the outcome of vertical ridge augmentation is difficult to predict due to a limited vascular and cellular supply. However, rhPDGF-BB stimulation may expedite angioneogenesis and cell migration in the grafted area.

A preclinical investigation evaluating the use of rhPDGF-BB with the presence or absence of a resorbable barrier membrane was investigated to assess its predictability for bone augmentation. Following dental extractions and surgical creation of ridge defects, bovine bone block with a collagen membrane, or bovine bone block infused with rhPDGF-BB, or bovine bone block infused with rhPDGF-BB with a collagen resorbable barrier membrane were used for vertical ridge augmentation. Histologic analysis indicated significant new bone formation and bone-to-implant contact in bone block and PDGF-BB-grafted sites. The absence of the barrier membrane positively contributed to the vertical bone regeneration, possibly due to better vascularization of the graft through the periosteum (Simion et al., 2006). This technique was recently assessed in humans. In a case report, the use of an rhPDGF-infused bone block was found to provide vertical augmentation. However, this technique was surgically demanding and the bone block structure may have been less than ideal (Simion et al., 2008).

In summary, studies completed in vitro, in vivo, and in clinical levels show strong evidence regarding the potency of PDGF-BB in regard to periodontal regeneration (Figure 8.2). Indeed, PDGF-BB is considered to be a well established biologic/ growth factor for periodontal regeneration. At this time there is limited but very promising evidence for guided bone regeneration.

Platelet Rich Plasma

The use of autogenous growth factors such as platelet rich plasma (PRP) have been investigated over the past decade. PRP is platelet aggregate obtained following blood centrifugation. It has been suggested that PRP has three times more growth factors such as TGF, PDGF, IGF, EGF compared to venous blood (Marx et al., 1998). Upon degranulation, platelet alpha-granules release growth factors that have stimulatory effects. Platelet counts and the presence of growth factors such as transforming growth factor-β (TGF-β) and PDGF are positively correlated in PRP concentration. Generally, PDGF is more than four times and TGF-β is more than three times more concentrated compared to venous blood. Both of these are well established osteogenic growth factors. However, the stimulation of osteoblasts by PRP was modest and only around 1.4 times more, compared to the control group (Okuda et al., 2003). The in vitro stimulation of human periodontal ligament cells, gingival fibroblasts, and keratinocytes by PRP resulted in variable effects of these cells. PRP stimulated periodontal ligament cells for collagen production four-fold in three days, and alkaline phosphatase, which indicates calcification in six days. PRP also decreased keratinocyte activity about 40% and did not significantly alter gingival fibroblasts (Annunziata et al., 2005). As mentioned above, PRP contains concentrated amounts of PDGF and TGF-β. Hence, human periodontal ligament cells were stimulated in vitro, with PRP obtained by centrifugation.

The creation of critical size rat or mouse calvaria defects is a classical animal model for evaluating bone graft effectiveness. PRP harvested from donor rats was applied in a collagen carrier matrix within rat calvaria defects. However, the PRP on rat calvaria model yielded variable results and was not significantly different than the control group (Pryor et al., 2005). In another investigation, PRP or platelet concentrate effects were evaluated on mini pig mandibles. Autogenous, xenogenous, and alloplastic bone grafts were also used in conjunction with PRP. No correlation between TGF and PDGF presence and platelet counts was present. Moreover, histomorphometric analysis in two, four, and eight weeks demonstrated no significant difference in bone formation with or without PRP presence (Jensen et al., 2005).

The application of PRP for human periodontal regeneration has produced a series of clinical case reports which indicate a positive but varied response. Periodontal regeneration with bovine bone in combination with PRP compared to open flap debridement in mandibular Class II defects demonstrated significant changes, especially for vertical and horizontal defect fill and clinical attachment level gains (Lekovic et al., 2003). Furthermore, GTR with bovine bone with or without PRP compared to GTR alone demonstrated modest effects for pocket depth reduction and clinical attachment level gain at six-month reentry results. This modest effect was not attributable to PRP since no significance was present between GTR with or without PRP. The combination with PRP compared to open flap debridement showed approximately 2 mm clinical attachment level gain (Camargo et al., 2003). Conversely in another investigation, PRP and bone graft with or without GTR showed a significant improvement for clinical attachment level. In this particular study, addition of GTR with a membrane did not make a significant difference (Lekovic et al., 2002). Furthermore, the application of PRP on intrabony defects in comparison to mineralized bone or bovine bone with membrane did not exhibit a significant advantage clinically after one year (Döri et al., 2007a,b).

Meanwhile, a lateral window maxillary sinus augmentation procedure may take between nine to 12 months before dental implant placement. Thus, addition of growth factors may be able to decrease this healing period. However, the addition of PRP to bone graft for lateral window maxillary sinus augmentation did not enhance the quality or the quantity of bone (Danesh-Meyer et al., 2001).

In summary, PRP was originally suggested to have three times more growth factors such as TGF, PDGF, IGF, EGF than venous blood, possibly leading to a modest increase in the bone density (about 25%) (Marx, 1998). However, the actual presence and concentration of cytokines in the PRP are not clear because there may be individual variations among patients. The state of platelets in the blood, whether they are stimulated for cytokine/growth factor expression at the time of blood withdrawal, are unknown. Moreover, isolation of PRP may directly affect the presence of cytokines simply because cytokines may not be expressed at the DNA level and consequently may not be synthesized at the protein level at any given time. Altogether, although PRP is conceptually a stimulator of a biological response, there may be several variables for clinicians to consider for predictable clinical results.

FUTURE OF PERIODONTAL REGENERATIVE THERAPY

Several concepts in regenerative therapy are in development. These include the application of recombinant human bone morphogenetic Protein-2 (rhBMP-2) and the more continuous application of signal molecules with gene therapy.

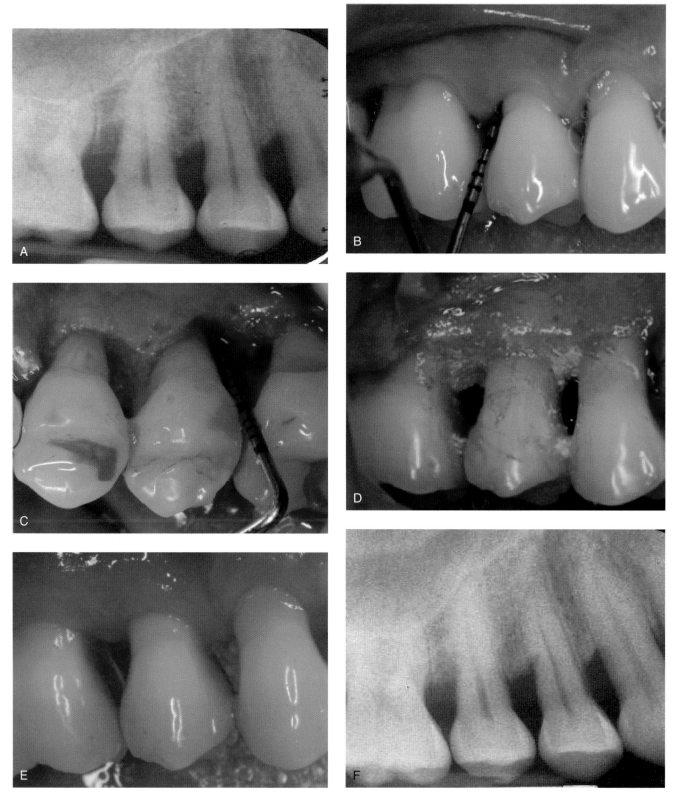

Figure 8.2. Guided tissue regeneration on upper right posterior sextant with recombinant human platelet-derived growth factor (rhPDGF). A, Periapical radiograph taken at the initial examination. Vertical bone defects as well as significant radiographic calculus are present in the area. B, Clinical picture after the completion of first phase of treatment. Probing depths up to 7 mm are present. However, the soft tissue profile is favorable for guided tissue regeneration. C, Clinical representation of bone defects following thorough debridement and degranulation during the GTR procedure. D, Application of rhPDGF with its carrier material (tricalcium phosphate) into the bone defects. E, Clinical healing eight months after the GTR procedure with probing depths not exceeding 3 mm. F, Radiographic healing eight months after the GTR procedure; bone fill is noticeable.

Bone morphogenetic proteins are involved in a wide variety of biologic activities, including embryogenesis. Except for BMP-1, which is an important factor for collagen synthesis (Uzel et al., 2001), the rest of the BMPs belong to the transforming growth factor family. In many biologic events different BMPs may work together. Among the numerous BMPs, BMP-2 and BMP-7 are known to stimulate periodontal regeneration.

The regeneration of the periodontal apparatus has been extensively investigated in preclinical models. rhBMP-2 periodontal regeneration in rodents was evaluated for early wound healing at 10 days and then 38 days. New bone formation was significantly increased 10 days after rhBMP-2 application on experimental periodontal wounds, as confirmed with histology. These exhibited new bone, cementum, and collagen fiber formation. Importantly, more cementum growth coronally was detected with rhBMP-2 application. Complete healing without any evidence of ankylosis occurred in all animals.

The application of rhBMP-2 for periodontal regeneration has been evaluated in canine and nonhuman primate studies. Various models, including naturally occurring or surgically induced, have been used to histologically assess the amount of regeneration. In general, new bone, cementum, and PDL were formed with the rhBMP-2. In addition, there were some indications of root resorption and anklyosis.

rhBMP-2 has been studied for its bone regenerative effects in preclinical and human studies. In a classical experimental model, calvaria were implanted with BMP/tricalcium phosphate (TCP) carrier in critical size defects in dogs. While rhBMP-2-stimulated sites demonstrated more than 90% new bone, the control group induced new bone formation below 10% (Urist et al., 1987). In animals, long bones were treated with rhBMP-2 in a collagen matrix carrier. Bone formation took place in a dose-related manner, while normal healing was observed for the control specimens (Yasko et al., 1992). Similar results were obtained in humans for long bone healing with rhBMP-2 (Johnson et al., 1988). Meanwhile, experiments on a calvaria model in Rhesus monkeys gave satisfying results, with critical size defect bone fill up to 100% with BMP-2 (Ferguson et al., 1987).

The clinical application of rhBMP-2 has involved bone and sinus augmentations (Figure 8.3). A randomized, masked, placebo-controlled, multi-center clinical study demonstrated that the novel combination of rhBMP-2 and a commonly used collagen sponge had a striking effect on de novo osseous formation for the placement of dental implants (Fiorellini et al., 2005). Two concentrations of rhBMP-2 were evaluated by using bioabsorbable collagen sponge vs. no treatment in a human buccal wall defect model following tooth extraction. Patients who required localized ridge augmentation for buccal wall defects and had more than 50%

bone loss of extraction sockets of maxillary teeth participated in the study. The patients were randomly selected to receive 0.75 mg/ml or 1.50 mg/ml rhBMP-2/ACS, placebo (ACS alone), or no treatment. The efficacy of rhBMP-2 was assessed by evaluating the amount of bone induction and the adequacy of the alveolar bone volume to support an endosseous dental implant. Patients treated with 1.50 mg/ml rhBMP-2/ACS had significantly greater bone augmentation compared to the other groups. Moreover, the adequacy of bone for the placement of a dental implant was approximately twice as great in the rhBMP-2/ACS groups compared to those with no treatment or placebo. In addition, bone density and histology revealed no differences between newly induced and native bone. In a follow-up study, the efficacy of different rhBMP-2 concentrations in the anterior maxilla for the volume of bone regeneration was assessed with computer assisted tomography. These evaluations demonstrated a significant difference in bone formation between subjects treated with a concentration of 1.5 mg/mL rhBMP-2 (Bianchi et al., 2004).

The safety of rhBMP-2 at regenerative doses was assessed in the sinus augmentation indication. Either rhBMP-2 and absorbable collagen sponge at 0.75 mg/ml and 1.50 mg/ml concentrations or with conventional bone graft were used. Alveolar ridge height, width, and density were measured by computer assisted tomography scans taken prior to treatment, four months after treatment, and six months following implant loading. Alveolar ridge height at four months was similar in all three groups, at approximately 10 mm. The use of rhBMP-2/ACS was safe in terms of not causing any side effects or harm to patients (Boyne et al., 2005).

rhBMP-2 was also assessed for its use around dental implants, mainly aiming to understand its effect on osseointegration. For that purpose, perforated dental implants were placed in beagle dogs. Then, rhBMP-2 in a gel was applied onto these perforations and implant osteotomy. Histological sections were evaluated for the extent of new bone formation within the through-and-through perforations. Data indicated that significantly more bone formation occurred with rhBMP-2-treated sites when compared to the control gel alone (Fiorellini et al., 2001).

A similar study in dogs evaluated a synthetic bioabsorbable carrier and rhBMP-2 use in osseous defects around dental implants. Following the extractions of mandibular teeth, implants were placed in standardized circumferential bone defects with or without rhBMP-2. In addition, half of the implants were submerged with a non-resorbable, expanded polytetrafluoroethylene (ePTFE) membrane. Specimens were obtained at four or 12 weeks for histomorphometric analysis, which included percent new bone contact with implant, area of new bone, and percent defect fill. Although all implants were clinically and radiographically successful, the amount of

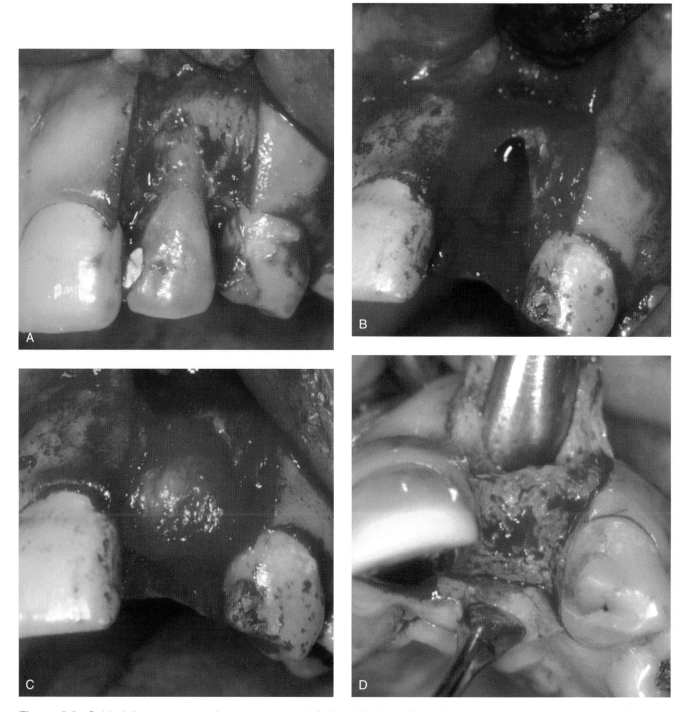

Figure 8.3. Guided tissue regeneration on an upper left lateral incisor site with recombinant human bone morphogenic protein-2 (rhBMP-2). A, The upper left lateral incisor is hopeless due to root caries. A significant dehiscence that contributed the etiology is present. B, The buccal plate is partially missing following extraction. C, rhBMP-2 with ACS (cellulose) carrier is used to augment the ridge. D, Complete bone regeneration is achieved three months after the guided bone regeneration with rhBMP-2.

new bone formation was dependent on rhBMP-2. The percent bone-implant contact was greater with rhBMP-2 in 12 weeks (Jones et al., 2006). However, membrane presence reduced bone formation.

Gene therapy approaches to bone tissue engineering have been widely explored. The maximum dose may be limited due to protein stability, half-life, and carrier properties. Even though topical application and/or delivery with carrier matrices are currently the best available clinical option, maintaining therapeutic protein levels at the surgical site may not always be possible. Gene therapy may become a viable option for continuous stimulation for periodontal regeneration.

Gene therapy is the alteration and manipulation of harvested target cells and redelivery of those cells into the target organ. A dose-dependent vector (adenovirus) was also used when critical size defects were on the femora of rats where the defects received different doses of plaque forming units of BMP-2 vector. Upon radiographic and histological evaluation, the high dose of vector bridged 100% of the femurs, while the medium-low dose did not exceed 25% (Betz et al., 2007). In addition, gene delivery using viral vectors may have some limitations for bone defects that need more time for healing. Thus, a condensing plasmid DNA with nonviral vectors such as polylactic/glycolic acid scaffolds were used for delivering plasmid DNA encoding for bone morphogenetic protein-4 into a cranial critical size defect for up to 15 weeks. Histomorphometric analysis revealed a significant 4.5-fold increase in total bone formation with a significant increase in both osteoid and mineralized tissue density for scaffolds incorporating condensed BMP-4 DNA in comparison to control (Huang et al., 2005). Neither of these more advanced techniques have been tried clinically. However, they certainly may have great use in larger sites such as lateral window maxillary sinus augmentation or vertical ridge augmentation as well as generalized periodontitis cases as indicated because these methods may significantly expedite healing.

In summary, BMP-2 is a potent mitogenic factor for periodontal and bone regeneration. The consensus is that animal and human studies show that bone regenerated with the application of BMP-2 resulted in bone density and histology no different than native bone. The application of rhBMP-2 for periodontal regeneration still requires human clinical evidence.

FUTURE REGENERATIVE THERAPY WITH rhPDGF

The topical administration of growth factors has been optimized for periodontal regeneration. Molecular biological techniques, such as gene therapy, have been used to demonstrate PDGF-BB effects on periodontal regeneration. PDGF-BB gene transfer was evaluated in rats for periodontal tissue regeneration in critical size alveolar bone defects. Several different gene combinations were used for PDGF-A and -B. Histomorphometric evaluations indicated that PDGF-B application stimulated cell proliferation compared to the control and PDGF-A. In addition, bone regeneration was four times greater for PDGF-B specimens compared to the other two groups. More importantly, gene expression remained active three weeks after PDGF-B application in periodontal defects (Zhu et al., 2001; Jin et al., 2004).

Although PDGF-A had low effects on periodontal regeneration for bone, its direct effects may be different on cementoblasts. Using a similar gene therapy technology, cementoblasts were altered with a PDGF-A gene. Gene-altered cementoblasts exhibited proliferation similar to that of continuous rhPDGF-AA protein application on native cementoblasts. RNA and protein analyses demonstrated significant presence for PDGF-A. This indicates gene delivery of PDGF-stimulated cementoblastic activity in addition to osteoblastic activity (Giannobile et al., 2001). The same group of researchers evaluated the effects of PDGF-A and PDGF-B gene transfer in human gingival fibroblasts in three-dimensional collagen lattices. An advantage to the 3D model is the possible quantification of defect fill. In this particular study, human gingival fibroblasts were altered with PDGF-A and PDGF-B genes. Findings of this study indicated that cell repopulation and defect fill was stimulated more than four times for the PDGF-B-gene-applied gingival fibroblasts, while PDGF-A and the controls exhibited similar diminished cellular activity (Anusaksathien et al., 2003).

While overall periodontal regeneration with rhPDGF-BB has been established, the clinical application of gene therapy may target specific cell types. In addition, the timing of protein expression may be critical to enhancing the clinical outcome. Gene therapy by turning on genes such as PDGF for sustained release will amplify the intensity and duration of periodontal regeneration. The findings for PDGF gene therapy confirm its potency for periodontal ligament cells and gingival fibroblasts as well as osteoblasts. As established for other systems, gene therapy is technically possible for periodontal regenerative treatment.

In summary, different treatment modalities have been introduced aimed at regenerating periodontal tissues lost secondary to the disease. The current regenerative options include the surgical placement of different bone grafts into the osseous defect sites, typically with a barrier membrane (Figure 8.4). Several biomaterials, agents, and growth factors for surgical procedures involving guided tissue regeneration have been developed. As reviewed, many studies support their clinical use. Certainly our goal as clinicians is to maximize the predictability of the prognosis of typically complex surgical procedures. Currently the additional benefits of growth factor proteins will enhance these patient-centered outcomes.

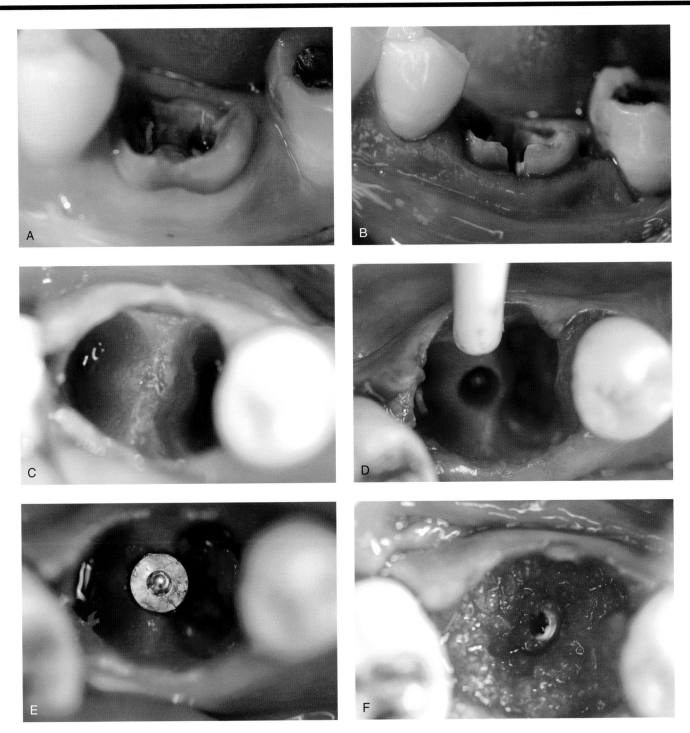

Figure 8.4. Guided tissue regeneration around the immediate molar implant placement. A, Lower left molar is hopeless due to the amount of recurrent decay around a PFM crown. Favorable intra-radicular bone and root convergence are present for an immediate implant placement. B, Sulcular incisions were made to preserve the maximal amount of soft tissue for the GTR procedure. The roots were sectioned for an atraumatic extraction. C, The extraction socket is favorable for an immediate implant placement and GTR. D, Osteotome prepared for a 4.5-mm diameter implant. An adequate amount of bone is present for initial stability and GTR. E, A 4.5 mm X 13 mm implant was placed in the prepared osteotome. F, Freeze-dried bone allograft (FDBA) was used to graft the remaining socket. G, A resorbable membrane was used to exclude epithelium and to contain the bone graft material. H, Primary closure of the soft tissue is essential for such a procedure. For that purpose, releasing incisions were done on the buccal aspect. In addition, simple interrupted and horizontal mattress suture techniques were used to minimize tension onto the flap and primary closure.

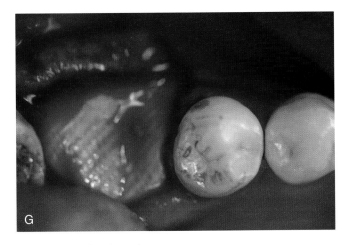
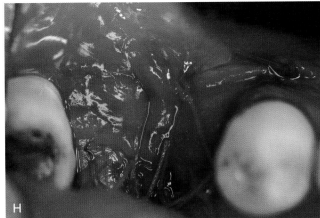

Figure 8.4. *Continued*

REFERENCES

Anderegg CR, Martin SJ, Gray JL, Mellonig JT, Gher ME. 1991. Clinical evaluation of the use of decalcified freeze-dried bone allograft with guided tissue regeneration in the treatment of molar furcation invasions. *J. Periodontol.* Apr;62(4), 264–8.

Annunziata M, Oliva A, Buonaiuto C, Di Feo A, Di Pasquale R, Passaro I, Guida L. 2005. In vitro cell-type specific biological response of human periodontally related cells to platelet-rich plasma. *J. Periodontal. Res.* Dec;40(6), 489–95.

Anusaksathien O, Webb SA, Jin QM, Giannobile WV. 2003. Platelet-derived growth factor gene delivery stimulates ex vivo gingival repair. *Tissue Eng.* Aug;9(4), 745–56.

Aukhil I, Pettersson E, Suggs C. 1986. Guided tissue regeneration. An experimental procedure in beagle dogs. *J. Periodontol.* Dec;57(12), 727–34.

Barkana I, Alexopoulou E, Ziv S, Jacob-Hirsch J, Amariglio N, Pitaru S, Vardimon AD, Nemcovsky CE. 2007. Gene profile in periodontal ligament cells and clones with enamel matrix proteins derivative. *J. Clin. Periodontol.* Jul;34(7), 599–609. Epub 2007 Apr 13.

Betz OB, Betz VM, Nazarian A, Egermann M, Gerstenfeld LC, Einhorn TA, Vrahas MS, Bouxsein ML, Evans CH. 2007. Delayed administration of adenoviral BMP-2 vector improves the formation of bone in osseous defects. *Gene Ther.* Jul;14(13), 1039–44.

Bianchi J, Fiorellini JP, Howell TH, Sekler J, Curtin H, Nevins ML, Friedland B. 2004. Measuring the efficacy of rhBMP-2 to regenerate bone: a radiographic study using a commercially available software program. *Int. J. Periodontics Restorative Dent.* Dec;24(6), 579–87.

Blom S, Holmstrup P, Dabelsteen E. 1994. A comparison of the effect of epidermal growth factor, platelet-derived growth factor, and fibroblast growth factor on rat periodontal ligament fibroblast-like cells' DNA synthesis and morphology. *J. Periodontol.* May;65(5), 373–8.

Boyne PJ, Lilly LC, Marx RE, Moy PK, Nevins M, Spagnoli DB, Triplett RG. 2005. De novo bone induction by recombinant human bone morphogenetic protein-2 (rhBMP-2) in maxillary sinus floor augmentation. *J. Oral Maxillofac. Surg.* Dec;63(12), 1693–707.

Camargo PM, Lekovic V, Weinlaender M, Vasilic N, Madzarevic M, Kenney EB. 2005. A reentry study on the use of bovine porous bone mineral, GTR, and platelet-rich plasma in the regenerative treatment of intrabony defects in humans. *Int. J. Periodontics. Restorative Dent.* Feb;25(1), 49–59.

Camelo M, Nevins ML, Schenk RK, Lynch SE, Nevins M. 2003. Periodontal regeneration in human Class II furcations using purified recombinant human platelet-derived growth factor-BB (rhPDGF-BB) with bone allograft. *Int. J. Periodontics Restorative Dent.* Jun;23(3), 213–25.

Caton JG, DeFuria EL, Polson AM, Nyman S. 1987. Periodontal regeneration via selective cell repopulation. *J. Periodontol.* Aug;58(8), 546–52.

Cortellini P, Pini Prato G, Tonetti MS. 1993a. Periodontal regeneration of human infrabony defects. I. Clinical measures. *J. Periodontol.* Apr;64(4), 254–60.

Cortellini P, Pini Prato G, Tonetti MS. 1993b. Periodontal regeneration of human infrabony defects. II. Re-entry procedures and bone measures. *J. Periodontol.* Apr;64(4), 261–8.

Cortellini P, Pini-Prato G, Tonetti M. 1994. Periodontal regeneration of human infrabony defects. V. Effect of oral hygiene on long-term stability. *J. Clin. Periodontol.* Oct;21(9), 606–10.

Cortellini P, Tonetti MS. 2007. Minimally invasive surgical technique and enamel matrix derivative in intra-bony defects. I: Clinical outcomes and morbidity. *J. Clin. Periodontol.* Dec;34(12), 1082–8. Epub Oct 22.

Danesh-Meyer MJ, Filstein MR, Shanaman R. 2001. Histological evaluation of sinus augmentation using platelet rich plasma (PRP): a case series. *J. Int. Acad. Periodontol.* Apr;3(2), 48–56.

Döri F, Huszár T, Nikolidakis D, Arweiler NB, Gera I, Sculean A. 2007a. Effect of platelet-rich plasma on the healing of intra-bony defects treated with a natural bone mineral and a collagen membrane. *J. Clin. Periodontol.* Mar;34(3), 254–61.

Döri F, Huszár T, Nikolidakis D, Arweiler NB, Gera I, Sculean A. 2007b. Effect of platelet-rich plasma on the healing of intrabony defects treated with an anorganic bovine bone mineral and expanded polytetrafluoroethylene membranes. *J. Periodontol.* Jun;78(6), 983–90.

Ferguson D, Davis WL, Urist MR, Hurt WC, Allen EP. 1987. Bovine bone morphogenetic protein (bBMP) fraction-induced repair of craniotomy defects in the rhesus monkey (Macaca speciosa). *Clin. Orthop. Relat. Res.* Jun;(219), 451–458.

Fiorellini JP, Buser D, Riley E, Howell TH. 2001. Effect on bone healing of bone morphogenetic protein placed in combination with endosseous implants: a pilot study in beagle dogs. *Int. J. Periodontics Restorative Dent.* Feb;21(1), 41–7.

Fiorellini JP, Howell TH, Cochran D, Malmquist J, Lilly LC, Spagnoli D, Toljanic J, Jones A, Nevins M. 2005. Randomized study evaluating recombinant human bone morphogenetic protein-2 for extraction socket augmentation. *J. Periodontol.* Apr;76(4), 605–13.

Galli C, Macaluso GM, Guizzardi S, Vescovini R, Passeri M, Passeri G. 2006. Osteoprotegerin and receptor activator of nuclear factor-kappa B ligand modulation by enamel matrix derivative in human alveolar osteoblasts. *J. Periodontol.* Jul;77(7), 1223–8.

Gestrelius S, Andersson C, Lidström D, Hammarström L, Somerman M. 1997a. In vitro studies on periodontal ligament cells and enamel matrix derivative. *J. Clin. Periodontol.* Sep;24(9 Pt 2), 685–92.

Gestrelius S, Andersson C, Johansson AC, Persson E, Brodin A, Rydhag L, Hammarström L. 1997b. Formulation of enamel matrix derivative for surface coating. Kinetics and cell colonization. *J. Clin. Periodontol.* Sep;24(9 Pt 2), 678–84.

Giannobile WV, Lee CS, Tomala MP, Tejeda KM, Zhu Z. 2001. Platelet-derived growth factor (PDGF) gene delivery for application in periodontal tissue engineering. *J. Periodontol.* Jun;72(6), 815–23.

Gottlow J, Nyman S, Karring T. 1992. Maintenance of new attachment gained through guided tissue regeneration. *J. Clin. Periodontol.* May;19(5), 315–7.

Gottlow J, Nyman S, Lindhe J, Karring T, Wennström J. 1986. New attachment formation in the human periodontium by guided tissue regeneration. Case reports. *J. Clin. Periodontol.* Jul;13(6), 604–16.

Hammarström L. 1997. Enamel matrix, cementum development and regeneration. *J. Clin. Periodontol.* Sep;24(9 Pt 2), 658–68. Review.

Hoffmann T, Richter S, Meyle J, Gonzales JR, Heinz B, Arjomand M, Sculean A, Reich E, Jepsen K, Jepsen S, Boedeker RH. 2006. A randomized clinical multicentre trial comparing enamel matrix derivative and membrane treatment of buccal class II furcation involvement in mandibular molars. Part III: patient factors and treatment outcome. *J. Clin. Periodontol.* Aug;33(8), 575–83.

Howell TH, Fiorellini JP, Paquette DW, Offenbacher S, Giannobile WV, Lynch SE. 1997. A phase I/II clinical trial to evaluate a combination of recombinant human platelet-derived growth factor-BB and recombinant human insulin-like growth factor-I in patients with periodontal disease. *J. Periodontol.* Dec;68(12), 1186–93.

Huang YC, Simmons C, Kaigler D, Rice KG, Mooney DJ. 2005. Bone regeneration in a rat cranial defect with delivery of PEI-condensed plasmid DNA encoding for bone morphogenetic protein-4 (BMP-4). *Gene Ther.* Mar;12(5), 418–26.

Jensen TB, Rahbek O, Overgaard S, Søballe K. 2005. No effect of platelet-rich plasma with frozen or processed bone allograft around noncemented implants. *Int. Orthop.* Apr;29(2), 67–72.

Jin Q, Anusaksathien O, Webb SA, Printz MA, Giannobile WV. 2004. Engineering of tooth-supporting structures by delivery of PDGF gene therapy vectors. *Mol. Ther.* Apr;9(4), 519–26.

Johnson EE, Urist MR, Finerman GA. 1988. Bone morphogenetic protein augmentation grafting of resistant femoral nonunions. A preliminary report. *Clin. Orthop. Relat. Res.* May;(230), 257–65.

Jones AA, Buser D, Schenk R, Wozney J, Cochran DL. 2006. The effect of rhBMP-2 around endosseous implants with and without membranes in the canine model. *J. Periodontol.* Jul;77(7), 1184–93.

Lekovic V, Camargo PM, Weinlaender M, Vasilic N, Aleksic Z, Kenney EB. 2003. Effectiveness of a combination of platelet-rich plasma, bovine porous bone mineral and guided tissue regeneration in the treatment of mandibular grade II molar furcations in humans. *J. Clin. Periodontol.* Aug;30(8), 746–51.

Lekovic V, Camargo PM, Weinlaender M, Vasilic N, Kenney EB. 2002. Comparison of platelet-rich plasma, bovine porous bone mineral, and guided tissue regeneration versus platelet-rich plasma and bovine porous bone mineral in the treatment of intrabony defects: a reentry study. *J. Periodontol.* Feb;73(2), 198–205.

Lynch SE, de Castilla GR, Williams RC, Kiritsy CP, Howell TH, Reddy MS, Antoniades HN. 1991. The effects of short-term application of a combination of platelet-derived and insulin-like growth factors on periodontal wound healing. *J. Periodontol.* Jul;62(7), 458–67.

Mariotti A. 2003. Efficacy of Chemical Root Surface Modifiers in the Treatment of Periodontal Disease. A Systematic Review. *Annals of Periodontology.* December, Vol. 8, No. 1, 205–226.

Marx RE, Carlson ER, Eichstaedt RM, Schimmele SR, Strauss JE, Georgeff KR. 1998. Platelet-rich plasma: Growth factor enhancement for bone grafts. *Oral Surg. Oral Med. Oral Pathol. Oral Radiol. Endod.* Jun;85(6), 638–46.

McGuire MK, Kao RT, Nevins M, Lynch SE. 2006. rhPDGF-BB promotes healing of periodontal defects: 24-month clinical and radiographic observations. *Int. J. Periodontics Restorative Dent.* Jun;26(3), 223–31.

Nevins M, Camelo M, Nevins ML, Schenk RK, Lynch SE. 2003. Periodontal regeneration in humans using recombinant human platelet-derived growth factor-BB (rhPDGF-BB) and allogenic bone. *J. Periodontol.* Sep;74(9):1282–92.

Nevins M, Giannobile WV, McGuire MK, Kao RT, Mellonig JT, Hinrichs JE, McAllister BS, Murphy KS, McClain PK, Nevins ML, Paquette DW, Han TJ, Reddy MS, Lavin PT, Genco RJ, Lynch SE. 2005. Platelet-derived growth factor stimulates bone fill and rate of attachment level gain: results of a large multicenter randomized controlled trial. *J. Periodontol.* Dec;76(12):2205–15.

Nyman S, Gottlow J, Karring T, Lindhe J. 1982a. The regenerative potential of the periodontal ligament. An experimental study in the monkey. *J. Clin. Periodontol.* May;9(3), 257–65.

Nyman S, Lindhe J, Karring T, Rylander H. 1982b. New attachment following surgical treatment of human periodontal disease. *J. Clin. Periodontol.* Jul;9(4), 290–6.

Okuda K, Kawase T, Momose M, Murata M, Saito Y, Suzuki H, Wolff LF, Yoshie H. 2003. Platelet-rich plasma contains high levels of platelet-derived growth factor and transforming growth factor-beta and modulates the proliferation of periodontally related cells in vitro. *J. Periodontol.* Jun;74(6), 849–57.

Pontoriero R, Lindhe J. 1995. Guided tissue regeneration in the treatment of degree II furcations in maxillary molars. *J. Clin. Periodontol.* Oct;22(10), 756–63.

Pontoriero R, Nyman S, Lindhe J, Rosenberg E, Sanavi F. 1987. Guided tissue regeneration in the treatment of furcation defects in man. *J. Clin. Periodontol.* Nov;14(10), 618–20.

Pryor ME, Polimeni G, Koo KT, Hartman MJ, Gross H, April M, Safadi FF, Wikesjö UM. 2005. Analysis of rat calvaria defects implanted with a platelet-rich plasma preparation: histologic and histometric observations. *J. Clin. Periodontol.* Sep;32(9), 966–72.

Schallhorn RG. 1977. Present status of osseous grafting procedures. *J. Periodontol.* Sep;48(9), 570–6.

Schlueter SR, Carnes DL, Cochran DL. 2007. In vitro effects of enamel matrix derivative on microvascular cells. *J. Periodontol.* Jan;78(1), 141–51.

Sculean A, Schwarz F, Miliauskaite A, Kiss A, Arweiler N, Becker J, Brecx M. 2006. Treatment of intrabony defects with an enamel matrix protein derivative or bioabsorbable membrane: an 8-year follow-up split-mouth study. *J. Periodontol.* Nov;77(11), 1879–86.

Selvig KA, Kersten BG, Wikesjö UM. 1993. Surgical treatment of intrabony periodontal defects using expanded polytetrafluoroethylene barrier membranes: influence of defect configuration on healing response. *J. Periodontol.* Aug;64(8), 730–3.

Simion M, Rocchietta I, Kim D, Nevins M, Fiorellini J. 2006. Vertical ridge augmentation by means of deproteinized bovine bone block and recombinant human platelet-derived growth factor-BB: a histologic study in a dog model. *Int. J. Periodontics Restorative Dent.* Oct;26(5), 415–23.

Simion M, Rocchietta I, Monforte M, Maschera E. 2008. Three-dimensional alveolar bone reconstruction with a combination of recombinant human platelet-derived growth factor BB and guided bone regeneration: a case report. *Int. J. Periodontics Restorative Dent.* Jun;28(3), 239–43.

Song AM, Shu R, Xie YF, Song ZC, Li HY, Liu XF, Zhang XL. 2007. A study of enamel matrix proteins on differentiation of porcine bone marrow stromal cells into cementoblasts. *Cell Prolif.* Jun;40(3), 381–96.

Urist MR, Nilsson O, Rasmussen J, Hirota W, Lovell T, Schmalzreid T, Finerman GA. 1987. Bone regeneration under the influence of a bone morphogenetic protein (BMP) beta tricalcium phosphate (TCP) composite in skull trephine defects in dogs. *Clin. Orthop. Relat. Res.* Jan;(214), 295–304.

Uzel MI, Scott IC, Babakhanlou-Chase H, Palamakumbura AH, Pappano WN, Hong HH, Greenspan DS, Trackman PC. 2001. Multiple bone morphogenetic protein 1-related mammalian metalloproteinases process pro-lysyl oxidase at the correct physiological site and control lysyl oxidase activation in mouse embryo fibroblast cultures. *J. Biol. Chem.* Jun 22;276(25), 22537–43.

Yasko AW, Lane JM, Fellinger EJ, Rosen V, Wozney JM, Wang EA. 1992. The healing of segmental bone defects, induced by recombinant human bone morphogenetic protein (rhBMP-2). A radiographic, histological, and biomechanical study in rats. *J. Bone Joint Surg. Am.* Jun;74(5), 659–70.

Zeldich E, Koren R, Nemcovsky C, Weinreb M. 2007. Enamel matrix derivative stimulates human gingival fibroblast proliferation via ERK. *J. Dent. Res.* Jan;86(1), 41–6.

Zhang L, Leeman E, Carnes DC, Graves DT. 1991. Human osteoblasts synthesize and respond to platelet-derived growth factor. *Am. J. Physiol.* Aug;261(2 Pt 1), C348–54.

Zhu Z, Lee CS, Tejeda KM, Giannobile WV. 2001. Gene transfer and expression of platelet-derived growth factors modulate periodontal cellular activity. *J. Dent. Res.* Mar;80(3), 892–7.

Zucchelli G, Mele M, Checchi L. 2006. The papilla amplification flap for the treatment of a localized periodontal defect associated with a palatal groove. *J. Periodontol.* Oct;77(10),1788–96.

Chapter 9 Surgical vs. Non-surgical Treatment of Periodontitis

INTRODUCTION

The goal of periodontal therapy can be defined as "to arrest the inflammatory disease process by removal of the subgingival biofilm and establish a local environment and microflora compatible with periodontal health" (Heitz-Mayfield, 2005). Biofilm can be removed and a favorable local environment can be established with non-surgical mechanical debridement and/or surgical debridement. This may be supplemented by local or systemic antibiotic or antiseptic modalities. Non-surgical and surgical therapies as well as adjunctive pharmacotherapies are described elsewhere in this volume. This chapter focuses on the issues relating to the relative effectiveness of non-surgical vs. surgical periodontal therapy.

It is generally accepted that mechanical debridement is at the core of any periodontal therapy (Van Dyke and Serhan, 2003). However, it should be noted that this view has been challenged (Mombelli, 2006), and may well change in the future as we gain a better understanding of the mechanisms underpinning the pathogenesis of periodontitis. (Van Dyke, 2007). Nevertheless, the question of whether mechanical debridement should be carried out using non-surgical or surgical techniques is obviously a very important one in clinical periodontology, and consequently has been studied and debated for decades. To date, a total of three systematic reviews/meta-analyses evaluating the relative effectiveness of non-surgical vs. surgical periodontal therapy have been published. This illustrates the importance of the clinical question and is also a reflection of the fact that a relatively large number of clinical trials have been conducted to investigate it.

EVIDENCE-BASED OUTCOMES

One of the first systematic reviews/meta-analyses published in the periodontal literature addressed the question of the relative effectiveness of surgical vs. non-surgical methods of treatment for periodontal disease (Antczak-Bouckoms et al., 1993). This review identified five studies that described similar treatment comparisons that were suitable for meta-analysis. The main conclusions of the study were that the relative effectiveness of surgical vs. non-surgical therapy depends on the initial, pre-surgical level of disease severity as measured by probing depth and on the outcome measure chosen (probing depth reduction vs. clinical attachment levels). For all levels of initial disease, surgical therapy results in greater pocket depth reduction compared to non-surgical therapy. However, the differences between surgical and non-surgical therapy in terms of mean probing depth reductions were generally around 0.5 mm or less. Furthermore, there was some evidence that the advantages of surgical therapy with regard to probing depth reduction became smaller with increased length of follow-up time (up to six years). For initially shallow and moderately deep pockets (up to 6 mm), non-surgical therapy results in better average outcomes in terms of clinical attachment levels, while surgical therapy performs better in initially deep pockets (greater than 6 mm probing depth). Again, the mean differences between treatment modalities were relatively small.

Two further systematic reviews/meta-analyses have been published since then (Heitz-Mayfield et al., 2002; Hung and Douglass, 2002), and the overall results are, perhaps not surprisingly, consistent with the first meta-analysis published by Antczak-Bouckoms et al. (Antczak-Bouckoms et al. 1993). A further review paper attempts to reconcile the minor differences between the results of the three published systematic reviews (Heitz-Mayfield, 2005). Figure 9.1 shows the results of the systematic review by Heitz-Mayfield (Heitz-Mayfield et al., 2002) for both probing depth reduction and clinical attachment levels as a function of initial probing depth. Although studies have suggested that non-surgical therapy has better outcomes in anterior teeth, this systematic review found similar relative effectiveness of non-surgical vs. surgical therapy in molar vs. non-molar teeth (Heitz-Mayfield et al., 2002).

Notwithstanding these limitations, the conclusions to be drawn from the available evidence are seemingly straightforward in that surgical therapy is the therapy of choice in severe disease (initial probing depths 7+ mm) or if the goal is probing depth reduction.

AUTHOR'S VIEWS/COMMENTS

As stated above, the goal of periodontal therapy may be defined as "to arrest the inflammatory disease process by removal of the subgingival biofilm and establish a local environment and microflora compatible with periodontal health" (Heitz-Mayfield, 2005). While this is a sensible definition in light of our current understanding of the pathogenesis of periodontitis, it does not lend itself to the assessment of success or failure of any periodontal intervention.

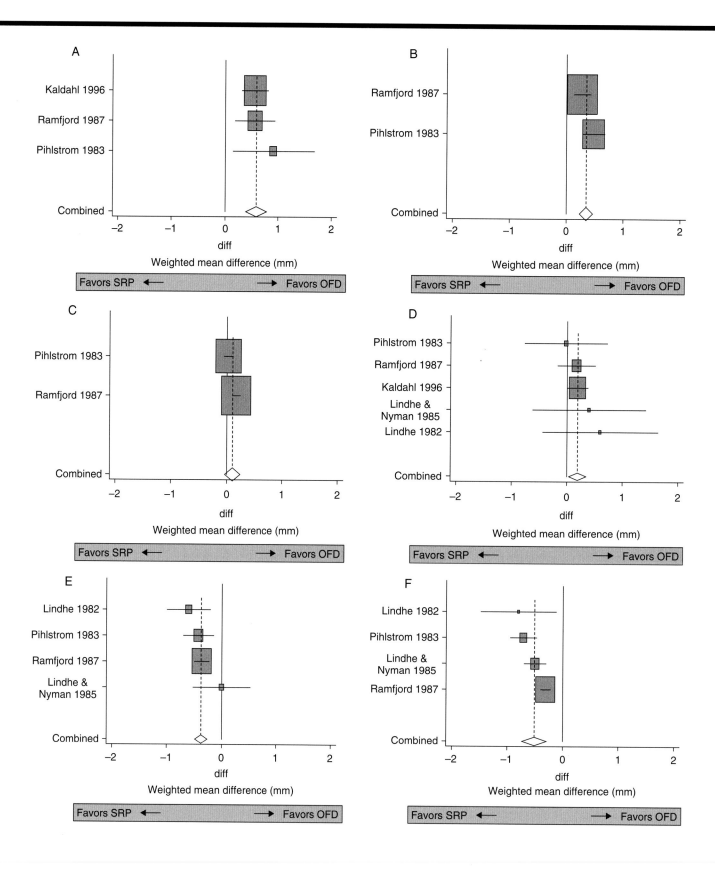

In terms of objective clinical periodontal outcomes, we may define the goals of periodontal therapy to be—at least in the short-term—the reduction or elimination of periodontal pockets and the prevention of further attachment loss. Periodontal pocket depth and attachment loss have several characteristics that, for dentists, make them almost intuitive endpoints to measure success or failure of periodontal therapy. First, periodontal pocket depth and attachment loss are literally defining signs of periodontitis, given that periodontitis is defined as a chronic inflammatory disease characterized by loss of attachment (and the associated pocketing). Second, the assessment of periodontal pocket depth and clinical attachment loss is relatively straightforward, both in clinical practice as well as in clinical studies. Third, clinical attachment level and in particular periodontal pocket depth are relatively sensitive to non-surgical or surgical periodontal interventions in the short-term, i.e., the clinician can almost immediately (i.e., within weeks to a few months) see an effect (benefit) of his or her intervention. It is therefore hardly surprising that the bulk of the available clinical trials on the effects of surgical vs. non-surgical periodontal therapy used periodontal probing depth and clinical attachment levels as outcome measures.

However, for patients suffering from periodontitis, probing pocket depth and attachment levels in and of themselves may be entirely irrelevant. They only become tangible when they cause symptoms such as recession, malodor, or bad taste, or when they result in tooth loss. A better definition of the goals of periodontal therapy would, therefore, make reference to patient-centered, tangible outcomes such as oral-health-related quality of life, or hard, tangible endpoints such as tooth loss. Therefore, probing pocket depth and clinical attachment level are what is called surrogate outcomes, because they are explicitly or implicitly used as surrogates for hard, tangible outcomes such as tooth loss.

Results from studies using surrogate endpoints generally must be cautiously interpreted, because they may not necessarily be generalized to the hard endpoints of interest (Hujoel, 2004). For example, serum cholesterol and blood pressure are surrogate endpoints for interventions to reduce cardiovascular disease risk. Because serum cholesterol and blood pressure are strong risk factors for cardiovascular disease, it would generally be expected that treatments effective in reducing serum cholesterol or blood pressure will also have beneficial effects on cardiovascular disease. While this may be true for many interventions, some interventions that effectively reduce serum cholesterol may actually increase cardiovascular disease risk through a different pathway. Hence, surrogate endpoints need to be carefully validated, and there may always be uncertainty as to whether the effectiveness of a specific intervention as assessed with a surrogate endpoint holds for a true endpoint.

Tooth loss is one tangible endpoint relevant to periodontal therapy, and based on common sense and clinical experience, one may argue that attachment levels and probing depth are valid surrogate endpoints for assessing the effect of periodontal therapy on tooth loss risk. Indeed, it is difficult to think of a scenario in which progressive attachment loss would not ultimately result in tooth loss. Therefore, if flap surgery is superior to non-surgical therapy in terms of both probing depth and attachment level in initially deep pockets (7+ mm), should one surely go for surgical therapy to reduce tooth loss risk? Unfortunately, it may not be that straightforward. For example, surgical therapy will result in more severe recession, which in turn may be associated with an increased risk for root caries and subsequent tooth loss. Furthermore, non-surgical therapy may be preferable over surgical therapy with regard to other tangible endpoints, such as esthetics (recession) and hypersensitivity.

Figure 9.1 A, Forest plot of studies investigating the difference in probing depth change between open flap debridement (OFD) and scaling and root planing (SRP) at sites with initial PPD > 6 mm. The rectangles represent the individual results for each study, in this case the weighted mean difference (WMD) in mm between open flap debridement vs. scaling and root planing. The size of the rectangle represents the weighting given to the study in the meta-analysis and is directly related to the precision of the study. The horizontal line extending from each square represents the 95% confidence interval (95% CI). The diamond at the bottom is the pooled value from the meta-analysis. The center of the diamond is the summary value and the horizontal points represent the 95% CI. When the diamond is to the left of the zero line the outcome is in favor of scaling and root planing. When the diamond is to the right of the zero line the outcome is in favor of open flap surgery. This analysis shows a 0.58-mm greater pocket depth reduction for surgery than scaling and root planing (95% CI: 0.38, 0.79, P < 0.001). B, Difference in the PPD change between OFD and SRP at sites with initial PPD: 4 mm to 6 mm. Fixed effects forest plot. C, Difference in the PPD change between OFD and SRP at sites with initial PPD 1 mm to 3 mm. Random effects forest plot. D, Difference in the CAL change between OFD and SRP at sites with initial PPD: >6 mm. Fixed effects forest plot. E, Difference in the CAL change between OFD and SRP at sites with initial PPD 4 mm to 6 mm. Fixed effects forest plot. F, Difference in the CAL change between OFD and SRP at sites with initial PPD 1 mm to 3 mm. Random effects forest plot. Reprinted from Heitz-Mayfield, 2005 with permission.

To further complicate things, when considering the evidence regarding the effectiveness of non-surgical vs. surgical periodontal therapy, the clinician faces the formidable dilemma that either form of treatment may be more efficient depending on whether probing pocket depth or clinical attachment level is chosen as the (surrogate) endpoint of interest. The conclusion that (1) surgical therapy provides a greater benefit than non-surgical therapy if the objective is reduction of probing depth, and (2) non-surgical therapy provides a greater benefit for shallow and moderate initial pockets (up to 6 mm) but not for deep pockets (7+ mm) in terms of attachment level, is hardly satisfying and not particularly helpful in decision making (Heitz-Mayfield, 2005). In fact, as discussed above, neither probing pocket depths nor clinical attachment levels are reasonable endpoints, and shouldn't be the objectives of periodontal treatment on which treatment decisions are based.

The scenario is equivalent to a hypothetical intervention that increases LDL cholesterol levels but lowers blood pressure. In this case a physician would have to choose whether he considers blood pressure or LDL cholesterol to be more important. While there may be a specific patient for whom a physician could make such a decision, the surrogate endpoints are clearly not useful in assessing the benefit of this hypothetical intervention with respect to cardiovascular disease. Such evidence could only come from a clinical trial using true disease endpoints. In any case, it is unlikely that an intervention that lowers blood pressure and increases LDL cholesterol would be a popular, first line treatment to prevent cardiovascular disease in patients with high blood pressure. Therefore, in the absence of robust evidence from clinical trials regarding the effects of surgical vs. non-surgical therapy on tooth mortality, it may not be justifiable to prescribe surgical therapy universally, even for deep sites.

It is often argued that probing depth reduction (and therefore surgical therapy) has priority because shallow sites are easier to maintain by the patient, hygienist, and dentist in the long term. While this may be true with respect to periodontal conditions, this does not necessarily translate into benefits with regard to tooth mortality. Again, robust trial evidence is needed to assess the validity of this assertion. Another important limitation of the available evidence is that studies have been exclusively conducted in university settings, i.e., under ideal conditions with few time constraints and often very frequent, intensive follow-up care. Hence, it is uncertain whether these conclusions can be generalized to general or periodontal practice settings.

Non-surgical therapy and flap surgery are, strictly speaking and in current periodontal practice, not true treatment alternatives, because non-surgical therapy is almost invariably performed initially, i.e., practically all patients diagnosed with periodontitis initially receive non-surgical periodontal therapy (American Academy of Periodontology, 2000). Accordingly, only some of the studies included in the systematic reviews compared non-surgical vs. surgical therapy without any pretreatment scaling, while the majority of studies conducted non-surgical treatment in all groups and then either compared surgery to no treatment or surgery to a second non-surgical treatment (Heitz-Mayfield et al., 2002). Hence, the title of this chapter, albeit reflecting what is often perceived as alternative approaches, is, strictly speaking, a misnomer.

In a given clinical situation, the relevant clinical question to be discussed with the patient would be whether or not the likely benefits of flap surgery outweigh the likely adverse effects when compared to continued maintenance therapy after non-surgical therapy. If the expected benefits of surgery outweigh the expected adverse effects, the next question to be discussed with the patient is whether the net benefit of surgery over maintenance justifies its additional cost.

This is not merely an academic discussion. Importantly, there is no need to make a decision for or against surgical therapy before initial therapy from a periodontal perspective. Rather, whether or not surgical therapy is necessary and if so, on what teeth, should be decided only after the results of non-surgical therapy have been evaluated. In this context it is important to remember that the conclusions drawn from clinical trials refer to population averages, i.e., periodontal surgery results in greater pocket depth reduction and better clinical attachment levels in deep pockets on average. For most treatment outcomes, considerable inter-individual variability exists, i.e., many patients respond unexpectedly well to non-surgical therapy, and additional surgery would not be expected to yield significant benefits (Figure 9.2.). In fact, it

Figure 9.2 37 yr old female patient, non-smoker, medically fit. A, Clinical and B, radiographic status at the time of presentation to the university clinic. Note the massive bone and attachment loss of maxillary incisors. The maxillary right central incisor has a 9-mm pocket mesially; pocket depths are up to 6 mm at the other incisors. The patient received non-surgical periodontal therapy with hand and sonic instruments combined with systemic antibiotics (375 mg amoxicillin and 250 mg metronidazole tds for seven days). The patient was recalled every three months for supportive periodontal therapy, at which time the sites with probing depths of 4 mm and bleeding on probing and all sites with probing depths of 5+ mm were instrumented with ultrasonic instruments. C, After 17 months of therapy no probing depths greater than 3 mm remain and D, there is radiographic evidence of bony repair. Case courtesy of Drs. Walter and Krastl, Basel, Switzerland. Full case report: Walter C and Krastl G. 2007. Quintessence, 58, 1085–1096.

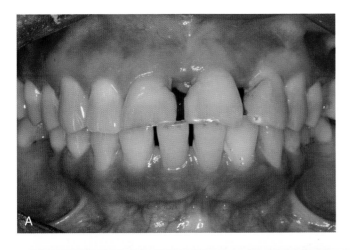

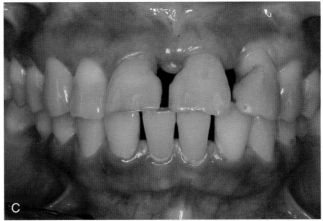

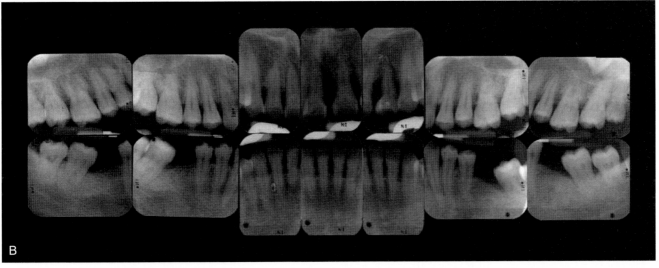

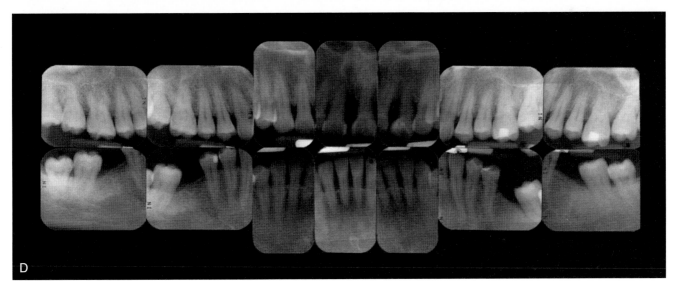

was shown more than 20 years ago that "there is no certain magnitude of initial probing pocket depth where non-surgical periodontal therapy is no longer effective" (Badersten et al., 1984). Others may respond unexpectedly poorly to non-surgical therapy and surgical therapy may have to be considered, even in shallow or moderately deep pockets.

The emerging evidence for an association between chronic periodontitis and systemic disease, particularly cardiovascular diseases, may also have implications on the choice of treatment in periodontitis patients. In the future, it may well become evident that surgical therapy may be advantageous for cardiovascular risk reduction. However, at present, it is uncertain to what extent the associations observed in epidemiologic studies represent a causal effect of periodontitis (Dietrich et al., 2008), and a benefit of periodontal therapy on cardiovascular disease risk has not been demonstrated, although recent studies suggest an effect at least on some surrogate cardiovascular endpoints (Tonetti et al., 2007).

In summary, the relative effectiveness of surgical vs. non-surgical periodontal therapy depends on the initial disease level (initial pocket depth). There is robust evidence from clinical trials that in the short term, surgical periodontal therapy results in better outcomes in terms of probing depth reduction and, in deep sites with initial probing depths greater than 6 mm, better outcomes in terms of clinical attachment levels, compared to non-surgical therapy. However, the relevance of these benefits in the long term with regard to tooth loss and other outcomes relevant to the patient, including any adverse effects of surgical vs. non-surgical therapy, is uncertain. In the absence of such evidence, it may be prudent to offer non-surgical therapy as a first line treatment to every patient with periodontitis, irrespective of initial disease levels, and to consider surgical therapy in cases in which the response to non-surgical therapy was unsatisfactory.

REFERENCES

American Academy of Periodontology. 2000. Parameter on chronic periodontitis with advanced loss of periodontal support. *J. Periodontol.* 71, 856–858.

Antczak-Bouckoms A, Joshipura K, Burdick E, Tulloch JF. 1993. Meta-analysis of surgical versus non-surgical methods of treatment for periodontal disease. *J. Clin. Periodontol.* 20, 259–268.

Badersten A, Nilveus R, Egelberg J. 1984. Effect of non-surgical periodontal therapy. II. Severely advanced periodontitis. *J. Clin. Periodontol.* 11, 63–76.

Dietrich T, Jimenez M, Krall Kaye EA, Vokonas PS, Garcia RI. 2008. Age-dependent associations between chronic periodontitis/edentulism and risk of coronary heart disease. *Circulation.* 117, 1668–1674.

Heitz-Mayfield LJ. 2005. How effective is surgical therapy compared with non-surgical debridement? *Periodontol. 2000.* 37, 72–87.

Heitz-Mayfield LJ, Trombelli L, Heitz F, Needleman I, Moles D. 2002. A systematic review of the effect of surgical debridement vs. non-surgical debridement for the treatment of chronic periodontitis. *J. Clin. Periodontol.* 29 Suppl 3, 92–102.

Hujoel PP. 2004. Endpoints in periodontal trials: the need for an evidence-based research approach. *Periodontol. 2000.* 36, 196–204.

Hung HC, Douglass CW. 2002. Meta-analysis of the effect of scaling and root planing, surgical treatment and antibiotic therapies on periodontal probing depth and attachment loss. *J. Clin. Periodontol.* 29, 975–986.

Mombelli A. 2006. Heresy? Treatment of chronic periodontitis with systemic antibiotics only. *J. Clin. Periodontol.* 33, 661–662.

Tonetti MS, D'Aiuto F, Nibali L, Donald A, Storry C, Parkar M, Suvan J, Hingorani AD, Vallance P, Deanfield J. 2007. Treatment of periodontitis and endothelial function. *N. Engl. J. Med.* 356, 911–920.

Van Dyke TE. 2007. Control of inflammation and periodontitis. *Periodontol. 2000.* 45, 158–166.

Van Dyke TE, Serhan CN. 2003. Resolution of inflammation: a new paradigm for the pathogenesis of periodontal diseases. *J. Dent. Res.* 82, 82–90.

Chapter 10 Supportive Periodontal Therapy

INTRODUCTION

"Supportive periodontal therapy (SPT)" is a term suggested by the 3rd World Workshop of the American Academy of Periodontology (AAP, 1989). It refers to the phase of treatment concerned with maintenance of patients following active periodontal therapy and includes maintenance of dental implants. This therapy has also been referred to as periodontal maintenance (Cohen, 2003). Such maintenance or supportive therapy is important to assess long-term success of periodontal therapies, prevent recurrence or continued progression of disease, and importantly, to facilitate timely interception and adequate treatment when recurrent disease becomes apparent. Implicit in the phrase is the understanding that the patient's own efforts to control periodontal disease are key, and that therapeutic measures from the dental team are necessary to maintain these in the long term.

This maintenance entails regular recall of patients at chosen intervals. The clinician would normally conduct an update of the medical and dental histories, extraoral and intraoral soft tissue examination, dental examination, periodontal evaluation, implant evaluation, radiographic review, removal of bacterial plaque and calculus from supragingival and subgingival regions, selective root planing or implant debridement if indicated, polishing of teeth, and a review of the patient's plaque removal efficiency (AAP, 2001).

In general terms, supportive periodontal therapy is considered a necessary condition of successful long-term management of periodontal disease after initial treatment. Teleologically, this maintenance is designed to control, over the longer term, the causes of periodontal disease. Historically, supportive periodontal therapy has largely focused on the control of bacterial plaque (Loe et al., 1965; Lindhe et al., 1975). As our understanding of the pathogenesis of periodontitis has grown substantially over recent decades, the importance of elements of host susceptibility in general, specific risk factors such as smoking and diabetes, and the individual composition of microbial flora has become evident. This has important implications for the scope of supportive periodontal therapy.

While maintenance of adequate plaque control remains important, it is clear that in supportive periodontal therapy, individual patients may require more or less maintenance than others, depending on their risk profile. Furthermore, risk factor modification and maintenance should be an integral part of supportive periodontal therapy (see Chapter 3). Inherent in the therapy, therefore, is the need to assess risk to patients on an individual basis. Otherwise, application of standardized protocols for treatment may permit supervised neglect and reinfection in some patients or overtreatment with poor cost effectiveness or unnecessary adverse effects in others. Although there is general agreement on these principles, evidence-based protocols for determining adequate recall intervals are lacking (Needleman et al., 2005).

INDICATIONS

Supportive periodontal therapy follows initial periodontal therapy. Initial therapy normally comprises a cause-related therapeutic phase, i.e., plaque control measures, smoking cessation therapy, and removal of local plaque retentive factors. This is often followed by a corrective phase comprising surgical and non-surgical periodontal management. Clearly, where initial cause-related therapy or corrective therapy has been unsuccessful, these elements may either require revisitation or treatment planning may need to reflect a more aggressive management of the periodontally involved dentition. Where therapy has been successful in controlling active disease, however, the patient enters the maintenance phase, SPT. Thus, SPT is an integral part of any periodontal therapy and should always follow initial non-surgical or surgical therapy.

TECHNIQUE

Risk Assessment

No single technique or recall interval for SPT is appropriate for every patient; therefore, each patient must be assessed on an individual basis and therapy prescribed accordingly. Such prescriptions should assess an individual's risk, and that is an important element of the treatment planning process. In principle it has been demonstrated that such an approach can produce stable results in long-term longitudinal studies (Axelsson et al., 1991).

A number of factors contribute to a patient's overall risk. It is useful to consider all factors simultaneously. Lang and Tonetti (2003) have developed a functional diagram to evaluate the risk of disease progression. They consider the following as important factors:

- Percentage of bleeding on probing sites

- Prevalence of residual pockets greater than 4 mm

- Loss of teeth from a total of 28

- Loss of periodontal support relative to patient age

- Systemic and genetic conditions

- Environmental factors, e.g., smoking

Each factor has its own scale describing risk as low, medium, or high.

It should be noted that for some of the risk factors, particularly the genetic factors, there is insufficient evidence to support their use in a clinical prediction tool. Furthermore, the contribution of each of these risk factors or risk factor domains is arbitrarily weighted to yield an overall risk score and the method has not been validated prospectively. Nevertheless, the proposal of such risk assessment tools illustrates the growing interest and need to individualize supportive periodontal therapy and at the very least, these tools may have value for patient motivation. However, in the absence of a validated tool, risk assessment during supportive periodontal therapy remains a matter of clinical judgment. While such a scale may be useful for patient motivation, decision making based on such risk assessment remains a matter of clinical judgment.

Measuring Baseline Values

A baseline measure of periodontal health should be recorded when the patient completes active periodontal therapy (Claffey, 1991). This should include details of the level of clinical attachment under such optimal circumstances. Continuous monitoring of such measurements over time can provide an indication of further attachment loss and thus active disease. Normally, baseline health values should be measured three months after initial periodontal therapy. It appears that after this time limited amelioration is possible (Becker et al., 2001).

Treatment Considerations

The American Academy of Periodontology offers guidance on SPT with its position paper on periodontal maintenance (Cohen, 2003). It includes a detailed checklist of items which may be included in a maintenance visit. With limited evidence available for appropriate management, such guidelines are to an extent anecdotal or based on evidence of limited quality. In the absence of clear evidence-based protocols for treatment it would appear reasonable to follow such guidelines as the considered opinion of an expert group. A précis of this guidance is presented below (see Box 10.1). Sensibly, the academy has suggested that the clinician's judgment should guide adaptation of such protocols to individual cases.

BOX 10.1. Example of an Ordinary Periodontal Supportive Therapy Appointment

A. Review and update of medical and dental history

B. Clinical examination

Intra- and extraoral examination.

C. Dental examination

General restorative, occlusal factors and mobility.

A detailed periodontal examination to include probing depths, bleeding on probing, levels of plaque and calculus, and any local factors such as furcation involvement and purulent exudates.

Gingival recession and attachment levels where indicated.

An examination of dental implants where present should include restorations present and an assessment of peri-implant tissues.

Where appropriate, good quality radiographs should be exposed when diagnostic yield is anticipated. Radiographs should never be exposed as routine and should always be reported appropriately.

D. Measurement of changes in baseline periodontal status

An assessment of stability or disease progression should be made based on the clinical findings.

E. Assessment of adequacy of plaque control

F. Treatment

Professional mechanical plaque removal.

Oral hygiene instruction and other behavioral modification, e.g., smoking cessation, maintenance visits.

Root planing where appropriate.

Occlusal adjustment.

Antimicrobial therapy and root desensitization.

Surgical intervention or discontinuation of SPT as appropriate.

G. Communication

Detailed advice should be given to the patient about the nature, progress, or stability of her periodontal disease status and the necessity for further treatment.

Referral to appropriate colleagues for aspects of treatment plan.

H. Planning

Further treatment planning should be on a case-by-case basis and is normally based on careful risk assessment and clinical judgment.

Recall Intervals, Duration, and Setting

The clinician should set recall intervals based on her risk assessment for each patient. The American Academy of Periodontology (Cohen, 2003) suggests that these should normally be about three months apart. This is a relatively arbitrary figure, however. Given that patients undergoing SPT have undergone cause-related and corrective periodontal therapy in the first instance, their risk should be regarded as moderate to high. Therefore, this recall interval may be reasonable. As time progresses, the clinician may reassess the patient's risk as lower and a longer time to recall may be more appropriate. Thus, the clinician's judgment on a case-by-case basis is the most important arbiter of setting such intervals.

The time spent on a recall visit appointment should be a matter of clinical judgment. Again, this should be based on risk assessment of the patient, previous maintenance needs, modifying factors such as systemic disease or smoking, plaque control, and patient motivation. Such visits may vary from 15 minutes to an hour in duration, depending on the patient's needs.

Recall appointments need not necessarily be with a periodontist at every stage. When risk is low to medium, such visits may be more cost-effectively managed by a patient's general dental practitioner.

Risk Factor Modification

Some of the risk factors for periodontal disease progression are lifelong and immutable. The periodontist cannot change a patient's genetic susceptibility to periodontal disease or previous loss of teeth and periodontal support. Additionally, a proportion of patients will have chronic lifelong diseases, e.g., diabetes, that will render them periodontally susceptible. There may be few risk factors, in fact, that can be changed by SPT recalls. In the main, these are bacterial colonization and smoking habits.

Good supragingival plaque control is an effective method of preventing periodontal disease (Axelsson and Lindhe, 1981). Indeed, supragingival plaque control can itself effect change on the subgingival flora to that of a less pathogenic nature (Hellstrom et al., 1996). Oral hygiene instruction and continued motivational reinforcement should therefore be an important element of SPT. Supra- and subgingival deposits of plaque and calculus should be removed. There is little evidence to support the use of specific clinical signs or diagnostic tests such as bleeding on probing to determine which sites benefit from reinstrumentation (Renvert et al., 2002). Clearly, bleeding on probing in itself is not an indication for mechanical subgingival debridement during SPT visits. It has been shown that such treatment in shallow sites, can, in fact, result in attachment loss (Claffey and Egelberg, 1995).

Smoking cessation therapy should be considered an important facet of periodontal risk control. Smoking cessation therapy has been shown by Preshaw et al. (2005) in a longitudinal cohort study of 49 smokers over a 12-month period to be a successful intervention in an SPT setting, with 20% of the cohort successfully remaining stopped. The study also demonstrated a significant reduction in probing pocket depths for those who stopped smoking. Although intervention studies on the periodontal benefits of a smoking cessation intervention in the dental setting are scarce, epidemiological studies on the association between smoking and periodontitis consistently show lower periodontitis prevalence or incidence and better treatment outcomes among non-smokers compared to current smokers (Heasman et al., 2006)

EVIDENCE-BASED OUTCOMES

Many studies report on the value of SPT in the management of periodontal disease, particularly the use of professional mechanical plaque removal (PMPR) to this end. In general terms, narrative reviews of such research are positive about the value of PMPR in controlling further disease (Cohen, 2003; Renvert and Persson, 2004). However, variable quality of research and its reportage along with heterogeneity of study design renders clinical decision making on the basis of available evidence difficult. The heterogeneity of studies additionally renders meta-analysis of these clinical trials inappropriate.

A number of good quality systematic reviews relevant to SPT are available in the current literature (Needleman et al., 2005; Beirne et al., 2007). The Cochrane systematic review by Beirne et al. updates a previous review from 2005 (Beirne et al., 2005) on the value of routine scaling and polishing for the prevention of periodontal disease. This review was designed to answer several questions: Is routine scaling and polishing (SP) at regular intervals beneficial or harmful for periodontal health? Is there a difference between providers (dentist or dental hygienist) on periodontal health?

Robust search strategies and inclusion and exclusion criteria yielded nine randomized, controlled trials suitable for inclusion in the review. All were regarded as being at high risk of bias. Two split-mouth studies provided data for comparing SP vs. no SP. One study (Glavind, 1977), which involved 28 patients undertaking SPT, found no statistically significant differences for plaque, gingivitis, and attachment loss between experimental and control units at each time point during a year-long trial. The second study (Lembariti, 1998) involved 136 Tanzanian adolescents with high existing levels of calculus and who had not received any dental intervention for at least five years. This study reported statistically significant differences in calculus and gingivitis (bleeding) scores between treatment and control units at six, 12, and 22 months (in favor of scale and polish units) following a single scale and polish provided at baseline to treatment units. Improvements in periodontal health were small following SP and were negligible following oral hygiene instruction in a cohort of the group. For this group, however, no pockets greater than 4 mm were present when high levels of calculus were present. Therefore, the participants could be regarded as low risk and the results should be seen in this context.

The authors of the study also question the value of such short-term interventions, which appear to be common in the developing world. The value of longer term PMPR vs. no measures cannot, be gleaned from such short-term trials. The systematic review also revealed that clinical trials of routine scale and polish that were provided at different time intervals provided some statistically significant differences in favor of scaling and polishing more frequently: two weeks vs. six months, two weeks vs. 12 months (for the outcomes of plaque, gingivitis, pocket depth, and attachment change), and three months versus 12 months (for the outcomes of plaque, calculus, and gingivitis). No evidence was available to compare the effects of routine scaling and polishing by dentists vs. PCD delivery.

Problematic in the review is the definition of the term routine scale and polish. This is not a precisely defined intervention in periodontal disease management. The term oral prophylaxis is often used in the United States and has been defined as "the removal of plaque, calculus and stain from exposed and unexposed surfaces of the teeth by scaling and polishing as a preventive measure for the control of local irritational factors" (AAP, 1992). Within the review, routine scale and polish was defined as scaling, polishing, or both of the crown and root surfaces of teeth to remove local irritational factors (plaque, calculus, debris, and staining), that did not involve periodontal surgery or any form of adjunctive periodontal therapy such as the use of chemotherapeutic agents or root planing. The definition, therefore, included both supragingival and subgingival scaling. Clinical trials were therefore excluded on the basis of involving antimicrobial therapy and/or surgical therapy or root planing. The review must therefore be viewed in this context. These elements might not be unreasonable additions to an SPT regime, though it may be argued that they represent a return to initial cause-related therapy.

In contrast, the systematic review by Needleman et al. (2005) was relatively more inclusive than the review of Beirne et al. (2007). This study evaluated the differences between PMPR and no PMPR and between different types of PMPR. Randomized controlled trials (RCT), controlled clinical trials (CCT), and cohort studies with comparison groups were considered as suitable for inclusion within the review. However, data were stratified according to study type. An initially stringent definition of PMPR (supragingival plaque removal by a healthcare professional) was relaxed somewhat after initial screening of articles. This included subgingival

instrumentation not intended to comprise scaling and polishing. An exhaustive literature search yielded 39 articles (representing 32 trials) suitable for inclusion in the review. With this review, heterogeneity of studies meant that meta-analysis was not possible.

The authors drew the following conclusions from the study:

- A limited body of evidence of treatment in adults suggests that PMPR, particularly if combined with oral hygiene instruction (OHI), may be more effective than no treatment in terms of the outcomes of interest. The outcomes assessed in studies were surrogate endpoints of periodontal disease prevention, including the reduction of plaque, gingival bleeding/inflammation, and pocket depth, and the maintenance of attachment levels.

- There was no clear evidence to suggest that PMPR with OHI was more successful than OHI alone. It is uncertain whether professionally delivered plaque removal on a regular basis is important to primary or secondary prevention of periodontal diseases.

- Data from clinical trials provided conflicting evidence on the benefit of PMPR for prevention of secondary and tertiary periodontal disease. Some trials revealed a significant benefit on recorded outcomes. Interestingly, this did not include tooth loss, which is arguably the most significant outcome that should be measured in trials of periodontal therapy. Other studies contradictorily suggest no difference between interventions and controls.

With regard to specific PMPR interventions, the authors made the following conclusions:

- Rubber cup polishing and air polishing showed no evidence of differences in efficacy outcomes. However, bleeding and gingival trauma were greater with air polishing, though this effect was only temporary.

- When rubber cup polishing was combined with PMPR, there were clinical benefits and patient satisfaction was greater.

- The review concludes that there are benefits to periodontal health with more frequent scaling intervals. This concurs with the review by Beirne et al. (2007), although the ideal frequency of such SPT cannot be determined from existing evidence.

It is important to note that this systematic review excluded studies that specifically included subgingival debridement, which is an important limitation because SPT would typically include subgingival debridement of active sites. Furthermore, only four of the studies that were included specifically dealt with supportive periodontal therapy, i.e., investigated the effects of PMPR in patients previously treated for periodontitis (Axelsson and Lindhe, 1981; Glavind, 1977; Nyman et al., 1975; Westfelt et al., 1983). Three of these four studies compared PMPR in SPT to no PMPR/SPT. One study failed to show any short-term (11 months) benefits of PMPR/SPT in terms of plaque levels, bleeding scores, or attachment levels (Glavind, 1977). However, two longer term studies indicated benefits of PMPR/SPT with regard to plaque levels, bleeding scores, probing pocket depth, and attachment levels after two to six years (Axelsson and Lindhe, 1981; Nyman et al., 1975). Only one study compared different frequencies of PMPR/SPT (two-, four-, or 12-week intervals). Although no statistical analysis of the data was provided, increased frequency of PMPR/SPT was associated with benefits in probing depth levels but increased attachment loss.

AUTHOR'S VIEWS/COMMENTS

The value of professional supragingival mechanical plaque removal as part of supportive periodontal therapy is currently unclear when the available evidence is considered. In particular, supragingival PMPR without oral hygiene instruction appears to be of very limited value indeed. In addition, the ideal frequency of recall intervals again is unclear. However, lack of robust evidence must not be mistaken for evidence for lack of effect. Hence, this lack of evidence does not necessa rily mean that PMPR in SPT or more frequent PMPR/ SPT is inappropriate, but is an indictment of the quality of evidence that supports it.

This is by no means a trivial problem. From a public health perspective SPT may be an expensive intervention:

- Approximately 13 million scale and polishes were provided in 1999-2000 for National Health Service (NHS) patients in England. The gross cost of this intervention to the NHS was around £122 million (Do, 2000).

- A survey of preventive recommendations by general dental practitioners in western New York state revealed that 86% of respondents would recommend scaling and polishing every six months for low-risk patients of all ages (Frame et al., 2000).

It appears sensible to limit such treatment, particularly when it is funded from the public purse, to where there is good evidence for health gain and cost effectiveness. Funding of high-quality research trials to investigate SPT and its efficacy therefore appear to be a priority for periodontal researchers and clinicians alike. Such studies should be meticulously designed to contribute to future systematic reviews or meta-analyses, with adequate power and longevity of follow up. Studies should be conducted in the most relevant environment, i.e., primary care. Outcomes of interest, such as tooth loss, quality of life, and economic analysis, should be reported rather than reliance on simpler surrogate endpoints. From a practical clinical perspective it appears that current research evidence should be regarded with caution when designing SPT programs for individual patients and that above all the clinician's judgment should supplant other considerations when making decisions about care.

REFERENCES

AAP. 1989. Clinical periodontics: 3rd World workshop: Discussions.

AAP. 2001. Periodontology AAo. *Glossary of Periodontal Terms*, 4th ed. Chicago: American Academy of Periodontology.

AAP. 1992. Periodontology AAo. *Glossary of Periodontal Terms*, Chicago: American Academy of Periodontology.

Axelsson P, Lindhe J, Nystrom B. 1991. On the prevention of caries and periodontal disease. Results of a 15-year longitudinal study in adults. *J. Clin. Periodontol.* 18, 182–9.

Axelsson P, Lindhe J. 1981. The significance of maintenance care in the treatment of periodontal disease. *J. Clin. Periodontol.* 8, 281–94.

Becker W, Becker BE, Caffesse R, Kerry G, Ochsenbein C, Morrison E, et al. 2001. A longitudinal study comparing scaling, osseous surgery, and modified Widman procedures: results after 5 years. *J. Periodontol.* 72, 1675–84.

Beirne P, Forgie A, Worthington HV, Clarkson JE. 2005. Routine scale and polish for periodontal health in adults. *Cochrane Database Syst. Rev:* CD004625.

Beirne P, Worthington HV, Clarkson JE. 2007. Routine scale and polish for periodontal health in adults. *Cochrane Database Syst. Rev.* CD004625.

Claffey N. 1991. Decision making in periodontal therapy. The re-evaluation. *J. Clin. Periodontol.* 18, 384–9.

Claffey N, Egelberg J. 1995. Clinical indicators of probing attachment loss following initial periodontal treatment in advanced periodontitis patients. *J. Clin. Periodontol.* 22, 690–6.

Cohen RE. 2003. Position paper: periodontal maintenance. *J. Periodontol.* 74, 1395–401.

Do H. 2000. *Modernising NHS dentistry—implementing the NHS plan.* In: Health Do, editor. HMSO; 2000.

Frame PS, Sawai R, Bowen WH, Meyerowitz C. 2000. Preventive dentistry: practitioners' recommendations for low-risk patients compared with scientific evidence and practice guidelines. *Am. J. Prev. Med.* 18, 159–62.

Glavind L. 1977. Effect of monthly professional mechanical tooth cleaning on periodontal health in adults. *J. Clin. Periodontol.* 4, 100–6.

Heasman L, Stacey F, Preshaw PM, McCracken GI, Hepburn S, Heasman PA. 2006. The effect of smoking on periodontal treatment response: a review of clinical evidence. *J. Clin. Periodontol.* 33, 241–53.

Hellstrom MK, Ramberg P, Krok L, Lindhe J. 1996. The effect of supra-gingival plaque control on the subgingival microflora in human periodontitis. *J. Clin. Periodontol.* 23, 934–40.

Lang NP, Tonetti MS. 2003. Periodontal risk assessment (PRA) for patients in supportive periodontal therapy (SPT). *Oral Health Prev. Dent.* 1, 7–16.

Lembariti BS, van der Weijden GA, van Palenstein Helderman WH. 1998. The effect of a single scaling with or without oral hygiene instruction on gingival bleeding and calculus formation. *J. Clin. Periodontol.* 25, 30–3.

Lindhe J, Hamp SE, Loe H. 1975. Plaque induced periodontal disease in beagle dogs. A 4-year clinical, roentgenographical and histometrical study. *J. Periodontal. Res.* 10, 243–55.

Loe H, Theilade E, Jensen SB. 1965. Experimental Gingivitis In Man. *J. Periodontol.* 36, 177–87.

Needleman I, Suvan J, Moles DR, Pimlott J. 2005. A systematic review of professional mechanical plaque removal for prevention of periodontal diseases. *J. Clin. Periodontol.* 32, Suppl. 6, 229–82.

Nyman S, Rosling B, Lindhe J. 1975. Effect of professional tooth cleaning on healing after periodontal surgery. *J. Clin. Periodontol.* 2, 80–6.

Preshaw PM, Heasman L, Stacey F, Steen N, McCracken GI, Heasman PA. 2005. The effect of quitting smoking on chronic periodontitis. *J. Clin. Periodontol.* 32, 869–79.

Renvert S, Persson GR. 2002. A systematic review on the use of residual probing depth, bleeding on probing and furcation status following initial periodontal therapy to predict further attachment and tooth loss. *J. Clin. Periodontol.* 29, Suppl 3, 82–9; discussion 90–1.

Renvert S, Persson GR. 2004. Supportive periodontal therapy. *Periodontol. 2000.* 36, 179–95.

Westfelt E, Nyman S, Socransky S, Lindhe J. 1983. Significance of frequency of professional tooth cleaning for healing following periodontal surgery. *J. Clin. Periodontol.* 10, 148–56.

Chapter 11 Dental Implants Therapy

INTRODUCTION

The history of implants and their surgical placement, indications, healing process, etc. have been discussed in great detail in a previous book (Dibart, 2007). The purpose of this chapter is a little bit more challenging. What evidence do we have that the treatments we are rendering are really necessary or effective? And if so, how effective? We looked at systematic reviews in our attempt to answer these questions in light of the most recent evidence-based research literature available. Such reviews of the existing literature can be found in various databases (MEDLINE, Cochrane, EMBASE). Several authors have described the value of systematic reviews in dental research, and as a result they have been recognized as powerful research tools in evidence-based dentistry. Systematic reviews are inherently less biased, more reliable, and more valid than narrative reviews (Carr, 2002; Bader, 2004). The treatment decisions we make need to be based on the scientific study of clinical outcomes taken from properly documented and executed clinical research.

INDICATIONS

Implant therapy is aimed at replacing natural teeth that have been lost in the past or had to be recently extracted, leaving an area edentulous. So let us look at a few reasons why we would need to extract natural teeth. The decision to extract is made when the restorability of the tooth is in doubt. The usual scenario involves incipient or recurrent caries, trauma, endodontic failure, root fracture, and periodontal disease.

EVIDENCE-BASED OUTCOMES

The Tooth Extraction Dilemma: Root Canal Therapy, Fixed Partial Denture, or Implant-supported Crown?

There are enormous benefits in retaining a natural tooth; we have to remember that we, as periodontists, have the duty to preserve the natural dentition as long as possible and that dental implants, as wonderful as they are, may never replace fully natural teeth. The advantages of retaining a natural tooth include:

- Preservation of the alveolar bone

- Preservation of the papilla

- Preservation of pressure perception

- Preservation of natural structures (crown, root)

- Lack of movement of the surrounding teeth

Torabinejad et al., in 2007, after a thorough systematic review of the literature, tried to compare the long-term success rate of endodontic treatment vs. fixed partial denture (FPD) or implant-supported crown (ISC). This proved to be an arduous task, because the evidence identified by the authors did not permit them to definitively answer all of the questions posed. The evidence available for answering the questions came from mainly indirect comparisons, hence the warning that these conclusions are tentative and that there is a need for additional studies.

The concept of success is also reported differently in the literature when we compare the outcomes of RCT, FPD, or implant-supported crowns (ISC). An implant that has had some marginal bone loss and is still functional is not generally considered a failure, whereas FPD's failure can be reported as presence of recurrent decay, root fracture, porcelain fracture, loss of retention, etc. The endodontic literature is far more precise in documenting/defining success and failure. Because RCT is aimed at treating an existing disease, the evaluation of a successful outcome via radiographic monitoring or patient's lack of symptoms is much easier.

In Torabinejad's analysis, looking at 6+ years follow-up, the weighted survival data indicated that in patients with periodontally sound teeth having pulpal and/or periradicular pathosis, root canal therapy resulted in a survival rate of 97% (Table 11.1). The same rate (97%) was also found for extraction and replacement of a missing tooth with an implant. On the other hand, an extraction and replacement with FPD had a survival rate of 82%, well below that of RCT and ISC at six years. The authors also reported that FPD success rates continued to drop steadily over time beyond 60 months. This was confirmed by another review of the literature, by Salinas et al. (2004), which stated that at 15 years the rate of survival of the FPD had dropped to 69%, whereas at 11 years the cumulative success rate for implants was 93% (Naert et al., 2000). This indicates that an implant-supported crown would be the better choice when deciding on how to restore a missing tooth in a dentition.

In 2007, Stavropoulou and Koidis conducted a systematic review of the literature to test the hypothesis that the placement of a prosthetic crown on an endodontically treated

Table 11.1. Comparative long-term survival rates of root canal treatment plus crown, root canal treatment without crown, implant-supported crown, and fixed partial denture.

Treatment option	6 years	10 years	11 years	15 years
Root canal treatment with crown	97%	81 ± 12%		
Root canal treatment without crown		63 ± 15%		
Implant-supported crown	97%		93%	
Fixed partial denture	82%			69%

Table 11.2. Failure rate comparison between immediate, immediate delayed, and delayed implants.

Study	Immediate	Immediate delayed	Delayed
Lindeboom, 2006 N=50	2/25 (8%)		0/25 (0%)
Schropp, 2003 N = 44		2/22 (9%)	1/22 (4.5%)

tooth was associated with improved survival rates. They found that the cumulative survival rates after 10 years for RCT with crowns and RCT without crowns were 81 ± 12% and 63 ± 15%, respectively. Hence, the necessity to crown the teeth that have been endodontically treated.

Author's Views/Comments: The longevity of the classical treatment—RCT, possible crown lengthening when needed, and prosthetic crown—depends on the quality of each of the steps performed by the general dentist or the specialists involved. Not all dentists are created equal, hence the variability of long-term success/survival. It is much easier and less technique-sensitive to remove a questionable tooth and place an implant followed by a crown.

Dental Implant Placement: Immediate, Immediate Delayed, or Conventional Delayed Placement?

Dental implants can be placed in fresh extraction sockets, just after tooth extraction. These are called immediate implants. They have the advantage of shortening the treatment time for the patient as well as reducing the number of surgical procedures. They also can be placed without raising a flap in most cases. The disadvantages are enhanced risk of infection and failure, the presence of a gap between the implant and alveolus, and the necessity sometimes of bone grafting (Rosenquist, 1997; Takeshita, 1997). An alternative is the immediate-delayed option. These implants are placed in the healing socket after four to eight weeks to allow for the soft tissue healing that will permit primary closure of the coronal gingiva when using a two-stage system. Finally, conventional or delayed implants are those placed several months after extraction in a partially or completely healed socket.

Esposito et al. (2008), after a very thorough review of the existing literature, found only two randomized control trials (Lindeboom, 2006; Schropp, 2003) that could be used to shed some light on which therapeutic conduct to adopt

(Table 11.2). They concluded that based on the outcome from these two well-designed and -conducted studies, immediate and immediate delayed implants were viable treatment options. Looking at the raw numbers, these groups both had more implant failures and complications than the delayed implant group. Esposito et al. mentioned that patients prefer immediate delayed implants, which may provide a better esthetic outcome, even though they might be associated with increased failures and complication rates. They also mentioned that there is not enough reliable evidence supporting or refuting the need for augmentation procedures at immediate implant placements in fresh extraction sockets and that there is no reliable evidence supporting the efficacy of platelet-rich plasma (PRP) in conjunction with implant placement. Finally, they emphasized the fact that these are only preliminary results and that more randomized, controlled trials are necessary to confirm these findings.

Author's Views/Comments: All of these options are viable, but immediate implants are quite technique-/operator-sensitive. They seem to be more prone to complication/failure when compared to the delayed implants. If one does not have much experience with implant placement, one should do many delayed placements before attempting the immediate implant placement.

Is Antibiotherapy Justified to Prevent Implant Failures?

We routinely give patients antibiotics to avoid complications, but with the alarming increase in antibiotic-resistant bacteria, is this reasonable? Are we really helping the patient or are we helping ourselves to a better night's sleep? Once again, let us look at the pertinent literature. Esposito et al. (2009), in the Cochrane database of systematic reviews of 2008, tried to identify suitable randomized, controlled trials to assess the effects of prophylactic antibiotics for implant placement vs. no antibiotics or placebo administration. They found no randomized, controlled trial that could pass rigorous scrutiny (some had flaws in the methodology, others had flaws in data extraction, etc.). They concluded that there is no appropriate scientific evidence to recommend or discourage the use of prophylactic systemic antibiotics to prevent complications and failures of dental implants. They stated, "It seems sensible to recommend the use of prophylactic antibiotics for patients at high and moderate risk for endocarditis, patients with immunodeficiencies, metabolic diseases, irradiated in the head and neck area and when an extensive or prolonged surgery is anticipated." This implies that every single healthy patient who receives an implant may not necessarily need to be premedicated and that antibiotherapy should be reserved for medically compromised patients and those undergoing long or traumatic procedures (multiple implant placement, external sinus lifts, guided bone regeneration, bloc grafts, surgery performed in infected sites, etc.).

In a 2009 update, Esposito et al. concluded that there was some evidence suggesting that 2 g of amoxicillin given orally on hour preoperatively significantly reduced failures of dental implants placed in ordinary conditions. Various prophylactic systemic antibiotic regimens are available, and the current recommendation is to keep the prophylaxis short (i.e., a single dose of amoxicillin—2 g—given one hour prior to surgery) with the understanding that with each administration, adverse events may occur, ranging from diarrhea to life-threatening allergic reactions.

Author's Views/Comments: I personally believe that we are too quick in prescribing antibiotics. But this is also a reflection on the type of litigious society we are living in—40% of the world's lawyers practice in the USA! In my opinion, a good presurgical intraoral rinse with chlorhexidine, followed by thorough cleansing of the skin (lips, nose, cheeks, etc.) and the use of surgical drapes and aseptic surgical technique should cut down on the use of antibiotics tremendously, especially when the patient is healthy and the procedure is short and atraumatic (i.e.. single implant placement).

When Should Implants Be Loaded?

Primary implant stability and lack of micro-movements are considered to be two of the main factors necessary for achieving predictable high success of osseointegrated oral implants (Albrektsson, 1981). The presence of micro-movements during the healing period may impair successful osseointegration of the implant by allowing a soft tissue interface to develop between the bone and the implant (Brunski, 1979), hence the original recommendation to keep the implants load-free during the healing period (three to four months for the mandible and six to eight months for the maxilla) (Branemark, 1977). With the current desire to reduce the length of treatment, achieve better esthetics, and reduce the annoyance of removable temporaries, we are restoring and loading the implants at a different pace. The immediately placed implant can be restored immediately (within 72 hours) and can be occlusally loaded or not (immediate provisionalization). The early loading of an implant takes place six to eight weeks after surgical placement; finally, the

conventional loading takes place according to Branemark's recommendations.

Whether implants can be loaded immediately after their placement or months later has important clinical repercussions. Patients like to leave the office with teeth, and do not enjoy wearing a transitional partial denture while waiting for the process of osseointegration to take place. Furthermore, in this fast-paced society, short treatment times are appealing to the patient and dentist alike—so is this a viable option? Esposito et al. (2007) conducted a systematic review of the subject and retained 11 articles out of the 20 originally selected. They found no statistically significant difference at six months to one year follow-up between the various loading regimens.

An interesting finding that is directly correlated to the success of immediate loading is the initial insertion torque of the implant. In fact, Ottoni et al. (2005) demonstrated a strong correlation between implant failures and the initial insertion torque of the implant. Nine of the 10 immediate nonocclusal load implants inserted with a 20 Ncm torque failed, vs. only one failure out of 10 placed with an insertion torque of 32 Ncm torque (90% failure vs. 10%!) (Table 11.3). This demonstrates the imperative need to have a high degree of primary stability at implant insertion for a successful immediate or early loading procedure.

Another question that comes to mind is: Is immediate nonocclusion loading safer than immediate occlusal loading, where there is full occlusal contact with the opposing dentition? Lindeboom et al. attempted to answer this question in a randomized, controlled trial in 2006. They concluded that there is no statistically significant difference nor clinical increased failure when comparing immediate occlusal loading and nonocclusal loading.

Author's Views/Comments: It is important to use caution when reading the above-mentioned findings, because the number of patients and trials is relatively small and the follow-up period short (six months to one year). There is a need for more randomized, controlled studies to gain the definitive answers. This being said, and reviewing the relevant current literature, one notices that in the very successful trials only the "ideal" patients were recruited, using stringent selection

Table 11.3. Correlation of insertion torque values and failure rates of immediate nonocclusal load implants (after Ottoni, 2005).

Torque value	Failure rate
20 Ncm	90%
32 Ncm	10%

criteria and being treated by very skilled operators. Therefore, the chances of failure were minimized. When less experienced operators were involved, failure rates could be as high as 42% (Tawse-Smith, 2002). One constant seems to be the necessity of a high degree of primary stability (torque value of at least 32 Ncm) for the immediate loading to be successful. This could be achieved during the surgical phase by "under preparing" the osteotomy site and inserting the implant slowly, avoiding unnecessary heating of the bone. Another critical component, in my opinion, is the control of the occlusion and the necessity of avoiding lateral forces and excessive load after provisionalization.

REFERENCES

Albrektsson T, Branemark PI, Hansson HA, Lindstrom J. 1981. Osseointegrated titanium implants. Requirements for ensuring a long lasting, direct bone to implant anchorage in man. *Acta. Orthopedica. Scandinavica.* 52(2), 155–70.

Bader JD. 2004. Systematic reviews and their implications for dental practice. *Tex Dent J.* 121, 380–7.

Branemark PI, Hansson BO, Adell R, Breine U, Lindstrom J, Hallen O, et al. 1977. Osseointegrated implants in the treatment of the edentulous jaw. Experience from a 10 year period. Stockholm: Almqvist and Wiskell International.

Brunski JB, Moccia AF, Pollack SR, Korostoff E, Trachtenberg DI. 1979. The influence of functional use of endosseous dental implant on the tissue-implant interface.1. Histological aspects. *J. Dent. Res.* 58(10), 1953–69.

Carr AB. 2002. Systematic review of the literature: the overview and meta analysis. *Dent. Clin. North Am.* 46, 79–86.

Dibart S. 2007. Practical Advanced Periodontal Surgery. Blackwell Publishing.

Esposito M, Grusovin MG, Talati M, Coulthard P, Oliver R, Worthington HV. 2008. Interventions for replacing missing teeth: antibiotics at dental implant placement to prevent complications. Cochrane Database of Systematic Reviews.

Esposito M, Grusovin MG, Talati M, Coulthard P, Oliver R, Worthington HV. 2009. Interventions for replacing missing teeth: antibiotics at dental implant placement to prevent complications. Cochrane Database of Systematic Reviews, Issue 2.

Esposito M, Grusovin MG, Willings M, Coulthard P, Worthington HV. 2007. Interventions for replacing missing teeth: different times for loading dental implants. Cochrane Database of Systematic Reviews, Issue 2.

Lindeboom JA, Tjiook Y, Kroon FH. 2006. Immediate placement of implants in periapical infected sites: a prospective randomized study in 50 patients. *Oral Surg. Oral Med. Oral Pathol.* 101(6), 705–710.

Naert I, Koutsikakis G, Duyk J, et al. 2000. Biologic outcome of single implant restorations as tooth replacements: A long term follow up study. *Clin. Impl. Dent. Relat. Res.* 2, 209.

Ottoni JM, Oliveira ZF, Mansini R, Cubral AM. 2005. Correlation between placement torque and survival of single tooth implants. *IJOMI.* 20(5), 769–76.

Rosenquist B. 1997. A comparison of several methods of soft tissue management following the immediate placement of implants into extraction sockets. *IJOMI.* 12(1), 43–51.

Salinas TJ, Block MS, Sadan A. 2004. Fixed partial denture or single tooth implant restoration? Statistical considerations for sequencing and treatment. *J. Oral Maxillofac. Surg.* 62(9), 2–16.

Schropp L, Kostopoulos L, Wenzel A. 2003. Bone healing following immediate versus delayed placement of titanium implants into extraction sockets: a prospective clinical study. *IJOMI.* 18(2), 189–199.

Stavropoulou AF, Koidis PT. 2007. A systematic review of single crowns on endodontically treated teeth. *Journal of Dentistry.* 35, 761–767.

Takeshita F, Tyama S, Ayukawa Y, Suetsugu T, Oishi M. 1997. Abscess formation around a hydroxyapatite coated implant placed into the extraction socket with autogenous bone graft. A histological study using light microscopy, image processing and confocal laser scanning microscopy. *J. Perio.* 68(3), 299–305.

Tawse-Smith A, Payne AG, Kumara R, Thomson WM. 2002. Early loading of unsplinted implants supporting mandibular overdentures using a one stage operative procedure with two different implant systems: a two year report. *Clinical Implant Dentistry and Related Research.* 4(1), 33–42.

Chapter 12 Inflammation and Bone Healing Around Dental Implants

The integration of dental implant materials with bone takes advantage of the fact that bone is able to heal with new bone following injury. Furthermore it can do so in very close apposition with certain metals and ceramics—for example, titanium or hydroxyapatite—without an intervening layer of less differentiated connective tissue. The implantation of titanium into bone initiates a wound healing process very similar to that which occurs when bone forms via the membranous pathway and later when bone remodels and repairs itself. This chapter reviews the basic processes in bone biology as they relate to bone formation, homeostasis, remodeling, and repair, and finally the events that occur at the bone-implant interface.

BONE FUNCTION AND STRUCTURE

Among the numerous functions now attributed to bone, structural integrity and protection remain central. Mature bone is made up of two distinct calcified compartments, an outer cortical or compact shell and an inner trabecular or cancellous core. Cortical bone is tightly organized in a series of concentric calcified rings or lamellae organized around a central canal containing blood vessels, lymphatics, nerves, and connective tissue. Embedded in islands or lacunae within these lamellae are osteocytes. Whereas cancellous bone is highly mineralized and poorly vascularized, trabelcular bone is much less mineralized but highly vascularized. Trabecular bone is composed of an interconnected lattice-work of mineralized trabeculae with the trabeculae organized parallel to lines of stress. Again, osteocytes are embedded in lacunae within the trabeculae. The outer layer of cortical bone is sheathed in a specialized connective tissue, periosteum.

Periosteum is composed of an outer fibrous layer and an inner cellular layer. While the outer layer has no osteogenic potential, the inner layer that is in contact with the bone is home to osteoblasts and their precursors as well as osteoclasts and their precursors. Similarly, the inner endosteal surfaces of trabeculae and cortical bone are also surrounded by a connective tissue layer, endosteum, that again contains osteoblasts and osteoclasts and their progenitor cells.

Bone Homeostasis

Appearances aside, bone is a dynamic organ undergoing constant remodeling and adaptation in response to mechanical, systemic, and local factors. This process involves the closely coupled destruction of existing bone by osteoclasts followed by deposition of new bone by osteoblasts. If either of these processes—destruction or formation—is interrupted, pathology is observed. Bone multicellular units (BMU) comprised of osteoblasts, osteoclasts, and osteocytes are responsible for maintaining bone homeostasis and for repair and regeneration following injury.

Osteoblasts and Osteocytes

Osteoblasts are derived from mesenchymal tissue along a tightly regulated pathway. Mesenchymal cells can form connective tissue fibroblasts, adipocytes, and bone. Differentiation of mesenchymal cell into osteoblasts occurs along a pathway involving regulation by autocrine, paracrine, and endocrine factors. Endocrine factors including parathyroid hormone, growth hormone, and insulin-like growth factor stimulate proliferation and in certain instances differentiation for pre-osteoblastic cells.

Critically, RUNX2, a nuclear transcription factor, must be expressed for a mesenchymal cell to differentiate along an osteoblastic lineage. The mechanisms by which expression of RUNX2 lead eventually to an osteoblast phenotype is beyond the scope of this chapter. However, it should be noted that bone morphogenetic proteins (BMPs) are critical for the induction of RUNX2 expression. BMPs are a member of the transforming growth factor family of proteins, and to date 30 have been identified. BMPs are present in bone and become soluble following demineralization. At that point they are able to exert inductive effects on differentiating cells in the osteoblast lineage. Thus, bone formation, at least in adulthood, is critically dependent on bone destruction occurring first. Several existing and emerging therapeutic approaches in bone grafting are intended to introduce autogenous BMPs, allogenic BMPs, or more recently, recombinant BMPs to a surgical site.

Once fully differentiated, osteoblasts synthesize an extracellular matrix principally composed of type 1 collagen but also containing other molecules. This matrix eventually becomes calcified and the osteoblasts are encased within the mineralized tissue. At that point the osteoblast is called an osteocyte. Osteocytes communicate with one another via dendritic processes, and the function of viable osteocytes with bone appears to be one of mechanosensation. Thus, bone that is not being mechanically stimulated tends to atrophy, while the converse is true of bone stimulated by exercise.

Osteoclasts

Osteoclasts are multinucleated cells of hematopoietic lineage, specifically of the monocyte/macrophage lineage. Differentiation of monocytes to osteoclasts requires physical contact with osteoblasts or stromal cells. Osteoblasts express receptor activator of nuclear factor $\kappa\beta$-ligand (RANKL) on their membrane surface, which binds to the RANK receptor on osteoclast precursor macrophages and induces them to differentiate and eventually fuse into multinuclear cells, called osteoclasts. Osteoblasts also produce monocyte colony stimulating factor (M-CSF), which stimulates proliferation of osteoclast precursors. Whereas RANKL binds to RANK and stimulates osteoclastogenesis, the soluble molecule and decoy receptor osteoprotegrin (OPG) competitively binds RANKL and inhibits osteoclastogenesis. The relative proportions of RANKL and OPG have been termed the RANKL/OPG axis and seem to be instrumental in inflammation-dependent bone loss. This is especially significant for maintaining long-term stability of bone levels around the osseointegrated implant. This will be discussed later in this chapter.

BMUs

Osteoblasts, osteoclasts, and osteocytes are organized into BMUs. These units are organized as cutting cones, which are led by osteoclasts that resorb bone and are trailed by osteoblasts that lay down new bone and eventually become osteocytes. BMUs have a limited life span and new units are continually formed to replace old, inactive ones. In good health, about 3% to 5% of an individual's skeleton is being replaced at any given time and there is a relative homeostasis between bone formation and resorption.

BONE HEALING FOLLOWING IMPLANT PLACEMENT

Osteotomy preparation for implant placement, and implant placement itself, results in the destruction of both trabecular and cortical bone. It should be noted that the proportion of each varies such that a much higher percentage of cortical bone is present in the anterior mandible vs. the posterior maxilla. Whenever an implant is placed, there will be regions where the implant is in direct contact with the bone and areas where there are gaps. The areas with gaps are initially filled with blood clot and bone debris, which eventually give way to bone formation. These gaps may be evident only at a microscopic level or, in the case of immediate implant placement, they may be 3 mm or more. It has been shown by Botticelli et al. (2004) and Paolantonia et al. (2001) that gaps of 2 mm and perhaps as large as 5 mm can be expected to heal with osseointegration, even in the absence of membranes or grafting materials.

The areas of bone implant contact provide initial primary stability. However, Roberts et al. (1988) have shown that there is at least 1 mm of necrotic bone adjacent to an osteotomy site, even with optimal surgical technique, and that bone initially in contact with the implant remodels before integrating. In humans, the remodeling cycle, or sigma, is about 4.5 months. In other words, 4.5 months are required for osseous resorption, osteogenesis, and subsequently resorption. Hoshaw et al. (1997) have shown that the rate of bone remodeling increases following implant site preparation. Initial implant loading protocols of four months in the mandible and six months in the maxilla were based on the concept of sigma (Branemark et al., 1977). However, the success of contemporary protocols that emphasize much shorter or even immediate loading suggests that complete remodeling is not a requirement for long-term implant success (Esposito et al., 2007).

Given that de novo bone formation is required along the length of the implant, Osborn and Newesely (1980) have described two ways in which this may occur. Contact osteogenesis describes the formation of bone in direct apposition to the dental implant, whereas distance osteogenesis describes formation of bone from the mineralized surface toward the implant surface (Davies, 2003) (Figure 12.1). Davies has discussed extensively the benefits of contact osteogenesis vs. distance osteogenesis (Davies, 2003). A series of papers from his group, as well as others, have shown that where gaps occur, fibrin adherence to the implant surface is critical for de novo bone formation on the implant surfaces—contact osteogenesis—and that this adherence is improved when the implant surface is textured as opposed to machined. Methods for texturing have included acid etching, sand blasting, electrolysis, plasma spray, and coating with hydroxyapatite. The relative advantages and disadvantages of each surface treatment are beyond the scope of this volume, but in terms of bone implant contact (BIC), all have been shown to be superior to machining (Cochran, 1999).

A matrix is required for bone to form. In non-endochondral bone formation, this matrix is usually preexisting bone. In the case of implant placement, it has been shown that fibrin can be used as a matrix. Osteoblasts migrate through fibrin to the implant surface and first deposit a thin layer of glycoprotein similar to a cement line seen at the junction of old and newly formed bone. Bone is then deposited on the surface of the implant itself; this is contact osteogenesis.

Conversely, no blood clot is present in areas where bone is initially in contact with the implant. Rather, the necrotic bone that results for the osteotomy preparation serves as the substrate for new bone formation. As a result, bone forms from the surface of the bone toward the implant. Distance osteogenesis is expected to predominate in cortical bone, given its more dense nature, vs. trabecular bone.

CONTACT vs. DISTANCE OSTEOGENESIS

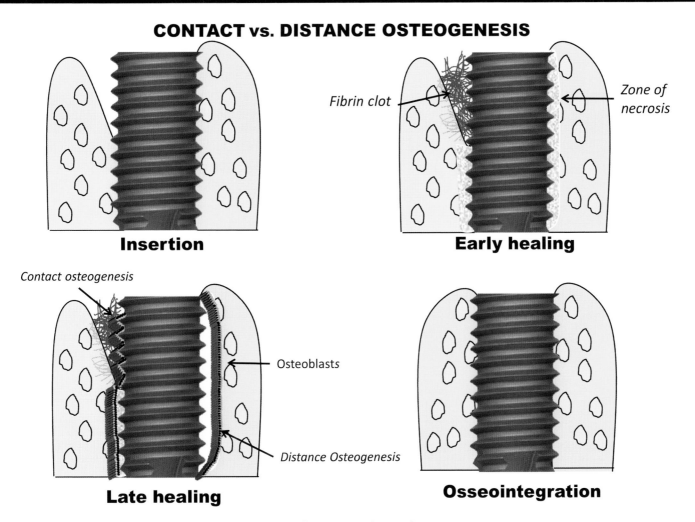

Figure 12.1. Contact vs. distance osteogenesis leading to osseointegration.

INFLAMMATORY BONE LOSS AROUND THE INTEGRATED IMPLANT

Whether by contact or distance osteogenesis, osseointegration is normally expected to result. However, bone is a dynamic structure and maintenance of integration is an ongoing dynamic process. Homeostasis and stability of bone around an implant is characterized by an absence of inflammation.

The precipitating causes of peri-implant bone loss are not entirely clear. Known periodontal pathogens have been localized to peri-implant lesions associated with a progressive crestal bone loss similar to periodontal disease, peri-implantitis. Excessive force or stress has been implicated at least in animal models in the loss of peri-implant bone, but this evidence is equivocal (Isidor, 1996; Kozlovsky et al., 2007; Heitz-Mayfield, 2008). Smoking and diabetes have been suggested as risk factors for peri-implantitis, as they are for periodontitis (Heitz-Mayfield, 2008). A very interesting study recently published by Heckmann et al. (2006) suggests that

the presence of both stress and inflammation together induce peri-implant bone loss more than either factor on its own.

While periodontal bone loss and peri-implant bone loss are not the same disease, there are important similarities. These include the presence of periodontal pathogens in both lesions, progressive bone loss over a long period of time and often in the absence of obvious local predisposing factors, and the presence of inflammation (Van Dyke and Sheilesh, 2005; Heitz-Mayfield, 2008).

Periodontal bone resorption has been shown to be caused by inflammation as opposed to bacterial lytic enzymes. The OPG/RANKL/RANK axis has been suggested as a mechanism for understanding the dynamics of bone formation and resorption, particularly as it relates to loss of bone around teeth, and this may have important implications for the management of bone loss around implants (Cochran, 2008). As discussed above, RANKL promotes the resorption of bone, whereas OPG interferes with this process by binding to RANKL and thus preventing the binding of RANKL to RANK

Inflammatory RANK-RANKL Axis

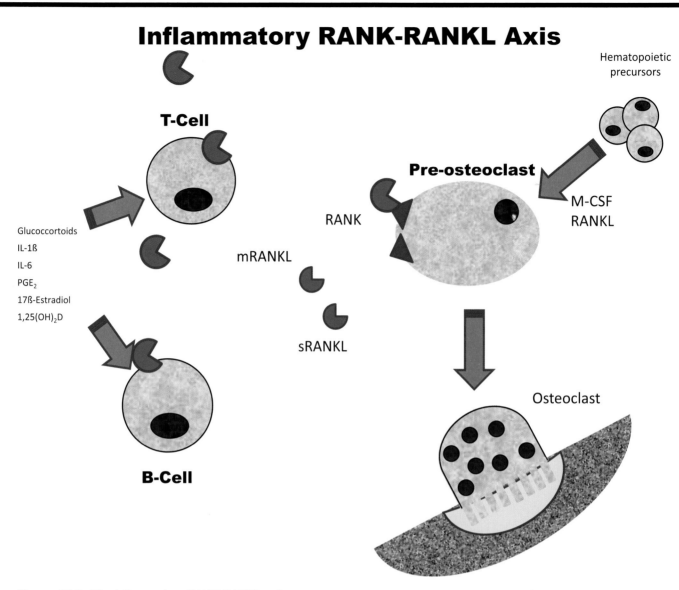

Figure 12.2. The inflammatory RANK-RANKL axis.

(Figure 12.2). In the absence of RANKL-RANK binding, osteoclast differentiation does not occur and osteoclast apoptosis increases. Stability of the ratio of OPG/RANKL is expected in homeostasis, where neither bone formation nor loss occurs. Increased bone formation is expected to be the result of an increase of OPG relative to RANKL, and an increase of RANKL relative to OPG is expected to result in an increase in bone loss. As was discussed earlier, in classical models, RANKL is produced by osteoblasts, then binds to RANK on osteoclasts, induces osteoclast differentiation and bone resorption, and inhibits osteoclast apoptosis. OPG, which is also produced by osteoblast, binds to RANKL, and in so doing prevents it from binding to RANK. This provides the coupling mechanism between bone formation and resorption in homeostatic conditions.

There is an alternative pathway for production of RANKL that does not involve osteoblasts and results in the net loss of

bone. It has been shown that T- and B-lymphocytes and fibroblasts also produce RANKL, and that this occurs in response to stimulation by pro-inflammatory molecules including IL-1, IL-6, PGE$_2$, and TNF-α. Production of RANKL by inflammatory processes such as these results in increased RANKL relative to OPG; osteoclast-mediated bone loss is stimulated in the absence of bone formation and the result is the net loss of bone.

Ongoing loss of peri-implant bone (Figure 12.3) may similarly be characterized not only by a state of inflammation but also by a failure of inflammation to resolve (Van Dyke, 2008). The most up-to-date research has begun to make it clear that the resolution of inflammation is an active process, just as is the development of inflammation, and that specific molecules including IL-4, -10, -12, -13, and -18 as well as Interferon-β (IFNβ) and -γ (IFN-γ) all play an important role in promoting this process. In addition, a new class of polyunsaturated fatty

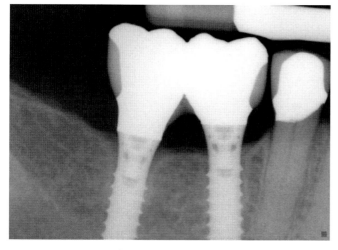
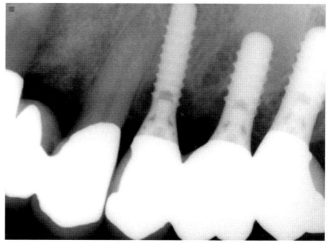

Normal Crestal Bone Height

Peri-Implant Bone Loss

Figure 12.3. Radiographs showing normal bone height (left) and bone loss around implants (right).

acids (PUFA) present in fish oil has been implicated in the resolution of inflammation. These molecules have been termed lipoxins, protectins, and resolvins, and have been shown in in vitro and in in vivo animal studies to promote resolution of inflammation (Serhan et al., 2008).

Early studies showed that using nonsteroidal antiinflammatories (NSAID) to interfere with the production of proinflammatory molecules such as PGE_2 mitigated periodontal bone loss in humans and animals (Jeffcoat et al., 1995). Unfortunately, undesirable side effects preclude the use of these medications over the long term. Lipoxins, protectins, and resolvins and our understanding of them has shed important new light on the dynamics of resolution of inflammation and hold special promise as the basis for a new class of therapeutic agents in the future. These may have a significant impact on the management of inflammatory bone loss in the oral cavity.

REFERENCES

Botticelli D, Berglundh T, et al. 2004. Hard-tissue alterations following immediate implant placement in extraction sites. *J. Clin. Periodontol.* 31(10), 820–8.

Branemark PI, Hansson BO, et al. 1977. Osseointegrated implants in the treatment of the edentulous jaw. Experience from a 10-year period. *Scand. J. Plast. Reconstr. Surg. Suppl.* 16, 1–132.

Cochran DL. 1999. A comparison of endosseous dental implant surfaces. *J. Periodontol.* 70(12), 1523–39.

Cochran DL. 2008. Inflammation and bone loss in periodontal disease. *J. Periodontol.* 79(8 Suppl), 1569–76.

Davies JE. 2003. Understanding peri-implant endosseous healing. *J. Dent. Educ.* 67(8), 932–49.

Esposito M, Grusovin MG, et al. 2007. The effectiveness of immediate, early, and conventional loading of dental implants: a Cochrane systematic review of randomized controlled clinical trials. *Int. J. Oral Maxillofac. Implants.* 22(6), 893–904.

Heckmann SM. Linke JJ, et al. 2006. Stress and inflammation as a detrimental combination for peri-implant bone loss. *J. Dent. Res.* 85(8), 711–6.

Heitz-Mayfield LJ. 2008. Diagnosis and management of peri-implant diseases. *Aust. Dent. J.* 53 Suppl 1, S43–8.

Heitz-Mayfield LJ. 2008. Peri-implant diseases: diagnosis and risk indicators. *J. Clin. Periodontol.* 35(8 Suppl), 292–304.

Hoshaw SJ, Fyhrie DP, Takano Y, Burr DB, Milgrom C. 1997. A method suitable for in vivo measurement of bone strain in humans. *J. Biomech.* May;30(5), 521–4.

Isidor F. 1996. Loss of osseointegration caused by occlusal load of oral implants. A clinical and radiographic study in monkeys. *Clin. Oral Implants Res.* 7(2), 143–52.

Jeffcoat MK, Reddy MS, et al. 1995. A comparison of topical ketorolac, systemic flurbiprofen, and placebo for the inhibition of bone loss in adult periodontitis. *J. Periodontol.* 66(5), 329–38.

Kozlovsky A, Tal H, et al. 2007. Impact of implant overloading on the peri-implant bone in inflamed and non-inflamed peri-implant mucosa. *Clin. Oral Implants Res.* 18(5), 601–10.

Osborn JF, Newesely H. 1980. The material science of calcium phosphate ceramics. *Biomaterials.* Apr;1(2), 108–11.

Paolantonio M, Dolci M, et al. 2001. Immediate implantation in fresh extraction sockets. A controlled clinical and histological study in man. *J. Periodontol.* 72(11), 1560–71.

Roberts EW. 1988. The oral surgeon-dental anesthesiologist team. *Anesth. Prog.* 35(1), 18.

Serhan CN, Chiang N, et al. 2008. Resolving inflammation: dual anti-inflammatory and pro-resolution lipid mediators. *Nat. Rev. Immunol.* 8(5), 349–61.

Van Dyke TE. 2008. Inflammation and periodontal diseases: a reappraisal. *J. Periodontol.* 79(8 Suppl), 1501–2.

Van Dyke TE, Sheilesh D. 2005. Risk factors for periodontitis. *J. Int. Acad. Periodontol.* 7(1), 3–7.

Appendix 1 A Little Slice of History: The Periodontal Condition of Napoleon's Grand Army—A Forensic Evaluation

INTRODUCTION

In June 1812, Napoleon Bonaparte engaged his Great Army in the campaign to invade Russia. This so-called "army of twenty nations" was made up not merely of French soldiers, but also largely of troops from other nations. Indeed, most present-day continental European states were represented in the Great Army of 1812.

Moscow fell, but Napoleon was unable to destroy the Russian forces which, fewer in number, refused to engage in battle directly. With its ranks already considerably thinned, the Great Army waited in Moscow for five weeks while vain negotiations were attempted with Tsar Alexander I. Before the first snows began to fall and it also became obvious that no capitulation was forthcoming, Napoleon took the decision to withdraw from Moscow on October 19.

The rigors of an early winter dogged the Great Army, decimating its forces and transforming the retreat into a disaster. On December 5, in the little town of Smorgonie on the Belarus side of today's border with Lithuania, Napoleon was informed of the attempted coup of General Malet and decided to leave his army and return to Paris. He entrusted the command to Murat, the king of Naples, but this departure had a disastrous effect on the morale of his troops, many of whom saw it as an abandonment or—worse still—a desertion in their time of need.

The regiments from Taranto and Capua, officially in charge of the army's retreat, were garrisoned in nearby Wilna (today's Vilnius). On December 9, in temperatures between −25° and −28°C, the rest of the army arrived in this town under the control of the French military authorities. The troops were exhausted and starving, the quartermasters delayed opening their stores, and the doors were soon knocked down. Pillage began spreading throughout the town but no sooner had all the columns of the bedraggled army entered the ramparts of the town than cannon fire opened up from the Russian troops positioned on the surrounding hills. Faced with mounting chaos, Murat decided to flout Napoleon's orders and to quit the town that very night. At 11:30 p.m. the army began its evacuation, leaving the streets full of stray soldiers and their comrades already dead of exhaustion or cold. According to Larrey's writings in 1817, between 20,000 and 25,000 wounded or dead soldiers were left in Wilna.

Writing his memoirs in 1848, Dr. Joseph Frank, founder of the chair of medicine at the University of Vilnius, noted,

> "40,000 corpses that were lying in and around Vilna, most of them in their uniforms, stiffened by the frost and remaining in the position in which death had surprised them…. This accumulation, I said, gave rise to the threat of a general infection at the slightest thaw. A mass burial place was thus ordered. To make sure it was properly made, Dr. Becu was put in charge of the work by field-marshal Koutousof as medical officer for the police. They used the trenches that the French had dug for their defense."

One of these mass graves, containing 3,269 corpses, was discovered in October 2001 in the course of urban development work. Among the many anthropological examinations subsequently carried out, one paleo-odontologic study included assessing the periodontal condition of the soldiers of the Great Army. Thus, we have an exceptional paleo-demographic sample representing a European military-style population (i.e., young males) in the early 19th century.

This present study sets out to evaluate the state of periodontal health by measuring the level of alveolar bone surrounding the teeth. Longitudinal analysis shows us the progression of osseous resorption over a period of almost 20 years in a young, masculine population with no supervision of oral hygiene and, more importantly, no access to healthcare. Thus we see the "natural" development of alveolar bone level in young adult subjects with and without periodontal disorders.

1. MATERIALS AND METHOD

1.1. Data Collection

From among the skeletons exhumed, we selected only those perfectly identified without any risk of confusion with other bones from the grave (Appendix Figure 1.1).

It also seemed important to us that the individuals studied from a dento-maxillary standpoint should also be examined generally to complete our data file and possibly allow cross-analysis. This was notably the case with the estimation of age and gender, carried out in collaboration with anthropologists. Standard anthropological methods were employed to determine age: epiphysary stages, changes in the pubic

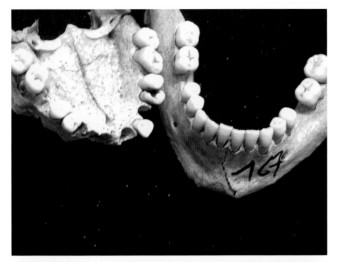

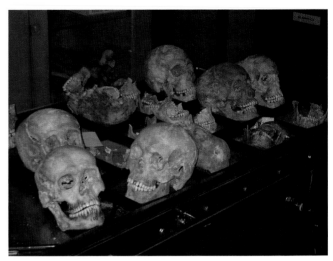

Appendix Figure 1.2. Individuals selected were sufficiently complete for the periodontal study.

Appendix Table 1.1. Distribution of sample by age categories.

Age categories	Strength	Percentage
18–25 Years	74	50%
25–35 Years	52	35%
>35 Years	22	15%

Thus, we selected individuals who had already undergone anthropological examination. This being the case, our study sample was random but excluded individuals whose dentomaxillary characteristics were considered insufficiently complete (Appendix Figure 1.2).

1.2. General Characteristics of the Sample Group

Our sample comprised 148 adults, identified as 146 male specimens and 2 women. After a precise estimation as possible of their age, we divided them into age categories similar to those generally used in present-day dental studies, thus allowing us to make comparisons (see Appendix Table 1.1).

These 148 individuals were used for an overall study including, notably, measurement of the prevalence of dental caries. For the periodontal study, on the other hand, one of the principal complications encountered during measurements was the state of preservation of the alveolar bone. The skeleton remains had been found in sandy—and thus acid—soil and, because of this, certain bone structures had been destroyed, making measurement impossible (Appendix Figure 1.3). Of the 148 subjects, 17 were withdrawn from our study group because the poor condition of the alveolar bone precluded accurate measurement.

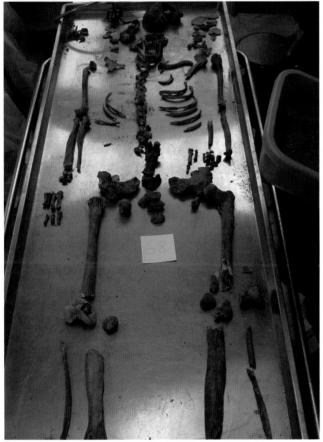

Appendix Figure 1.1. Identification of skeleton after exhumation.

symphysis, and closure of cranial sutures (Thillaud, 1996; White et al., 2000). Age was also estimated according to the appearance of the dentition and in accordance with Miles' table of dental abrasion (1963). Gender differentiation was done anthropomorphologically by observing the morphology of the hip bones and skulls and odontologically by examining the shape and arrangement of the teeth.

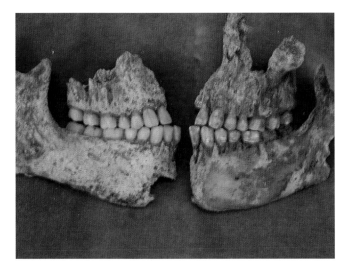

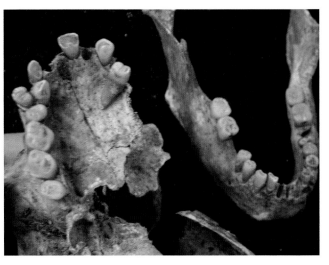

Appendix Figure 1.3. Lying on his left side, the subject illustrates the erosion caused by acid sediments. His right side, in comparison, is relatively unscathed. The green spot was left by copper leaching from a uniform button.

Appendix Figure 1.4. «pme» = post-mortem extraction, «a» = ante-mortem extraction, and «x» = entire tooth/socket section missing.

Our study thus focused on 131 subjects, on whom measurements were carried out as follows:

- 1 individual (i.e., 1%): 12 measurements (6 each on 2 teeth)

- 23 subjects (i.e., 17%): 18 measurements (6 each on 3 teeth)

- 12 subjects (i.e., 9%): 24 measurements (6 each on 4 teeth)

- 30 subjects (i.e., 23%): 30 measurements (6 each on 5 teeth)

- 65 subjects (i.e., 49%): 36 measurements (6 each on 6 teeth)

Data loss was highest for mandibular incisors (only 94 teeth examinable in 131 subjects (i.e., 71%), but gradually decreased for maxillary molars (108 measurements; i.e., 82%), maxillary incisors (111 measurements), mandibular premolars (114 measurements), mandibular molars (115 measurements), and finally, maxillary premolars (117 measurements (i.e., a substantial 89%)).

1.3. Special Characteristics of the Sample Group

For each subject retained, we replaced the loose teeth in their sockets and glued back broken bone fragments where necessary and possible. Certain bone fragments had been lost, however, and we identified the teeth corresponding to these missing fragments in our database with the code «x». After reconstruction of the maxillaries, certain tooth sockets remained empty because the corresponding teeth had not been found. In the absence of cicatrization, we considered

that these teeth had been in place before the subject's death. It seemed probable to us that these teeth had been lost during handling in the course of the excavation work. The teeth belonging to these empty sockets were coded as «pme», meaning post-mortem extraction.

Thus, in the absence of a tooth, and contrary to a study carried out on a living population, we had three possibilities: «x», meaning that the whole alveolar-dental section was missing, «pme» for an empty socket left by a fallen tooth, or «a», our code for a cicatrized socket indicating an ante-mortem extraction (Appendix Figure 1.4).

This peculiarity in dental studies of mass grave sites is one of the major difficulties in statistical processing of results, notably when comparing results with those from a living population.

1.4. Evaluation Methodology for Periodontal Pathology

Alveolar bone loss can be calculated by measuring the distance between the cementoenamel junction (CEJ) and the crest of the alveolar bone. With periodontitis, this distance increases and the measurement can thus be used as a marker for periodontal health. In order to estimate the periodontal condition of all the dental arches and to compare our results with those from living subjects, we adopted Ramfjord's (1967) approach for measurement of the periodontal disease index, or PDI. This method consists of taking six measurements from six teeth distributed over both arches. These are teeth #3, 9, and 12 for the maxilla and 19, 41, and 44 for the mandible. Where a tooth is missing, Ramfjord suggests that the measurements be taken on its neighbor. Our

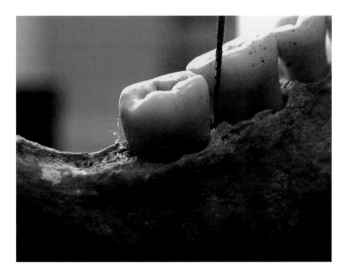

Appendix Figure 1.5. Measurement of the disto-lingual distance between the cemetoenamel junction (CEJ) and bone crest on tooth #19.

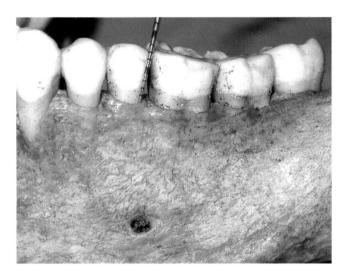

Appendix Figure 1.6. Measurement of the disto-buccal distance between the CEJ and bone crest.

measurements were made with a graduated periodontal probe (15UNC Color Coded Probe; Hu-Friedy, Chicago, USA) at the mesio-vestibular, vestibular, disto-vestibular, mesio-lingual, lingual, and disto-lingual positions (Appendix Figures 1.5, 1.6).

According to a consensus of the American Academy of Periodontology (1996), bone destruction is considered the most important criterion for assessing the severity of periodontal disease. This measurement is generally taken indirectly or from X-rays, but whatever the method, measurement of bone level remains difficult or imprecise and most observers use other criteria such as gingival bleeding or periodontal pocket/sulcular depths, which, as indices, provide scale

ratings of periodontal affection. Because of this difficulty in measuring bone level, very few indices have been developed to correlate bone loss with periodontal health. Carranza (1996) refers to the "historical interest" of the indices drawn up by Dunning and Leach (1960) or Sheiham and Striffler (1970). In none of these cases do we find any index for bone level measured at six points by a direct method.

In addition to the epidemiological aspect of periodontal disease, this study also allows us to establish a database for the CEJ/bone-crest distance in a young population, collected by direct—and thus very precise—measurement.

Reminder of Periodontal Anatomy

In a young subject with a healthy periodontium, we have a physiological system of attachment of the gingiva to the base of the tooth. This system extends from the bottom of the gingivodental furrow to the summit of the bony crest. It is composed of a connective tissue attachment, running from the alveolar rim to the CEJ, and an epithelial tissue attachment to the enamel. This overall site is referred to as the biological space. The dimensions of this biological space, according to the four stages of the passive eruption of the tooth, were studied for the first time by Gargiulo et al. (1961) and the results of their study remain a reference. The general width for the biological space is 2.04 mm. This distance is relatively constant and serves as a reference point when estimating bone level in living subjects. In our study, no measurement of soft tissue was possible and the CEJ/bone-crest distance can be considered solely for distinguishing the physiological from the pathological.

For Aubrey (2002), average annual bone loss varies from 0.07 to 0.14 mm in subjects aged 25 to 65 with cases of chronic periodontitis. According to a consensus of the American Academy of Periodontology (1996), the physiological resorption of the alveolar bone represents 0.1 mm a year. In the mass grave of the Great Army, when an individual showed a measurement between the crest of the bone and the CEJ in excess of 2 mm, we classified this as a pathological process. Understanding the limitations of this approach, we also considered that if the number of affected sites was less than 30%, we were in the presence of localized disease, and if above 30%, generalized periodontitis (Armitage, 1999).

1.5. Measurement of Tartar Deposits

The quantity of tartar was assessed subjectively by a single observer. Each subject was assigned to one of three categories:

- Low tartar (Appendix Figure 1.7)

- Average tartar (Appendix Figure 1.8)

- High tartar (Appendix Figure 1.9)

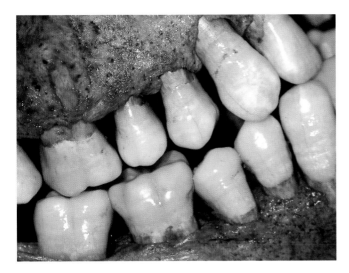

Appendix Figure 1.7. The presence of low tartar on the teeth.

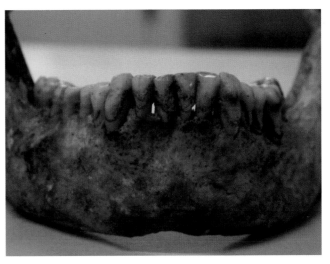

Appendix Figure 1.9. The presence of high tartar on the teeth.

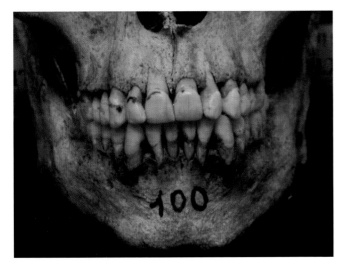

Appendix Figure 1.8. The presence of average tartar on the teeth.

Appendix Table 1.2. Number of individuals according to the cemetoenamel junction CEJ/alveolar bone crest distance.

Distance CEJ/ alveolar bone crest (mm)	1–2	>2 and ≤3	>3 and ≤4	>4 and ≤5	>5
Number of individuals	63	46	16	5	1
%	48%	35%	12%	3.8%	0.8%

2. RESULTS

2.1. *Average Distance CEJ/Alveolar Bone Crest Per Individual*

The individuals in our study were classified according to the mean CEJ/alveolar bone crest distance to situate the extent of bone resorption for all subjects (Appendix Table 1.2). This approach gave us an idea of the periodontal health condition of this special population (Appendix Figure 1.10).

The average of the distances measured per individual gave an average of between 1 mm and 2 mm, and thus the absence of any pathological process, for practically one person in two. Thirty-five percent of our population showed a moderate distance of between 2 mm and 3 mm, i.e., a very limited bone resorption. Surprisingly, only 4.6% of cases showed severe ratings of more than 4 mm. All in all, the overall periodontal health condition of the Great Army was relatively good.

2.2. *Average Distance CEJ/Alveolar Bone Crest According to Teeth*

To give a more precise estimate of the resorption zones, the CEJ/alveolar bone crest distance was calculated for each tooth measured (Appendix Table 1.3).

The distance between the CEJ and the alveolar bone crest was not systematically the same for all teeth; we found it greater for the molars and the mandibular incisors. The difference according to the type of tooth is the same as that found in living subjects today.

2.3. *Average Distance CEJ/Alveolar Bone Crest at Each of the Six Measurement Points*

In order to determine whether bone resorption is uniform around each of the six teeth observed per subject, we calculated the average distances recorded for each of the measurement points (Appendix Tables 1.4, 1.5, and 1.6).

Appendix Table 1.3. Mean CEJ/alveolar bone crest distance for each observed tooth.

Tooth	Distance CEJ/alveolar bone crest
9	1.8 mm
25	2.4 mm
28	1.9 mm
12	2 mm
19	2.4 mm
3	2.9 mm

Average distance for each individual represented by a point on the ordinate axis

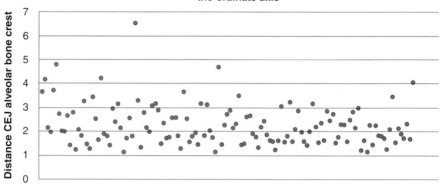

Appendix Figure 1.10. Classification of individuals according to the mean CEJ/alveolar bone crest distance.

Appendix Table 1.4. Mean distance for every probing point around teeth #25 and 9.

	Lower incisors (94 measurements)						Upper incisors (111 measurements)					
	25 MB	25 B	25 DB	25 ML	25 L	25 DL	9 MB	9 B	9 DB	9 ML	9 L	9 DL
Average	2.3	2.8	2.1	2.3	2.7	2.3	2.0	2.3	1.9	1.5	1.7	1.5
Standard deviation	1.3	1.3	1.2	1.2	1.1	1.2	0.9	1.0	1.0	0.7	0.8	0.7

Appendix Table 1.5. Mean distance for every probing point around teeth #28 and 12.

	Lower premolars (114 measurements)						Upper premolars (117 measurements)					
	28 MB	28 B	28 DB	28 ML	28 L	28 DL	12 MB	12 B	12 DB	12 ML	12 L	12 DL
Average	1.8	2.8	1.8	1.6	2.0	1.6	1.9	2.4	1.8	1.8	2.5	2.0
Standard deviation	1.2	1.4	1.1	1.2	1.2	1.0	1.0	0.9	0.9	1.0	1.0	0.9

Appendix Table 1.6. Mean distance for every probing point around teeth #19 and 3.

	Lower molars (115 measurements)						Upper molars (108 measurements)					
	19 MB	19 B	19 DB	19 ML	19 L	19 DL	3 MB	3 B	3 DB	3 ML	3 L	3 DL
Average	2.3	2.5	2.2	2.4	2.7	2.4	2.6	3.0	2.8	2.8	3.4	2.8
Standard deviation	1.2	1.3	1.2	1.2	1.4	1.4	1.4	1.2	1.3	1.5	1.5	1.4

The results indicated that, for each tooth, the proximal measurements (mesial and lingual) were practically identical and slightly lower than the vestibular and lingual readings.

2.4. Distance CEJ/Alveolar Bone Crest per Age Category

Even in the absence of pathology, the phenomenon of bone resorption around the teeth is a constant factor with aging. The presence of a periodontal pathology simply accelerates the process. Within the scope of this study, we were able to equate this progression of the CEJ/alveolar bone crest distance with the aging of our individuals (Appendix Table 1.7).

2.5. Identification of Periodontitis

The mean CEJ/alveolar bone crest distance gives a general picture of the state of the alveolar bone and, in our case, Ramfjord's (1967) approach was perfectly adapted for visualization of bone resorption over time. Distances exceeding 2 mm must be recorded on each of the teeth to estimate the prevalence of cases of periodontitis. In our sample of 131 individuals, 92% showed at least one measurement exceeding 2 mm on one of their teeth. This percentage was recalculated for the sample of 66 individuals for whom all measurements had been possible (i.e., six teeth) and remained the same.

As mentioned above, present-day classification of periodontal diseases sets a dividing line of 30% of affected teeth to distinguish between localized and generalized periodontitis (Armitage, 1999). This being so, a calculation based on six teeth seemed to us insufficient to indicate the prevalence of generalized, as opposed to localized, periodontal disease in an age category. By using only those individuals possessing

Appendix Table 1.7. Distance CEJ/alveolar bone crest per age category.

Age category	15–25 years	25–35 years	>35 years
Strength	N = 67	N = 46	N = 18
Mean distance CEJ/alveolar bone crest (mm)	2 ± 0.6	2.3 ± 0.7	3.1 ± 1.3

the six test teeth, however, we were able to note that the number of affected teeth increased in accordance with the age categories. We found that few individuals were wholly free from periodontal illness (11% in the 15 to 25 age bracket and only 5% in the 25 to 35 bracket). In the 35 to 44 age bracket, on the other hand, all the individuals showed indications of periodontitis on at least half the teeth observed and on all six teeth for 60% of the subjects (Appendix Figure 1.11).

2.6. Tartar Observed

The classification according to tartar observed (see section 1.5 above) gave the following results:

- Low tartar level: 67 subjects
- Medium tartar level: 35 subjects
- High tartar level: 29 subjects

Tartar distribution is thus uneven with a majority tendency toward absence of tartar insofar as more than one subject out of two (51%) had a very low tartar level and 27% had average readings (Appendix Figure 1.12).

2.6.1. Quantity of Tartar Correlated with Age

The quantity of tartar observed increased progressively with age (Appendix Table 1.8). In the 15 to 25 age bracket, 58% of subjects were in the low tartar category and only 19% of subjects were in the high category, whereas in the 35 to 44 age bracket, equal numbers of subjects were found in each of these categories.

2.6.2. Tartar Correlated with Bone Loss

Average bone loss is correlated with the quantity of tartar. As is shown in Appendix Table 1.9 below, the greater the quantity of tartar, the greater the bone loss.

3. DISCUSSION

The periodontal approach via measurement of alveolar bone level is relatively novel for, unlike studies on a living population, it is based on direct, unobstructed observation of gingival tissue. The bone level in a living subject cannot be seen

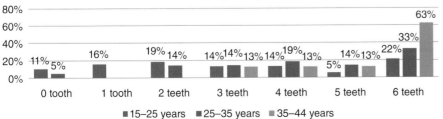

Percentage of teeth with periodontal desease among the six teeth studies and by age categories

Appendix Figure 1.11. The number of sites with bone resorption (distance greater than 2 mm) increases with age. It could be a progressive generalization of the periodontal disease.

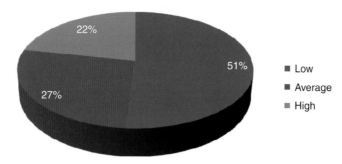

Appendix Figure 1.12. Distribution of individuals according to the quantity of tartar observed.

Appendix Table 1.8 Distribution of individuals in functions of the quantity of tartar in the different age categories.

Tartar observed

Age categories	Low	Average	High	Total
15–25 Years	39 (58%)	15 (22%)	13 (19%)	67
25–35 Years	21 (46%)	15 (33%)	10 (22%)	46
35–44 Years	7 (39%)	5 (28%)	6 (33%)	18
L	67	35	29	131

Appendix Table 1.9. Increasing distance CEJ/alveolar bone crest according to the quantity of tartar.

Tartar observed

	Low	Average	High
Means distance CEJ/ alveolar bone crest	2 ± 0.6	2.3 ± 0.7	2.9 ± 1.1

other than by retroalveolar X-ray, which poses a certain number of problems. Firstly, unless the X-rays are perfectly orthocentered, they induce deformations which alter the measurement. Second, X-rays only allow two measurements per tooth (mesial and distal), leaving the operator with no indications of vestibular and lingual bone levels.

In clinical studies, the attachment loss is measured to quantify bone resorption and, hence, periodontal pathology. This corresponds to a CEJ/alveolar bone crest distance of more than 2 mm. This 2-mm zone is occupied by the entire biological space (connective tissue attachment and epithelial tissue attachment; Gargiulo et al., 1961). A great number of studies use this 2-mm distance between CEJ and alveolar bone crest as the threshold for periodontitis (Gjermo et al., 1984; Perry and Newman, 1990). Indeed, any apical migration of this attachment is generally correlated with alveolar bone loss, indicating that a periodontal pathology has set in. In our study, 92% of subjects showed at least one measure-

ment exceeding 2 mm, notwithstanding a generally excellent state of periodontal health, as indicated by the fact that the average distance measured remained around 2 mm for most individuals. This percentage of 92 remained the same for the entire group and for the reduced group of 66 complete subjects.

If we calculate the average for measurement on all teeth per age bracket, we find a difference of 1.1 mm between the 15 to 25 age group and the 35 to 44 age group. This increase in the average general bone loss is accompanied by an increase in the number of teeth affected with age. This indicates that, in parallel with slow resorption of alveolar bone, localized pathological processes set in and tend to become generalized with time. As is the case with caries, the first sites affected are usually the molars. This is clearly noted in all modern studies, but without any generally admitted explanation. Certain authors bring up the fact that the first molar is one of the first teeth to appear on the dental arch and thus remains longer exposed to bacterial assault; others mention receptors at the level of this tooth which "attract" certain pathogenic bacteria.

This periodontitis then develops toward a more generalized form with an increase in the number of affected sites. This is the pattern also noted for contemporary populations. The loss of alveolar bone according to age brackets indicates very slowly progressing resorption which corresponds to the resorption levels generally measured. Papapanou (1989) estimated the average annual loss of alveolar bone at between 0.07 and 0.14 mm. For Benn (1990), it takes between seven and 10 years to detect a bone loss of 1 mm using standard X-rays.

A new AAP classification in December 1999 mentions "chronic periodontitis," defined as a pathology affecting teeth, developing slowly yet constantly. This symptomatology is described as possibly appearing independently of age but progressing over time if not treated, which is what we found in our study. The soldiers of the Great Army thus represent the standard clinical picture of untreated periodontal disease.

This study allows a very sensitive estimate of the prevalence of periodontal disease for two reasons. The first is that, owing to the directly visual method applied, it precludes any of the possibly inaccurate measurements that may be found in clinical studies with live patients. Based on gingival soundings, these studies may be skewed by various factors such as the depressibility of the gingiva, incorrectly applied pressure on the probe, or difficulties of access in proximal zones. These factors may in turn lead to over- or underestimation. The second reason is that the results of these different studies indicate that the teeth most sensitive to periodontal disease are the incisors and molars. By taking measurements of the alveolar bone around the molars and incisors on each face of the two dental arches, the results obtained are highly significant in the case of periodontal illness.

Our study remains limited, however, by the absence of soft tissue, notably in the vestibular measurements. We were unable to determine whether an increase in distance resulted from a periodontal pocket or a dehiscence.

Despite our precautions in the pre-selection process, unfavorable conditions of preservation may have led to bone loss along the alveolar ridges in those cases in which the bone was too fine, notably along the vestibular edge. This in turn may explain the increased distance measured when compared with the proximal readings.

Our main difficulty in this study was that of comparing it with others made on present-day populations. Other than those drawn from retro-alveolar X-rays, none use the same reference points that we did. These studies are often carried out on children, however, and the age brackets are in any case incompatible with those of the soldiers of the Great Army.

Tartar was long considered, erroneously, as a direct etiological factor in periodontal disease. This conclusion was drawn from observation of an improvement in the clinical signs of the periodontium after elimination of tartar deposits. According to Albandar et al. (1999), however, there is no scientific evidence for tartar being a direct causal factor in gingivitis and periodontitis. For Listgarten (1988), tartar is neutral and acts as a retaining factor for dental plaque. In our study, we noted that the quantity of bone loss was proportional to the quantity of tartar observed. This is normal, for the greater the quantity of tartar, the longer the bacterial assault caused by plaque and the greater the resulting bone loss. The quantities of tartar recorded were nevertheless low when we consider the lack of healthcare.

The reason for these low ratings may well lie in the patients' diet. Indeed, hard and non-sticky foodstuffs prevent stagnation of plaque on dental surfaces and its subsequent mineralization which transforms it into tartar. The 18th and 19th century diet was largely composed of bread, and military rations did not escape this rule. Pigeard (2000) indicates that the departmental order of 25th Fructidor of the year IX (i.e. September 12th, 1801) fixed the daily rations for French troops at 750 g of bread, 550 g of hardtack, 250 g of fresh meat or salt beef, 30 g of rice, 60 g of legumes, and 1/60 of a kilo of salt. The bread was distributed every four days and was often of poor quality. The hardtack was baked to be brittle and dry. All these foodstuffs were therefore hard and low in carbohydrates (sugars). These diet factors were common to all of the European population. Solid foodstuffs of this nature required a good deal of mastication (as witnessed by the severe wear on the occlusal surfaces of many subjects), which in turn produced a self-cleaning effect for

the dental surfaces and increased saliva flow. When tartar did form, it is possible that certain individuals used instruments like little wooden sticks to dislodge it.

This measurement of tartar was carried out somewhat empirically because of the limited time frame allowed for the study; the soldiers' remains were reburied shortly after their exhumation. As mentioned previously, the assessments were made by one single person, using simple criteria.

4. CONCLUSION

The aim of this study of an early 19th century population was to describe its state of health, notably bone health, and compare it with that of modern western populations. What we have described echoes Kelly's findings in 1979, with roughly similar percentages of periodontal disease in the American population (33.9%). This seems to prove that the incidence of periodontal illness and its development within a population has been a fixed constant over a long period for humanity. The absence of healthcare was compensated by diet, which once again proves its importance in bucco-dental health. The specific character of our sample population may also explain the quality of its periodontium insofar as we have young subjects, pre-selected with respect to natural defenses by the hard school of military life at that time.

Our study came up against a certain number of fixed limits and our results thus require confirmation from other studies of this nature on a larger number of subjects.

REFERENCES

Albandar JM, Kingman A. 1999. Gingival recession, gingival bleeding, and dental calculus in adults 30 years of age and older in the United States, 1988–1994. *J. Periodontol.* 70, 30–43.

American Academy of Periodontology. 1996. World workshop in periodontics. *Ann Periodontol.* 1, 1–947.

Armitage GC. 1999. Development of a classification system for periodontol diseases and conditions. *Ann Periodontol.* 4, 1–6.

Aubrey S, Gopalakrishnan SN. 2002. Periodontal Disease in Europe. *Periodontology 2000.* 29, 104–121.

Benn DK. 1990. A review of the reliability of radiographic measurement in estimating alvéolar bone changes. *J. Clin. Periodontol.* 17, 14–21.

Carranza FA, Newman MG. 1996. *Clinical Periodontology*, 8th Edition. *Saunders Company*. Philadelphia, Pennsylvania. Section two: 66–67.

Dunning JM, Leach LB. 1960. Gingival Bone Count: A method for epidemiological study of periodontal disease. *J. Dent. Res.* 39, 506.

Frank J, Jrank JP. 1848. Mémoires bibliographiques de Jean-Pierre et Joseph Frank. Bibliothèque de l'université de Vilnius.

Gargiulo AW, Wentz FM, Orban B. 1961. Dimensions and relations of the dentoginjival junction in humans. *J of Periodontology.* 32, 261–267.

Gjermo P, Bellini HT, Peneira Santos V, Martins JG, Ferracyoli JR. 1984. Prevalence of bone loss in a group of Brazilian teenagers assessed on bite wing radiographs. *J Clin Periodontol*.

Kelly JE, Harvey CR. 1979. Basic dental examinations findings of persons 1–74 years, United States 1971–1974. Publication no (PHS) 79-1662, series 11, no. 214 Hyattville, MD, USA. Public Health Service, US Department of Health, Education and Welfare, National Center for Health Statistics.

Larrey D. 1812–1817. Mémoire de chirurgie militaire et Campagnes. Paris.

Listgarten MA, 1988. Why do epidemiological data have no diagnostic value? In: Guggenheim B, ed. *Periodontology Today*. Basel: *Karger*. 59–67.

Papapanou PN. 1989. Patterns of alveolar bone loss in the assessment of periodontal treatment priorities. *Swed. Dent. J. Suppl.* 66, 1–45.

Perry DA, Newman MG. 1990. Occurance of periodontitis in an urban adolescent population. *J Periodontol*. 61, 185–188.

Pigeard A. 2000. *L'Armée de Napoléon. Organisaton de la vie quotidienne. Editions Tallandier*. Paris. 232–233.

Ramfjord SP. 1967. Indices for prevalence and incidence of periodontal disease. *J. Periodontol.* 30, 51.

Sheiham A, Striffler DF. 1970. A comparison of four epidemiological methods of assessing periodontal disease. *J. Periodont. Res.* 5, 155.

Thillaud PL. 1996. *Paléopathologie humaine. Kronos B.Y.*: Sceaux, 61–71.

White DT, Folkens PA. 2000. *Human Osteology, Academic Press*, London: 340–359.

Appendix 2 How to Write and Read a Scientific Paper

Dentistry is a healing art that is well founded in science. Demands from within and outside the profession require that standards of practice be increasingly based on scientific evidence. Such evidence is acquired largely through published peer-reviewed research reports, commonly referred to as "the literature." This chapter, which is adapted from the author's postdoctoral course in research writing, discusses how scientific papers are structured according to the principle components of the research process.

> The literature in a scientific field consists of various types of written communications, of which the primary sources of knowledge are peer-reviewed publications, called original reports.

One of the tenets of research is that the work be communicated publicly. A research report is the primary way to disseminate the findings of a study once it has been completed (after the fact). Similarly, a research proposal is written prior to beginning a study to obtain funding and/or permission to conduct the work (before the fact). Research reports and proposals have similar formats designed to explain to readers what the investigators did and found, or what the investigators will do and think that they will find, respectively.

Several types of research reports are found in the scientific literature. The predominant type is the original report, often referred to as a paper or article. Original reports typically are publications narrowly focused on a specific research question or idea that adds new knowledge, or confirms existing knowledge, in a particular scientific discipline. Most readers are familiar with the standard format used in original reports; namely, introduction, methods, results, and discussion, as described in detail below.

Another type of research report is the review, which summarizes sets of original reports in a scientific discipline. For the most part, reviews traditionally have been written by experts who often provide their own interpretation of the collected findings, and are therefore referred to as narrative reviews. Increasingly, however, a related type of review known as the structured review is being published, in part, to minimize the potential bias that may be associated with narrative reviews. Structured reviews follow stringent criteria regarding how articles are included and analyzed. These publications are particularly useful in documenting solid evidence in a field and also in identifying gaps or misperceptions that may exist.

Structured review articles can be both qualitative and quantitative in format. Qualitative structured reviews often use evidence tables to present summaries of articles that have been reviewed. Evidence tables are comprehensive listings of the salient aspects of each article that has been included in the review. These evidence tables allow the reader to judge the relative merit of the available evidence comprehensively and efficiently. Quantitative structured reviews additionally provide what is called a meta-analysis, which is a computational method for analyzing the data reported in a set of published papers. In essence, meta-analysis allows the reviewer to treat data compiled from individual studies as if such data were from one larger study. This is an extremely powerful technique to establish the strength of evidence, or lack thereof, in a scientific discipline.

Other examples of research reports include abstracts or proceedings of scientific conferences, which can be in the form of posters or oral presentations. A graduate dissertation or thesis is also a type of research report. Chapters in textbooks and monographs also can be categorized as research reports. Opinions of experts expressed in editorials or letters in journals can sometimes be considered as a type of scientific publication, although there are obvious limitations to how such information should be interpreted and used.

The predominant type of research proposal is the grant application. To be successful, grant applications must clearly describe the rationale, importance, and feasibility of a proposed research study. Grant applications also must clearly describe how the study will be performed, what results are anticipated, and how the results will be analyzed.

Increasingly, research proposals in the biomedical sciences have multiple levels of investigation: human, animal, and in vitro. By using humans as research subjects, investigators can identify clinical evidence of a particular disease or condition and can test new interventions or treatments. Animal models allow specific ideas or interventions to be tested that would not be feasible to do in humans. This is especially true in research activities that have little or no known benefit and relatively high risk for subjects. In vitro cellular, molecular, genetic, biochemical, and biophysical analyses are useful in identifying or confirming biological mechanisms that explain a particular condition, risk factor, or treatment outcome. As part of the grant application process, investigators often must apply for institutional permission to use humans, animals, and certain hazardous materials such as radioisotopes, recombinant nucleic acids, or toxic chemicals. Such applications themselves are proposals that must justify the particular permission being sought.

ORIGINAL REPORTS REFLECT THE BASIC FORMAT OF THE RESEARCH PROCESS

Research can be defined as any focused, systematic inquiry or activity designed to contribute to generalizable knowledge and enhanced understanding of a particular subject (Centers for Disease Control and Prevention, 1999). It is critical that the activity be systematic; that is, it must follow set rules or patterns designed to produce valid conclusions and allow repetition and confirmation. Often called the scientific method, this approach ensures that the knowledge in a scientific discipline is based on objective facts rather than on unsupported opinions. The criterion of generalizability further ensures that such knowledge can be applied to populations or conditions outside the sample group or condition being studied within a particular research investigation. The research process follows a logical sequence. Typically, research begins with an idea or observation that forms the basis of a hypothesis that can be tested and subsequently evaluated. The process is cyclical in that subsequent systematic investigations modify the accumulated knowledge base as new evidence is obtained (Appendix Figure 2.1).

Research writing, like the research that it describes, also is a process having a logical structure. Scientific reports and proposals both follow a formulaic pattern designed to communicate the various components of a particular research endeavor. As indicated in Appendix Figure 2.2, research writing is designed to answer the following questions in original reports (or grant proposals).

- What did (or will) you do?
- Why did (or will) you do it?
- How did (or will) you do it?
- What did (or will) you find?
- What does (or will) it mean?
- What might you do next (or do if you hit a roadblock)?
- Who helped (or will help) you, including paying for it?

These questions form the basis of the standard format used in original reports or grant proposals. The essential components of a scientific report or proposal often are presented as separate sections of the written work, but also can be collapsed and combined as deemed appropriate. The remainder of this appendix discusses these various components.

Research process

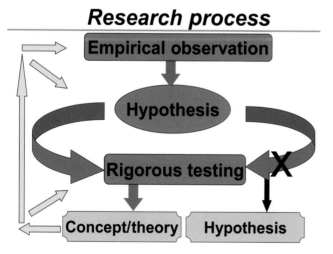

Appendix Figure 2.1. Algorithm for the general sequence of events in the research process. Research typically begins with an interesting observation or idea that is then developed into a hypothesis that can be tested. If the results are consistent and repeatable, then the initial idea may become part of an accepted concept or theory, which is subsequently modified as new knowledge is gained in the future. Without rigorous testing of the hypothesis, the original interesting idea remains speculative.

General Format of Reports/Proposals

	Reports ("did")	Proposals ("will")
What ___ you do? ⟷	Purpose	Specific Aims
Why ___ you do it? ⟷	Introduction	Background
How ___ you do it? ⟷	Methods	Experimental Design
What ___ you find? ⟷	Results	Preliminary Data
What ___ it mean? ⟷	Discussion	Relevance
What next? ⟷	Future Directions	Contingency Plans
Who to thank/ask? ⟷	Acknowledgments	Collaborators

Appendix Figure 2.2. Component questions addressed by research writing. Scientific papers attempt to convey to the reader the significance of the research, why and how it was conducted, and what the most likely interpretation and conclusion should be. Similarly, grant proposals seek to prove to the funding agency why the work should be done, provide the grant reviewers with some evidence that the proposed study can actually be done, and indicate what the investigators will do if unforeseen problems arise. In both published papers and grant applications, respectively, it is important to acknowledge those who have provided or will provide significant help with the project.

Research Question

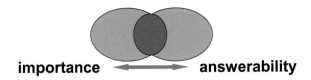

importance ⟷ answerability

- Is it important ?
- Can it be answered ?
- What is the best approach/modality to answer the question ?
- How much $$ will it cost to do ?

Appendix Figure 2.3. Balance between the significance of a research study and the feasibility of realizing the study's objectives. A research question that is easily answered may not be deemed important by the scientific community, and likely would not advance knowledge in any meaningful way. On the other hand, potential scientific, logistical, or financial constraints may render a research study overly ambitious and practically impossible to conduct. Thus, investigators seek to find a middle ground that allows them to actually answer a research question of reasonably high importance.

> The initial idea for an original report is developed into a justifiable and testable hypothesis through review of the existing literature (the "Introduction").

The introduction section of original reports generally states the purpose of the study, and also describes the background information that supports why the study was conducted. In performing the study, the researchers had to establish a balance between how interesting or important the research question was and how feasible it was to test, in terms of time, resources, and available methodologies. As suggested in Appendix Figure 2.3, a research question that is easily answered oftentimes may lack significance. On the other hand, an important research question may not be testable due to scientific or logistical constraints.

Any interesting research idea needs to be developed and refined so that it can be tested; otherwise, it remains merely an interesting idea with little practical merit. The process has analogy to the popular riddle: Which comes first, the chicken or the egg? In other words, one needs to know at least something about an area to come up with an interesting research question in the first place. The research question may be too broad or ill-defined at first, which then requires one to review the literature in the field to focus the question. This becomes a repetitive, iterative process until the nascent

Steps for Developing the Hypothesis

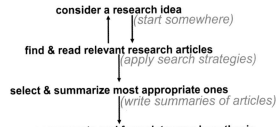

Appendix Figure 2.4. The generation and refinement of a research hypothesis is an iterative process. It begins with a nascent idea that is developed through a targeted search of the literature. Oftentimes, the question is modified based on evidence that may or may not be found in the literature. Articles are read and summarized in the context of the investigator's hypothesis. That is, articles are used strategically to produce "a story" that is rational, convincing, and scientifically exciting. The hypothesis then represents a reasoned justification for conducting the proposed study.

idea is transformed into a precise hypothesis worthy of investigation; that is:

> The research question is *developed* from a review of the available literature.
>
> ↑ ↓
>
> The review of the available literature is *focused* on the research question.

The key point to be made is that the steps taken to develop a research question into a testable hypothesis are the same as the steps taken to conduct a focused review of the existing knowledge base for that same research question (Appendix Figure 2.4).

THE HYPOTHESIS

The hypothesis is a clear and concise statement of the research idea that is to be tested. Often, the hypothesis is presented as the purpose of a particular study with specific aims or objectives that list how the purpose was (or will be) achieved. Hypotheses are built according to relatively simple logical patterns: if/then, cause/effect, and intervention/outcome. In simplest terms, a hypothesis of any clinical study has the following structure:

Appendix Table 2.1. Examples of hypotheses formulated using the PICO format.

	Problem/patients (P)	Intervention/treatment /risk factor (I)	Comparisons (C)	Outcomes (O)
Example 1	Among adults …	… does moderate-to-severe periodontal disease …	… compared to mild or no periodontal disease …	… lead to increased myocardial infarctions?
Example 2	In patients with fixed orthodontic appliances …	… would use of an electric toothbrush …	… compared to a manual toothbrush …	… lead to improved plaque removal?
Example 3	In patients with aggressive periodontitis …	… does flap surgery …	… compared with scaling and root planing …	… decrease the need for extraction during the maintenance phase?
Example 4	Among adults with type 2 diabetes …	… is periodontal treatment…	… compared with no treatment …	… associated with improved glycemic control?
Example 5	Among adults who smoke …	… do tapered implants…	… compared with cylindrical implants …	… demonstrate identical success rates?

Given A, B, and C (the current state of knowledge), if subjects do or have X (an intervention, treatment, or a risk factor), then they are expected to demonstrate Y (an outcome or effect) in comparison with subjects without X.

Such a structure points out four key factors to be considered in focusing the research question into a testable hypothesis: (1) **P**roblem and patients, (2) **I**ntervention, treatment, or risk factor, (3) **C**omparison intervention or group, and (4) **O**utcomes or effect. The acronym PICO describes this well accepted format for framing hypotheses (Richards, 2007). Each of these four factors addresses the following questions, respectively:

1. What is the problem of interest and the patients or subjects it concerns?

2. What is the main intervention, treatment, or risk factor being considered?

3. What is the main alternative to which the intervention, treatment, or risk factor will be compared? To what group will patients or subjects of interest be compared?

4. What do the researchers hope to accomplish? What do they realistically expect to see? To what will the risk or exposure lead? What outcome would be particularly worrisome?

Some examples of PICO-formatted research questions are listed in Appendix Table 2.1. It is important to note that by following this format each example makes clear not only what will be tested but also what general methods or measurements most likely will be used.

PUBLICATION DATABASES AND SEARCH STRATEGIES

There is little doubt that the biomedical literature has burgeoned during the past several decades. Increasing numbers of original reports are being published in increasing numbers of journals. This presents a considerable challenge for researchers interested in focusing a research question; that is, how to identify relevant publications efficiently and effectively without missing important ones and without obtaining ones that are not directly relevant. An important first step is to recognize that the literature is organized in several electronic databases that can be searched.

The most popular data base is MEDLINE, which is produced by the National Library of Medicine (NLM) in Bethesda, Maryland. MEDLINE is a comprehensive bibliographic database of citations to published journal articles in the biomedical sciences. It covers all aspects of health care: dentistry, medicine, nursing, allied health fields, biomedical and pre-clinical sciences, pharmacy, psychiatry, etc. MEDLINE indexes approximately 4,800 journals containing more than 15 million citations, dating from 1950 to the present. MEDLINE is free, open to the public, and available 24 hours/day, 7 days/week on the Web from any computer worldwide. This database is dynamic, with citations updated weekly. It can be readily accessed online through the PubMed portal (PubMed): http://www.ncbi.nlm.nih.gov/entrez/.

MEDLINE is not the only database available to biomedical and social scientists. Others include Biosis; CINAHL (Cumulative Index to Nursing and Allied Health Literature); Cochrane Central Register of Controlled Trials; Cochrane Database of Systematic Reviews, Genetics, Genomics and Proteomics Databases; PsycINFO; TOXLINE; TOXNET; and the Web of Science databases known as Science Citation Index and Social Sciences Citation Index. These databases would also be searched depending upon the particular research question being asked.

After an appropriate database has been identified, it next becomes necessary to execute an effective strategy to search for relevant publications. In this regard, it is useful to recognize that databases are compiled by library science personnel who read and catalogue the articles according to set criteria. For MEDLINE, these criteria constitute a controlled vocabulary thesaurus known as medical subject headings (MeSH), which represent the subject content of each article. MEDLINE uses more than 50,000 MeSH terms (also referred to as subjects) with more than 30 subheadings that are attached to the MeSH to further describe a particular subject. MeSH subjects also are grouped in hierarchies called trees that organize the relationships among diverse subject headings. A tree progresses from the most general (broad) term to the most specific (narrow) term. The indexers at the National Library of Medicine assign eight to 20 MeSH for each article, which can then be used by researchers in their literature searches.

The literature search process is generally organized into successive steps that result in the retrieval of a manageable number of relevant articles. The first step is to use various search terms (or fields) as needed. The MeSH terms are frequently used, as are specific text words from an article's title or abstract. The key words listed in articles are also useful terms. Searches can also be conducted according to the names of known authors or specific titles of journals. Once a first pass through the available literature is completed, the search is then either widened or narrowed, depending on the initial results. This is referred to as exploding or focusing, respectively. So-called limits can be applied to large sets of articles to reduce the number of articles identified and refine the search. These limits can be according to subject age or gender, type of publication, years of publication, language, dental specialty, or other criteria. The search results can be combined to include only articles that contain more than one of the search elements. Once these are done, the most efficient next step is to review the title and abstract of each individual article, without reading the entire article, to determine if the retrieved article is relevant to the topic. This entire process then repeats until the researcher is satisfied with the search results.

It should be noted that universities appoint professional searchers, typically library staff, to assist researchers in developing their research agenda. These individuals are experts in information recovery and generally provide ongoing training for researchers in need of assistance. Such training is very useful in improving the efficiency and effectiveness of one's literature searches.

SUMMARIZING THE LITERATURE

The net result of the literature search is to establish a set of articles with the most relevance to the intended research investigation. These articles must then be read and summarized so that they can form the basis for justifying why the intended investigation is necessary, and what is hoped to be accomplished. This constitutes the introduction section in an original report (or the background/significance section in

grant proposals). How these articles are actually summarized is usually a matter of preference of the individual researcher. However, to be useful, each article retrieved from the search process should be summarized with the following questions in mind:

1. What was the authors' research question?

2. How did the authors attempt to answer that question (i.e., research design and methods)?

3. What were the results?

4. What is the article's relevance to my own research question or project?

    a. Does it help indicate the current state of knowledge?

    b. Does it help argue the case for my own research question?

Once reviewed and summarized, the information reported in selected literature is compiled into a narrative that provides general background information and the details of the current state of knowledge in the relevant area. Arguments are then presented defending the need to answer the specific research question, which is formulated as a testable hypothesis. As indicated in Appendix Figure 2.4, these summaries are organized into a hopefully convincing story that provides the rationale for the intended research investigation.

CITATIONS AND CITATION MANAGEMENT

The format of citations in original reports is specified by the scientific journal in which they are published. In the biomedical literature, these tend to follow the Uniform Requirements for Manuscripts Submitted to Biomedical Journals (International Committee of Medical Journal Editors, 2007). Typically, one of two general formats is used: the numbering method for citing articles or the name and year method for citing articles. As the name implies, the numbering method cites references according to the order in which they appear in the publication. These are then listed in ascending numerical order at the end of the paper. In contrast, the name and year method cites references by indicating the name of the author(s) and the year in which the reference was published. These are then listed alphabetically at the end of the paper. Although each journal has its own rules, typically only up to three authors' names are listed in the body of the text, whereas all authors are listed at the end of the paper. An excellent resource that describes citation management can be found at The Writing Center, University of Wisconsin-Madison (The Writing Center).

It also should be noted that several software programs to facilitate the management of references are commercially available. These help organize one's personal electronic database of articles to which future articles can be added. These software programs allow citations to be easily inserted into the text of manuscripts that are being prepared for publication. A useful advantage is that the citations can then be listed at the end of the paper according to the varying formats specified by different journals; these formats come preset within the software program.

> The hypothesis is tested systematically using relevant protocols in established study designs (the "Methods").

In discussing the methods used in research studies, it is helpful to distinguish between the general design of a particular investigation and the specific protocols used to generate data.

STUDY DESIGNS

The design of a study refers to the general format of how the investigation is conducted. Several formats are commonly used in clinical studies, as reviewed in Callas (2008). These formats are based on several defining characteristics: the timing of data acquisition, the extent of influence or direct action by the researchers, and the amount of involvement and risk for the study subjects.

In the broadest sense, research study designs are either descriptive or explanatory. Descriptive studies are those that identify and report various characteristics of interest such as age, gender, race, geographic location, and incidence or prevalence of a particular disease, as examples, without testing a specific hypothesis. Descriptive studies are useful in generating information that can be subsequently used to develop hypotheses that can be tested. Clinical case reports, specifically those reported as case series, are examples of descriptive studies.

Explanatory studies (also referred to as analytical studies) are designed to answer and explain specific questions; that is, to actually test research hypotheses. These studies can be either prospective or retrospective: prospective studies collect and analyze data going forward from the start of an investigation, whereas retrospective studies collect data after an outcome has occurred or they analyze existing data that have been collected previously. Explanatory studies can be further classified as observational or experimental (also referred to as interventional). As the name implies, observational studies are those in which "natural" changes or differences in one characteristic (variable) are studied in relation to changes or differences in another variable(s), without any direct intervention by the investigator. In contrast, experimental studies are those in which the investigator actively inter-

venes by changing a particular variable and then measures what happens to other variables.

Observational studies can be further classified as cohort studies (also referred to as longitudinal), case-control studies, and cross-sectional studies. In cohort studies, groups selected by the presence or absence of a risk factor or other characteristic suspected of being a precursor for an outcome of interest are followed prospectively over time and the outcome is subsequently measured. In case-control studies, two groups are analyzed retrospectively to determine possible causes or risk factors for a particular outcome of interest. The two groups are defined by the presence (case) or absence (control) of the relevant outcome. In cross-sectional studies, data are collected at one point in time and then analyzed for the concurrent presence or absence of a factor suspected to be associated with a particular outcome characteristic. If data are compared between groups of subjects with and without the outcome characteristic, then the cross-sectional study is considered to be explanatory. If data for only one group of subjects is reported, then the cross-sectional study is more aptly considered to be descriptive.

Experimental or interventional studies are collectively referred to as clinical trials, which are designed to produce cause-and-effect relationships among variables of interest. In clinical trials, subjects are assigned into either experimental (test) or control groups. The experimental group is actively subjected to a suspected causal variable or intervention, while the control group is not, and predetermined outcome variables are then measured prospectively. There are several types of clinical trials that are characterized according to how subjects are assigned into the study groups and the nature of the control group.

The randomized clinical trial (RCT) has long been considered the gold standard in clinical research design. In the RCT, subjects are randomly assigned into either the experimental or the control group. Randomization is very important from a design standpoint because the process ensures that the two comparison groups are as similar as possible in multiple characteristics (for example, age, gender, health status), except for the suspected causal variable or intervention.

Nonrandomized clinical trials also can be found in the literature, but these studies are not considered as strong as the RCTs. Studies that compare two different groups (i.e., experimental and control) within the same study are considered stronger than those in which each research subject serves as its own control (called self-controlled trials, in which subjects participate in both the experimental and control groups at different times during the study). Along the same lines of reasoning, studies that compare two different groups within the same study are considered much stronger than studies in which the experimental group is compared with an external control group, either the general population itself or different groups studied in previous research investigations (called historical controls).

As described above, a systematic review is a type of literature review that attempts to identify, pool, and interpret available evidence on a specific research question, usually from RCTs, so that the strengths and weaknesses of the evidence can be made clear.

The various study designs can be summarized as follows:

Case Series Description: Did you see something interesting? These are a grouping of anecdotal observations about a particular outcome that helps to generate initial research ideas.

Case-Control Studies: What happened? In this type of study design one group of subjects already has a particular outcome (cases), as compared to another group that does not (controls).

Cross-Sectional Studies: What is happening? Groups are examined at one point in time for the presence or absence of a particular outcome.

Cohort (Longitudinal) Studies: What will happen "naturally"? Groups are followed over time for the occurrence or non-occurrence of a particular outcome.

Clinical Trials: What will happen "experimentally"? One group (experimental) is subjected to a specific manipulation while another group (control) is not; both groups are examined at a future point in time for the presence or absence of a particular outcome.

Systematic Reviews/Meta-Analyses: How can existing data in separate studies be critically summarized so that the "real" answer to a research question is identified? A systematic review uses rigorous, objective criteria to retrieve, evaluate, and summarize published scientific papers that are relevant to a topic. A meta-analysis is a statistical method used in certain systematic reviews that allows quantitative data published in different scientific papers to be evaluated and combined as if they were all from one large study.

HIERARCHY OF EVIDENCE

One of the fundamental goals of biomedical research is to discover and advance knowledge for alleviating human abnormalities and diseases and improving overall quality of life. Thus, research study designs have been ranked according to how directly applicable their respective findings may be to the human population and how well potential sources

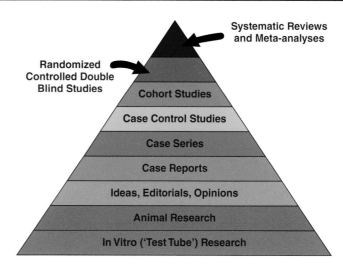

Appendix Figure 2.5. The evidence pyramid. Available evidence can be ranked according to its relative strength in clinically relevant contexts. In general, this ranking reflects how directly applicable the evidence may be to the human population, and to how well potential sources of bias or error have been reduced. It is important to point out that all types of evidence have intrinsic value but that only the study designs listed in the upper levels of the pyramid provide evidence that may be of immediate use for the practicing clinician. (Reprinted with permission of Dr. Andrea Markinson, Evidence Based Medicine Course, State University of New York Downstate.)

of study bias or error have been reduced. This ranking is often referred to as the hierarchy of evidence and includes in vitro, animal, and human clinical studies. This hierarchy can be illustrated by an evidence pyramid, as shown in Appendix Figure 2.5. The figure is available from the online Evidence Based Medicine Course at the Medical Research Library of Brooklyn, State University of New York Downstate Medical Center. This is an excellent tutorial on evidence-based medicine that can be accessed freely (Markinson).

The different types of evidence are labeled in the figure, with the least clinically relevant at the bottom and the most clinically relevant at the top. The top five layers indicate evidence generally considered strong enough to be clinically relevant (i.e., directly influencing clinical decisions). The bottom layers have considerable merit in terms of providing scientific information, but do not provide sufficient strength of scientific evidence to warrant direct relevance to humans. As illustrated, systematic reviews and meta-analyses are considered to be the highest level of evidence in biomedical research. These serve to increase the credibility and power (discussed below) of individual studies, and are extremely useful in helping busy practitioners distinguish between reality and hype, so to speak, regarding diagnostic and treatment interventions.

STUDY-SPECIFIC PROTOCOLS

These are intuitively understood as constituting the methods of a study. In a periodontal clinical study, for example, measurements of attachment loss, probing pocket depth, recession depth, gingival index, plaque index, or bleeding on probing would each be done according to specific protocols. Researchers determine a priori what measurements would be made, how many teeth or sites would be evaluated (for example, Ramfjord teeth) (Fleiss et al., 1987), by which instruments (for example, manual vs. electronic periodontal probe), and how often (for example, number of post-treatment recall visits). Oftentimes, these protocols are well established and commonly used across many different studies. In such instances the protocol is merely indicated by a published citation without much description of the details of the technique. A classic example of this is the highly cited Gingival Index (GI) of Loe and Silness (1963). On the other hand, if a well accepted protocol has been modified, or if a new method has been developed for the particular research study, then it is expected that a more detailed description will be provided. Thus, a balance is established between clarity and brevity in published reports. Appendix Figure 2.6 provides some examples of study-specific methods. The list is for illustrative purposes only and is not meant to be comprehensive. Moreover, many of these are applicable to human subjects and animal models, depending on the objectives of the research study.

> There are a number of important scientific principles to be considered when designing and conducting a research investigation.

SAMPLING, SAMPLE SIZE, AND POWER

The concepts described in this section are shown in greater detail in the Research Methods Knowledge Base (Trochim, 2006). Because it is highly impractical, if not impossible, to study all individuals in a population, researchers select a representative subset to study (i.e., the sample). This subset must be truly representative if valid conclusions are to be drawn from the research findings. Consequently, the methods section of a published scientific paper often describes how the research subjects were chosen and recruited. The reader should be confident that the subjects represent the full range of individuals who present with a particular condition, or who are exposed to a particular risk factor, or who require a particular intervention.

It is also important that inclusion and exclusion criteria are clearly identified. Inclusion criteria are those characteristics that subjects must demonstrate to be accepted into the study. In studies of periodontal disease, for example, subjects must often present with a minimum amount of attachment loss on a predetermined number of teeth prior to enrollment. Exclusion criteria are based on subject characteristics that, when present, would likely interfere with interpretation of the research data. In studies of periodontal disease, again for example, concurrent or recent use of systemic antibiotics due to a medical condition often would cause a prospective subject to be deemed ineligible.

Thus, appropriate sampling strategies for clinical studies are critical for ensuring that comparison groups are well-matched and that subjects do not present with characteristics that could diminish the strength of the research (Trochim, 2006). Several sampling strategies are commonly used to recruit subjects in clinical trials. In random sampling, as the name implies, subjects are selected at random. In consecutive sampling, all potential subjects who meet the inclusion criteria over a specified period of time are recruited. In convenience sampling, subjects who are easily accessible are recruited. Stratified and cluster sampling strategies are similar in that a population is subdivided according to demographic or geographic characteristics, respectively, and then random samples are taken from the subgroups.

In addition to using appropriate sampling methodologies, it is important for researchers to determine how large of a

Examples of Some Specific Protocols/Techniques

Clinical	Animal	Laboratory
Plaque score	Birth weight	H & E stain
Gingival index	Food Intake	Cell counts
Caries	Caries	RNA expression
Pulp vitality	Pulp vitality	Protein Levels
Intercanine distance	Behavior	Bond strength
Fluorosis	Sedation	Leakage
Use of Services	Sacrifice	Moment of Inertia
Attitudes	Phlebotomy	Stress/Strain

Appendix Figure 2.6. Some types of measurements or procedures that may be found in research studies. Each would be described in varying detail within scientific papers or grant proposals, depending on how well known and accepted the particular measurement or procedure may be to the scientific community. Intuitively, measurement protocols that are standardized and frequently used can be described by a simple citation, whereas novel techniques or common techniques that have been significantly modified should be described in detail. The important point to note is that the scientific community should be provided sufficient technical details to allow the study to be repeated. Such repetition by different groups of investigators is critical for confirming the validity of findings presented in the literature.

sample must be studied (i.e., the sample size) (Whitley and Ball, 2002). If the sample is too small, there is uncertainty about how much the findings are due to random chance instead of the study design. If the sample is too large, extra effort and costs are incurred unnecessarily. In both instances the possible risks to human subjects are unacceptably increased. Researchers are therefore obligated to calculate the sample size that is appropriate for their study. Although formulae and tables for calculating sample size are readily available, these require several pieces of information that should be known or estimated before the study is conducted.

One important estimate is the variability (variance) of the measures to be made in the study. In simplest terms, this represents the "natural" measurement error of a particular technique. Such an estimate can be determined from the available literature or from general consensus from practitioners in the field. For example, measures of probing pocket depth using a manual probe in clinical periodontics are generally accepted as ±1 mm. If this variance is unacceptably high for a proposed study, the use of an electronic probe would be required to reduce this inherent variability in the measure of pocket depth.

Another important determination is how large or small a difference between sample groups will be considered to be real. Intuitively, if the difference to be found is small, then larger samples must be measured to find the difference. On the other hand, large or gross differences between sample groups may be detected with smaller sample sizes. In the example of probing pocket depth measured with a manual probe, a difference of ≥3 mm pocket depth between two sample groups would be much easier to detect than would a 1 mm difference.

A third important parameter in calculating sample size is power (Danya International Inc., 2005). Power refers to the ability of a research study to detect a difference between comparison groups when such a difference does, in fact, really exist. Power, variance, difference, and sample size are interrelated. A study that is underpowered would not be able to adequately test a hypothesis because (1) the variance is too large, given the sample size and difference to be detected, (2) the difference to be detected between the groups is too small, given the variance and sample size, or (3) the sample size is insufficient for detecting the specified difference, given the variance and difference to be detected. To adequately test a hypothesis, therefore, a study must be appropriately powered. Increasingly, journals are requiring investigators to provide justification for their sample size and/or a power calculation in the methods section. This assures the reader that the work was worth the effort and expenditure of resources, and also that the potential risks to research subjects were acceptable. Without adequate power, the findings of a particular study will not be generalizable, which is one of the main goals of research.

RELIABILITY AND VALIDITY

The terms reliability and validity describe different aspects of what may generically be called the credibility of a study and its results (Colorado State University). Reliability is concerned with accuracy and precision of the actual methods, procedures, tests, instruments, etc. in a particular study. Specifically, reliability is a function of how well the measures reflect relevant characteristics or variables of interest, and how consistent these measures are over time. Validity is concerned with the degree to which the research study itself accurately tests the hypothesis. Validity is a function of how well the study is designed to answer the research question; that is, that the study actually measures what it is supposed to measure. Therefore, for a study to be considered valid it must not only have reliability of its measures, but also these reliable measures must be appropriate for testing the stated hypothesis.

A simple example can be used to illustrate the relationship between reliability and validity. Let us suppose that a particular investigation is evaluating the hypothesis that susceptibility to periodontal disease is related to the degree of surface mineralization of teeth. In this imaginary example, clinical attachment is measured at six sites in all teeth and periodontal disease is defined as clinical attachment loss of more than 3 mm in at least four teeth per subject. To test the hypothesis, the investigators designed a cross-sectional study that uses standard shade guides to evaluate the color of natural crowns in subjects with periodontal disease. After all data have been collected, the investigators will look for any associations between tooth shade and periodontal disease. Here, both attachment levels and tooth shade are reliable measures because they can be obtained with high accuracy and repeatability, when necessary, by an experienced clinical investigator. However, the study probably would not be valid even if an association was found between tooth shade and periodontal disease because tooth color per se does not necessarily reflect the surface mineralization status of either the crown or root.

In this example the investigators could generate lots of accurate and consistent data, but those data would probably have little to do with testing the relationship between surface mineralization and periodontitis. Despite any statistically significant associations that may be found, this study would have failed to test its hypothesis. Instead, the study would actually have tested a different hypothesis than intended; that is, that periodontal disease is associated with the color of natural crowns.

Several types of reliability have been described (Colorado State University). Publications of clinical studies often provide information about interrater reliability. This is the extent with which two or more investigators demonstrate agreement when measuring a particular characteristic or variable. Interrater reliability defines how well calibrated the clinical examiners may be, and this is often reported in scientific papers as the Kappa statistic. Intrarater reliability describes how consistent one clinical examiner is with herself over time. Internal reliability describes the extent to which two or more measures assess the same outcome; that is, the consistency of the tools that are measured by reliability tests such as Cronbach's Alpha and Spearman-Brown Split Half Coefficient. Stability reliability describes the extent to which the same measures remain consistent over time and is measured by the test-retest method. Equivalency reliability is the extent to which two or more outcomes co-occur; that is, the consistency of finding an association between measures. Importantly, equivalency reliability does not describe causal relationships but instead describes coincidental associations or correlations that are reported as correlation coefficients (r).

Several types of validity have also been described, but these generally fall into two main categories: internal validity and external validity (Colorado State University). Internal validity is concerned with how good the results of a study actually are in testing the hypothesis and, consequently, relates to factors inside the experiment or study design. One group of factors constitutes what may be viewed as the "rigor" of the study. These involve critical elements such as the appropriateness of the study design, whether or not correct decisions were made about what or what not to measure, and whether or not the methods and technical aspects of the study were carefully applied. Internal validity also establishes whether or not any cause-effect relationships have been identified and explained correctly, and if alternative explanations exist.

In contrast to internal validity, external validity is concerned with how well the results of the study can be generalized or transferred to larger groups or different populations. Consequently, external validity defines the applicability of the results beyond or outside the particular research investigation (i.e., generalizability). In simplest terms, the various types of validities can be considered as components of a logical hierarchy. The validity of a study increases as it answers the following levels of questions:

1. Is there a relationship between characteristic or variable X and characteristic or variable Y?

2. If yes, is this relationship causal (i.e., "if X, then Y")?

3. If yes, can this causal relationship be generalizable?

CHANCE, BIAS, AND CONFOUNDS

The validity of a study can be diminished by a number of factors. Again, these generally fall into two main categories:

internal validity-related and external validity-related. Internal validity is decreased when the study is not sufficiently controlled to be internally consistent. The main factors are chance, bias, and confounds (Colorado State University). Chance can be considered to be random error or experimental "noise." Causal associations may be found, or not found, merely due to chance error that can be reduced but never completely eliminated in research studies. The often published significance level of ≤0.05 is commonly interpreted to mean that the reported findings have only at most a 5% probability that they are due to chance alone. In other words, there is at least a 95% probability that the findings are real. Typically, the effect of chance on diminishing validity is not overly important in well designed and controlled studies.

In contrast with chance, factors that introduce bias into research studies are important to identify and eliminate or minimize. These affect the rigor of the study and lead to conclusions that deviate from reality. Bias can involve any aspect of the research process. Hawthorne-type effects are the well known biases related to performance of the research subject, wherein the subject responds in certain ways due to self-awareness of being in a research study (i.e., placebo effect). Subjects also can exhibit recall bias, which is a systematic error due to differences in accuracy or completeness of their memory of past experiences. Repeated-order effects are biases introduced when subjects learn a test that is repeated the same way over time, which produces data on how well subjects learn to take the test instead of the knowledge that the test is intended to identify. Investigator bias can also be introduced due to the selective gathering of data, either subconsciously or consciously on the part of the investigator. Loss to follow-up bias often occurs in long-term prospective studies when subjects drop out and do not complete participation in the study for whatever reason.

Confounding factors are those that negatively affect the cause-effect determination of the study. In the "if X, then Y" scenario, outcome Y depends on characteristic X. Confounding factors are additional variables that coexist coincidentally along with the independent variable X that is being studied. These extraneous factors are sometimes readily identifiable and controlled, but they can also be poorly known or measurable variables that may be unrelated or related to the independent variable. If, for example, smokers were on average younger than nonsmokers in a study examining the effect of smoking on the outcome of periodontal guided tissue regeneration, then age might confound the results. In other words, it might be possible that the younger age (and putatively better healing potential) could offset the factor of smoking, unless the analysis is adjusted for age. When confounding factors are not adequately accounted for, it becomes highly likely that something else caused the effect that the investigators measured so reliably.

External validity is decreased when the study is based on a sample of the population that is not sufficiently accurate to allow generalizability. This occurs due to sampling errors such as selection bias, or errors in the study due to systematic differences in characteristics between study participants and non-participants. Generalizability is also indirectly influenced by publication bias, which is the unwillingness of most journals to publish negative results.

Finally, it is important to point out that researchers use a number of methods to reduce bias and confounds in study designs. Many of these methods are commonly known, for example, the use of double-blinding in clinical trials to reduce both subject and investigator bias. The use of placebo groups helps facilitate the generalizability of a study. Drop-outs in long-term prospective clinical trials can be handled by an intent-to-treat analysis, which is a statistical method that allows incomplete data on a subject to be retained and analyzed rather than being discarded (i.e., lost to follow-up).

One way to control extraneous factors is through random assignment of subjects/samples to the experimental and control groups. Randomization is arguably the most important method to reduce selection bias and mitigate the effects of confounding variables, because any factor that participants bring to the study that might influence the outcome are randomly distributed across the groups. Researchers, and particularly statisticians, use a number of different randomization schemes to control for nuisance variables and ensure that experimental and control groups are equally matched except for the variable, intervention, or treatment of interest.

> There are also a number of important regulatory considerations in designing and conducting a research investigation.

INSTITUTIONAL REVIEW BOARDS

The use of humans as research subjects in university and industry studies is highly regulated. Federal and state regulations mandate that institutional review boards (IRB) review and approve all research that involves human subjects. The regulations specify the composition of the IRB, which must include scientific/medical experts, nonscientists, and outside consultants as needed. The IRB is charged with protecting the rights and welfare of human research subjects.

Protocols submitted to the IRB are judged according to three ethical principles: beneficence, justice, and respect for persons (U.S. States Department of Health and Human Services). Beneficence refers to activities or actions that maintain or improve the well-being of subjects. The principle of beneficence obligates researchers to prevent harm and promote good. The principle of justice obligates researchers to ensure that both the risks and benefits of research are distributed fairly across different groups and are not disproportionately borne by any one particular group. Respect for persons obligates researchers to treat individual research subjects as autonomous agents allowed to make informed choices freely. The primary expectation is that subjects will be respected as fellow human beings and not be viewed merely as means to an end.

The IRB determines whether risks to subjects, be they physical, psychological, sociological, or economic, are reasonable and justified given the potential benefits of the study. These benefits may be applicable to the individual research subject, to others in the larger population, and/or to the advancement of general knowledge. The IRB ensures that the consent process is clear, fair, and free from coercion. It also ensures that consent forms are written so that a lay person with a 7th- or 8th-grade education can understand exactly what he will undergo as part of the study. In addition, the IRB makes a judgment on how well subject confidentiality will be maintained. Privacy is an important consideration mandated by the federal Health Insurance Portability and Accountability Act (HIPAA), which regulates research activities as well as clinical practice.

It is interesting to note that the use of placebos as a method to control for bias and confounding factors in clinical trials is being questioned for ethical reasons. Such questions arise when researchers and IRBs consider the ethics and fairness of withholding treatment to subjects in the placebo or sham group, or continuing treatment in the experimental group, solely for the sake of the study. In drug trials, for example, the research is often discontinued before the study is completed when a drug is found to be effective. In such instances all subjects, including those in the placebo group, are then offered the use of the drug. On the other hand, drug trials are also terminated prematurely when a particular drug is found to be grossly ineffective or unacceptably dangerous. These decisions are made by the IRB, study-specific independent entities known as data safety and monitoring boards (DSMB), or data safety committees (DSC) during interim analyses performed at various times during the study. This illustrates how the protection of human subjects is a dynamic, ongoing process.

Journals require scientific papers to indicate that IRB approval was obtained for any research involving humans. This information typically is provided in the methods section of original reports.

INSTITUTIONAL ANIMAL CARE AND USE COMMITTEE

Universities and industry are sensitive to the ethical issues involved in using animals as research subjects. Federal, state, and local regulations ensure the humane treatment of animals in research studies, in particular non-human primates and other vertebrate animals. All universities are mandated to have an institutional animal care and use committee (IACUC) charged with overseeing such research (Office of Animal Care and Use). Like the IRB, the IACUC is composed of individuals having mandated expertise and interest in animal welfare. Specifically, the IACUC must include at least one doctor of veterinary medicine with training or experience in laboratory animal science, one practicing scientist experienced in research involving animals, one non-scientist layperson, and one individual who is not affiliated with the institution in any way other than as a member of the IACUC. Protocols submitted to the IACUC are reviewed for scientific merit and clear justification for the number and species of animals for which authorization is being requested. The IACUC is the legal mechanism through which institutions give researchers permission to purchase, house, and use animals specifically for research purposes.

Investigators submitting applications to the IACUC are required to demonstrate compliance with the three R's of animal research: reduction, refinement, and replacement. Reduction refers to decreasing the number of animals actually used in the study. Investigators must provide sample size and power calculations that justify the number of animals to be used, and they should use the fewest number of animals possible without compromising the statistical power of the study. Refinement refers to modifications in the research plan that lower the incidence or severity of pain and distress in the animals. The IACUC is especially concerned with animal pain and distress for practical as well as ethical reasons; animals respond to pain and distress with changes in their normal physiology that may skew any data being collected. Replacement refers to the substitution of nonsentient material for animals, or to the substitution of a lower species that might be less sensitive to pain and distress than a higher species. The replacement strategy also has a practical aspect; lower species tend to be less expensive to purchase, house, and feed.

As with human subject research, journals require scientific papers to indicate that IACUC approval was obtained for any research involving animals. This information typically is provided in the methods section of original reports.

LABORATORY SAFETY

Universities and industry are required to follow established regulations and standards for laboratory safety. These are designed not only to protect the researchers but also ancillary and noninvolved personnel. Radiation safety committees, for example, oversee the use of radioactive materials and modalities, including radiographs and CT scans when performed for research purposes rather than routine clinical

care. Biological safety committees ensure that dangerous microbes and recombinant genetic material are handled safely in approved settings. Investigators are required to be up to date with chemical safety (including material safety data sheets, or MSDS), fire safety, and infection control protocols. Although not usually indicated in scientific papers, it is presumed that the study has followed all applicable regulations.

Testing of the hypothesis generates findings that are compiled, analyzed, and presented systematically (the "Results").

DATA COMPILATION

The specific aims and design of a particular study dictate how data are acquired. In all research investigations, the results must be collected systematically to minimize bias and ensure consistency and integrity. The collection process often follows pre-determined rules for recording the data and also for sorting or reducing the data so that they can be managed effectively. This is especially true for large clinical trials that may be conducted across multiple locations.

The standard instrument for data collection in clinical trials is the case report form (CRF). Typically, these are paper or electronic forms specifically designed so that an investigator can record necessary information in an organized format that has a logical flow related to a specific visit or procedure for the research subject. For example, an important use of CRFs is to verify and document the eligibility (inclusion criteria) or ineligibility (exclusion criteria) of research subjects during the recruitment and enrollment phase of a study. CRFs are also designed to facilitate data transfer into electronic databases or spreadsheets for subsequent analysis. A large clinical study may use several different CRFs, depending on the number of variables or study characteristics that need to be measured and recorded. Appendix Figure 2.7 lists some examples of CRFs that might be used in clinical trials. Additional information on CRFs can be found in Incorporating Cancer Clinical Trials into Your Practice (Module 3) (National Cancer Institute).

DATA ANALYSIS

Data analysis, like data collection, must also be done systematically to ensure consistency and integrity of the research study. Myriad statistical methodologies, ranging from simple to complex, are available for analyzing data. These are described in original reports under the standard heading of "statistical analysis." The plan for statistical analysis follows pre-determined rules for accepting or rejecting the data, characterizing the data, and identifying which statistical

Examples of Case Report Forms

General CRFs	Study-specific CRFs
• P.I. Verification Form	• Biomarker Forms
• Subject Enrollment Form	• Apoptotic Index
• Eligibility Form	• Cell Differentiation Biomarkers
• Subject Randomization Form	• Inflammatory Cytokines
• Medical History	• DNA Ploidy Analysis
• Physical Examination	• Inflammatory Cell Infiltrate
• Clinical Laboratory Data	• Intracrypt Apoptotic Index
• Compliance	• Nucleolar Morphometry
• Concomitant Medication	• PGE2 Levels
• Adverse Events	• Proliferation Analysis
• Off Study	• Nuclear Morphometry
• Death	

See also: http://cme.cancer.gov/c02/s02/c3_4b_01.htm

Appendix Figure 2.7. Some types of case report forms (CRFs) that may be found in research studies. CRFs provide research investigators with standardized formats with which to record relevant data. These can be paper or electronic forms specifically designed to have a logical flow related to a specific visit or procedure for a given research subject or a particular test or laboratory measurement. Large clinical studies often use several different CRFs, depending on the number of variables or study characteristics that need to be measured and recorded. (Adapted from the public access Web site/online tutorial Incorporating Cancer Clinical Trials into Your Practice, National Cancer Institute, National Institutes of Health.)

methods will be used. The use of professional statisticians is usually highly recommended, if not required, in complicated or large-scale research investigations. It is also important to note that data may be both quantitative and qualitative. Quantitative data are represented by actual numbers and are, consequently, considered to be objective in nature. Qualitative data are considered subjective in nature and are represented by comments, opinions, or impressions that may be collected from study participants in focus groups or by surveys, for example. Although a comprehensive discussion of statistical methodologies is beyond the scope of this chapter, it is useful to review some fundamental knowledge regarding quantitative data.

Quantitative data are characterized by a hierarchy according to their properties (TheReasearchAssistant). These properties constitute a commonly described four-level scale: nominal, ordinal, interval, and ratio. Nominal data have the property of identity; that is, each number has a meaning such as "1" for female and "2" for male. Numbers in the nominal scale have no inherent magnitude, order, or linear relationship to each other. In contrast, ordinal data have both identity and magnitude; that is, the numbers can be ordered by size such as "mild," "moderate," or "severe." Although numbers

in the ordinal scale can be ranked relative to each other, they have no quantitative linear relationship to each other. Numbers in the interval scale have fixed equal differences between them, for example height in inches or attachment loss in millimeters. The ratio scale is identical to the interval scale with the additional property of having an absolute or true zero within the scale. That is, the number zero represents the absence of the characteristic that is being measured.

The properties of numbers determine which statistical tests may be applicable. For purposes of conducting statistical analyses, the four scales just described are collapsed into two types of data: categorical and continuous. Categorical data comprise those measured in categories or classes, and include those numbers that are nominal and ordinal. Continuous data comprise those measured on a numeric scale, thus representing a true quantity. Continuous data include interval and ratio numbers and are further classified as having a normal (bell curve) distribution or a non-normal (skewed or multi-modal) distribution.

Both categorical and continuous data can be described by two general statistical approaches: descriptive and inferential. As the name implies, descriptive statistics are those that use procedures for describing or summarizing data, and are also called summary statistics. Inferential statistics use procedures for actually making inferences or drawing conclusions about the data.

Inferential statistics allow analyses to be made according to three levels: comparisons, associations, or predictive relationships. Statistical tests of comparison evaluate the properties or characteristics of two or more groups of variables to determine if there is a difference between the groups. Tests of association identify the existence of a relationship between two or more variables. Tests of prediction determine if one or more variables can be predicted by one or more other variables. Tests of prediction are also used to quantify the association between two or more variables. Inferential statistics are further classified as parametric and non-parametric. Parametric statistical procedures are those used for continuous data and generally require that the data be normally distributed. Non-parametric statistical procedures are those used for categorical data or non-normally distributed continuous data.

Appendix Tables 2.2 and 2.3 list the common descriptive and inferential statistical tests, respectively, used in research studies (TheResearchAssistant).

DATA PRESENTATION

The development of the personal computer and a large variety of graphics software has led to an unfortunate tendency to overcomplicate figures by emphasizing the visual

Appendix Table 2.2. Common types of descriptive statistics (used for data summarization).

Type of Data	Statistical measure	
	Measures of central tendency	Measures of dispersion
Continuous— for normally distributed continuous data	Mean: the numerical average of the observations	Range: the difference between the largest and smallest observation (i.e., the spread)
	Mode: the value corresponding to the most frequently occurring observation	Standard deviation: measures the spread around the mean
Continuous— for non-normally distributed continuous data	Median: the numerical value at which half of the observations occur above and half of the observations occur below this value (i.e., the 50th percentile)	Interquartile range: the spread occurring around the middle 50% of the observations (i.e., between the 25th and 75th percentiles)
	Mode: may also be used to describe non-normally distributed continuous data	
Categorical— for ordinal data	**Statistical measure**	
	Mode: again, the most frequent observation	
	Median: again, the middle observation; half the observations are smaller and half are larger	
	Frequency: quantifies the various observations according to occurrence	
	*Frequency expressed as counts: summarize the number of observations in each category	
	*Frequency expressed as proportions: summarize the percentage of total observations for each category	
Categorical— for nominal data	Mode: as above	
	Frequency: as above (both counts and proportions)	
	(Note: the use of the median is not appropriate for nominal data)	

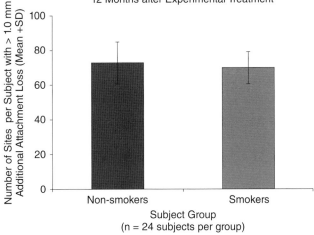

Disease Progression in Humans with Agressive Periodontitis 12 Months after Experimental Treatment

Appendix Figure 2.8. Presentation of findings from an imaginary study of periodontal disease progression measured in smokers and non-smokers one year after completion of a new type of experimental procedure. Although the data can be presented by several different graphical formats, the graphic illustrated here effectively conveys the results. It should be noted that some investigators prefer graphics that show the actual range and scatter of data points, in addition to the mean score. Similarly, some investigators advocate the use of illustrations that minimize the "ink area" in the graphic. The graphic layout illustrated here is one type commonly seen in scientific papers.

display over the data per se, which many times are relatively simple sets of numbers. As a consequence, the use of many different graphic effects can give the appearance that the data convey more information than actually may exist. An example of this is the increasing use of 3-dimensional or "depth" effects in published figures. The author of this chapter believes that figures in scientific reports should display data simply and efficiently. The noted statistician and expert in informational graphics, Edward Tufte, has succinctly noted

that "What is to be sought in designs for the display of information is the clear portrayal of complexity" (Tufte, 1983). Thus, the graphics should be the means to clearly and simply point out to the reader what important relationships may exist in the data.

Appendix Figure 2.8 presents data from an imaginary study of periodontal disease progression, measured in both smokers and non-smokers one year after completion of some new type of experimental procedure. The figure may be viewed as visually plain, but it is quite effective in conveying important findings. Even without a figure legend to provide details about the study, the reader can quickly and easily evaluate the results that are displayed. The title at the top of the figure indicates that the graph depicts disease progression measured at a specified time after treatment has been provided in a clinical study on humans. The label of the Y-axis at the left of the figure specifies how disease progression was defined in this study; that is, sites that exhibited more than 1 mm of additional attachment loss during the post-treatment follow-up period. The label also indicates that the data are being reported as the average number of sites per subject in each group with disease progression, plus or minus the standard deviation. The label of the X-axis indi-

Appendix Table 2.3. Common types of inferential statistics (used for data analysis).

Type of data	Types of Test		
	Tests of comparison (reported as the particular test statistic, ex. t, χ^2 [Chi-squared], or U)	Tests of association (reported as the correlation coefficient [r] or the ratio value)	Tests of prediction (reported as the regression value [R2])
Parametric—for normally distributed continuous data	t-test (Students): compares two means *One-sample t-test: compares the mean from your observations to a standard or norm value *Two-sample t-test: compares the means from your observations of two independent groups *Paired t-test: compares the means from two independent observations from one group Analysis of variance (ANOVA): compares three or more means either between or within groups	Pearson correlation coefficient: measures the relationship between two variables or observations within one group	Linear regression: used when the outcome (i.e., dependent) variables are continuous (either normally or non-normally distributed) or ordinal
Non-parametric—for ordinal or non-normally distributed continuous data	Wilcoxon signed-ranks test: compares median from your observation to a standard or norm value Mann-Whitney U test: compares medians from two independent groups Wilcoxon matched-pairs signed-ranks test: compares two independent medians from one group Kruskal-Wallis test: compares medians from three or more independent groups Friedman test: compares medians for three or more observations from one group	Spearman's rho: measures the relationship between the ranks of two variables or observations within one group Kendall's tau: similar to Spearman's correlation coefficient	Linear regression: used when the outcome (i.e., dependent) variables are continuous (either normally or non-normally distributed) or ordinal
Non-parametric—for nominal data	Binomial sign test: compares counts or proportions for your observation with a population standard Chi-square test: compares counts or proportions for data from two or more independent groups (including a standard or norm value) Fisher's exact test: compares counts or proportions for data from two or more independent groups (including a standard or norm value) McNemar test: compares counts or proportions for two observations from one group Cochran Q test: compares counts or proportions for three or more observations from one group	Relative risk: the chance of an outcome occurring relative to the presence of a risk or predisposing factor; used with cohort or clinical trial studies in which patient is followed over time Odds ratio: the chance that a group with a particular outcome was exposed to a particular risk or predisposing factor; used with case-control or cross-sectional studies	Logistic regression: used when the outcome (i.e., dependent) variables are nominal; often used when outcome data are dichotomous (ex. bleeding-on-probing positive and bleeding-on-probing negative)

cates that the two groups have been differentiated on the basis of smoking status, and also indicates how many subjects are included in each group. Of course, the figure does not provide all relevant information, nor is it necessarily expected to do so. The reader would need to review the methods section of the scientific paper, or the figure legend that may accompany the illustration, to learn additional information such as the age, gender, or racial characteristics of the subjects, how the smoking status was defined, and what comprised the experimental treatment.

Nonetheless, the figure readily illustrates that the two groups of subjects, smokers and non-smokers, had little difference in disease progression. The figure effectively communicates research findings without unnecessary fanfare.

> The results of a scientific investigation are explained according to the available literature and within the limitations of the study design (the "Discussion").

The discussion section of a scientific paper is often the most difficult section to write, especially for newer investigators. Whereas the introduction provides the background literature to justify the study, the discussion focuses primarily on the prior literature that supports and/or contradicts the findings of the present study. Thus, the discussion section serves to explain the results in the context of existing knowledge about the research topic.

Although scientific journals have varying guidelines governing the length, extent, and logical flow of discussion sections, most require that certain key components be presented. The majority of the discussion presents the authors' own interpretation of their results, including reasons for agreement or disagreement with the published findings of other investigators. Important relationships among the results are emphasized, as well as the perceived usefulness. The discussion describes how the present results confirm existing knowledge or, due to the use of newer or improved techniques, indicate that previously published findings need to be reinterpreted. Well written discussion sections also discuss the critical factors that influenced the study's findings, specifically those variables that may have diminished reliability and validity.

The appropriateness of the study design in answering the research question is often described, as are potential limitations of the techniques and measurements performed in the study. Some investigators prefer to restate briefly the most significant findings of their study, usually in the opening paragraph of the discussion. This is not necessarily required but, when provided, does help focus the reader on data having the most relevancy or generalizability. This is especially true

for high-impact studies that provide evidence for a novel concept or new scientific field. Alternatively, the authors may choose to present the most important findings as topic sentences in separate paragraphs throughout the discussion. Discussion sections typically end with concluding remarks that present the "take home message" of the study, and that may identify additional work that should be performed in the future.

> The results often may have more than one interpretation, or lead to additional questions that might warrant further investigation.

If the study design and specific protocols are both appropriate and well executed, and if the data are appropriately evaluated, the results of any given study will be credible regardless of whether the results are expected, unexpected, or even disappointing to the researchers. That is to say, the data themselves "are what they are" and should be unequivocal. What may be equivocal, on the other hand, is how such data are interpreted. Caution is required in reading the discussion section of original reports because this is where the authors interpret their results according to their own professional opinions. Alternative viewpoints may be possible and equally viable, so that many times the research data may be interpreted in more than one way.

Let us return to Appendix Figure 2.8. Such graphics usually indicate if the measurements exhibit statistically significant differences, for example, by an asterisk drawn above the bars. Because no asterisk or other indication is shown, we can reasonably conclude that the two groups of subjects, smokers and non-smokers, had no difference in disease progression. This would be the primary finding that the figure serves to illustrate. However, other information can also be gleaned from the figure. On closer inspection it appears that subjects in both groups continued to demonstrate aggressive disease, because some 60 to 70 sites per subject had disease progression measurable one year after treatment. Assuming that each tooth was measured at six sites in 28 teeth, then a range of about 10 to 28 teeth per subject had additional attachment loss.

The experienced reader would wonder why these subjects were so prone to continued disease. Was the experimental treatment grossly ineffective? Was there a control aggressive periodontitis group that received no treatment at all (and would withholding treatment be ethical)? Was there something particularly unique about the subjects in this study? Could the findings be explained by the presence of a very aggressive (i.e., extremely downhill) subset of subjects, who just happened to be recruited into the study by chance? If so, could this subgroup account for most of the continued disease progression measured in the study? Could the definition of disease progression be too stringent? Would a cut-off value of 2 mm or 3 mm possibly show a difference between smokers and non-smokers? These are the types of questions that are intended to be asked when the reader is exhibiting the important, albeit overused, notion of critical thinking. Critical thinking is the hallmark of so-called evidence-based dentistry or medicine. Stated simply, critical thinking implies that the informed reader decides for herself how to interpret the data.

Let us consider another imaginary example. A study reports retrospective data on patient mortality rates following cardiac bypass surgery in three different hospitals, A, B, and C. The data is reported in terms of absolute numbers of deaths and show that hospital C has the highest number of patient deaths after the procedure.

Assuming that the study is appropriately designed, powered, and evaluated, what can be concluded about hospital C? It is tempting to conclude that hospital C is worse than hospitals A or B; specifically, that the surgeons and the post surgical care are not as good as in the other two hospitals. But, do we have sufficient information to support this conclusion? Would our interpretation be different if we knew that hospital C performs many more procedures than hospitals A or B? That is, how do the numbers of deaths compare to the overall case loads in the three different hospitals, when expressed as a percentage of total procedures? Would our interpretation again be different if we knew that hospital C performs the procedure primarily on very sick patients not usually treated at hospitals A or B? That is, what would we conclude about hospital C if the data were normalized to the patient status and show that hospital C has markedly lower percent death rates for the sickest patients than do the other two hospitals? Perhaps our take-home message would be that the surgeons and the post surgical care at hospital C are actually better than in the other two hospitals, especially when patients are severely compromised.

These examples point out the widely accepted view that a good study leaves one with more questions than answers, provided that the hypothesis, study design, and methodology have been appropriate.

> Research requires intellectual, technical, and financial resources that must be planned for and acknowledged (the "Acknowledgements").

The cliché that nothing in life is free certainly is applicable to biomedical research. Research investigations have inherent costs that must be paid for somehow. Typically, funding for research in dental schools is derived from both intramural and extramural sources. Intramural funds are those provided to the researchers by the school or university to help establish a laboratory or clinical research center and to allow preliminary work that will allow the researchers to compete for extramural funding. Extramural sources are government, industry, and philanthropic organizations. It is widely appreciated that a good deal of researchers' time and energy are devoted to the arduous task of securing financial support for their research endeavors. As a consequence, these sources of support are gratefully acknowledged in published reports.

Extramural funding helps to defray both direct and indirect expenses of a study. As the name implies, direct costs are those incurred in the actual conduct of the study. These include a number of large- and small-scale expenses such as labor, materials, subject-related payments, consultant fees, statistical analyses, publication costs, travel to professional conferences, and even photocopying and mailing expenses. Indirect costs are those associated with overhead expenses incurred due to facilities-related costs, such as electricity, heating, and air conditioning, and to administrative costs such as grants management personnel, within the dental school and university. Not surprisingly, these indirect expenses are referred to as facilities and administration (F and A) costs and, although not directly related to a particular research question, must also be accounted for when conducting research. Thus, the total cost of a research study is the sum of direct and F and A costs.

Significant non-financial support is also acknowledged. This type of support may be quite varied, and could include collaborative arrangements with other investigators for the use of equipment, supplies, and technical help. Intellectual support, in the form of advice and technical training from colleagues, is also acknowledged. Many times, key administrative personnel on a research study are given a special "thank you" by the authors.

CONCLUSION

The research process typically begins with a proposal to obtain funding for the work, and ends with a published report to communicate the findings of the work. Research writing is the modality by which the research process and outcomes are communicated to the profession. This chapter has described the key components involved both in the research process and in the writing and reading of a scientific paper. The underlying aim has been to point out the necessity of critical thinking in evaluating the scientific merits of any given research study.

In conclusion, it should be added that good studies are those worthy of being reported by the researchers and read by the practicing professionals. Good studies are those that have addressed an important question and have provided valuable insight into a particular area. In turn, a well-written paper offers the reader a sense of excitement and a desire for even more knowledge in the subject area.

REFERENCES

Note: All online citations were accessed on or before September 14, 2008.

Callas PW. 2008. Searching the biomedical literature: research study designs and critical appraisal. *Clin. Lab. Sci.* 21(1), 42–8.

Centers for Disease Control and Prevention. 1999. Adapted from Guidelines for Defining Public Health Research and Public Health Non-Research. United States Department of Health and Human Services, revised October 4, 1999. http://www.cdc.gov/od/science/regs/hrpp/researchdefinition.htm.

Colorado State University. Overview: Reliability and Validity, an online writing course. http://writing.colostate.edu/guides/research/relval/.

Danya International, Inc. 2005. Computing Sample Size for Scientific Studies: A Non-Technical Overview." In: "TheResearchAssistant," a comprehensive web-based resource developed by Danya International, Inc., through the Small Business Innovation Research Program funded by the National Institute on Drug Abuse, National Institutes of Health (Contract No. N44DA-8-5060); revised August 22, 2005. http://www.theresearchassistant.com/tutorial/4-power.asp#.

Fleiss JL, Park MH, Chilton NW, Alman JE, Feldman RS, Chauncey HH. 1987. Representativeness of the "Ramfjord teeth" for epidemiologic studies of gingivitis and periodontitis. *Community Dent. Oral. Epidemiol.* 15(4), 221–4.

International Committee of Medical Journal Editors. 2007. Uniform Requirements for Manuscripts Submitted to Biomedical Journals: Writing and Editing for Biomedical Publication. Revised October 2007. http://www.icmje.org/.

Loe H, Silness J. 1963. Periodontal disease in pregnancy. I. Prevalence and severity. *Acta. Odontologica. Scand.* 21, 533–51.

Markinson A. Evidence Based Medicine Course. State University of New York Downstate. http://library.downstate.edu/EBM2/2100.htm.

National Cancer Institute. Incorporating Cancer Clinical Trials into Your Practice (Module 3). National Institutes of Health. http://cme.cancer.gov/c02/s02/c3_4b_01.htm.

Office of Animal Care and Use. Animal Care and Use. U.S. Department of Health and Human Services. http://oacu.od.nih.gov/.

PubMed. Home page. U.S. National Library of Medicine and National Institutes of Health. http://www.pubmed.gov.

Richards D. 2007. Creating a DEBT. *Evidence-Based Dentistry.* 8 (2), 35–6. Editorial in Evidence-Based Dentistry. 8, 2. doi: 10.1038/sj.ebd.6400484. http://www.nature.com/ebd/journal/v8/n2/full/6400484a.html.

TheResearchAssistant. Statistical Support on the Web. http://www.theresearchassistant.com/research/link.asp.

The Writing Center. University of Wisconsin-Madison home page. http://www.wisc.edu/writing/.

Trochim WM. 2006. "The Research Methods Knowledge Base," 2nd Edition. revised October 2, 2006. http://www.socialresearch-methods.net/kb/. This is a comprehensive web-based textbook that covers the entire research process including formulating research questions, sampling, measurement, research design, data analysis, reliability of measures, study validity, ethics, and writing the research paper.

Tufte ER. 1983. The Visual Display of Quantitative Information. Graphics Press. Page 191.

U.S. States Department of Health and Human Services. IRB Guidebook. Office for Human Research Protections. http://www.hhs.gov/ohrp/irb/irb_guidebook.htm.

Whitley E, Ball J. 2002. Statistics review 4: sample size calculations. *Crit. Care.* 6(4), 335–41. Epub May 10, 2002.

Index

A

AAP. *See* American Academy of Periodontology

Abscesses
  pericoronal, 20
  periodontal, 20

Abstracts, 147

Accessory pulp canals, in furcation area of molars, 88–89

Acid etching, 132

Acquired neutropenia, 18

Acrylic, allergic reactions to, 13

Actinobacillus Actinomycetemcomitans, localized aggressive periodontitis and, 15

Actinomyces species, 47

Acute necrotizing ulcerative periodontitis, in HIV-positive patient, *19*

Acute periodontal abscess, indications for, in periodontology, 72, 72*t*

ADA. *See* American Dental Association

Adult periodontitis. *See* Chronic periodontitis

Advanced glycation end products (AGE), 29

Aggregatibacter (Actinobacillus) actinomycetemcomitans, localized juvenile periodontitis and, 70

Aggressive periodontitis, 15–17
  defining diagnosis for, 15
  generalized, 15–16
  indications for, in periodontology, 72, 72*t*
  localized, 15

Aging process, periodontal diseases, 26–27

AIDS
  bone destruction and tooth loss with, 19
  periodontal diseases and, 30–31

Air polishing, 124

Alambadar, J. M., 145

Alexander I (tsar of Russia), 137

Allergic reactions, gingival disease and, 13

Allograft, 99, 100 (box 8.1)

Alloplasts, 99, 100 (box 8.1)

Alveolar bone
  periodontal regeneration and, 99
  surgery's effect on, 86

Alveolar bone anatomy, physiologic and pathologic, 77–78

Alveolar bone crest. *See also* CEJ/ alveolar bone crest
  of dry human mandible, *84*
  surgical exposure of, around maxillary incisors during crown lengthening procedure, *78*

Alveolar bone loss, calculating, Napoleon's grand army study and, 139

Amelogenin, 99, 102

American Academy of Periodontology, 7, 69, 121, 140
  recall intervals recommended by, 123
  SPT guidance through, 122

American Dental Association, evidence-based dentistry defined by, 3

American Heart Association, 72

Amoxicillin, 71

Analytical studies, 152

Angle Class I occlusal relationship, moving teeth toward, 64

Animal research, 147
  in evidence pyramid, *153*
  institutional animal care and use committees for, 157–158

Antczak-Bouckoms, A., 115

Anterior areas with no prosthetic involvement, indications and contraindications to surgical therapy in case of, 80*t*

Anterior areas with prosthetic involvement, indications and contraindications to surgical therapy in case of, 80*t*

Anterior disclusion, group function and, 58–59

Anterior guidance, 66

Anterior vertical overlap, steep, 66

Antibiotherapy, implant failure prevention and, 128–129

Antibiotics
  dental procedures and cardiac conditions for which antibiotic prophylaxis is required, 73*t*
  evidence-based outcomes relative to, 69–72
  indications for, in periodontology, 72, 72*t*
  regenerative procedures and, 71

regimens for periodontal conditions, 74*t*

Anti-convulsant drugs, gingival diseases and, 9

Anti-depressant therapy, 39

Antimicrobials, 69–74
  author's views and comments on, 74
  evidence-based outcomes on, 69–72
  indications for, 72
  local delivery systems and, 72, 74*t*
  localized juvenile periodontitis and, 70
  regimens for dental procedure, 73*t*
  resistance to, 69
  techniques, 72, 74

Antioxidants, periodontal health and, 32

Antiseptic mouthwashes, 71

Application steps, evaluating, 4–5

Appraisal results, applying to clinical practice, 4

Artefacta gingivitis, 7

Articles, 147

Articulators, 64–65
  programming for negative or positive error, *65*
  rehabilitation with complete dentures, 65
  rehabilitation with fixed prosthodontics, 64–65

Artificial crown, with poor biomechanics, *62*

Ascorbic acid deficiency gingivitis, 10

Aspirin-induced chemical injuries, to palate and gingiva, *13*

Atrophic candidosis, gingival diseases and, 11

Attachment level changes, summary of, following SRP, *47*

Attachment loosing sites, osseous resective surgery and, 87–88

Aubrey, S., 140

Augmentin, 16

Autogenous graft, 99, 100 (Box 8.1)

Azithromycin, 71

B

Back-action chisel, 82

Bacteria, as etiologic agents of periodontal disease, 69

Balanced articulation, 55, 57
  classical balanced, *57*
  fixed prosthodontics and, 57

Superman bone file, *95*
Supportive periodontal therapy,
121–125
  author's views/comments, 125
  economic costs and, 125
  evidence-based outcomes, 123–125
  example of ordinary appointment, 122
    (Box 10.1)
  indications for, 121
  overview, 121
  technique, 121–123
    measuring baseline values, 122
    recall intervals, duration, and
      setting, 123
    risk assessment, 121–122
    risk factor modification, 123
    treatment considerations, 122
Supragingival plaque control, 32–33,
  123
Surgical *vs.* non-surgical methods, for
  periodontal disease, systematic
  reviews/meta-analyses on, 115
Surrogate outcomes, probing pocket
  depth, clinical attachment level
  and, 117
Suturing, osseous resective surgery and,
  83
Syphilis, gingival lesions and, 10
Systematic reviews, 153, *153*

T
Tagger, M., 90
Tannerella Forsythensis, 47, 48, 70
Target lesions, with erythema
  multiforme, 13
Tartar deposit measurements
  Napoleon's grand Army study, 140
    distribution of individuals according
      to quantity of tartar observed,
      144
    distribution of individuals in
      functions of quantity of tartar in
      different age categories, 144t
    18th and 19th century diet and
      military rations and, 145
    increasing distance ECJ/alveolar
      bone crest according to tartar
      quantity, 144t
    presence of average tartar on teeth,
      141
    presence of high tartar on teeth,
      141
    presence of low tartar on teeth,
      141
    tartar correlated with bone loss,
      143

tartar observed, 143
    tartar quantity correlated with age,
      143
Temporary restorations, root resection
  therapy and, 91–92
Tests of association, 159
Tests of prediction, 159
Tetracycline, localized aggressive
  periodontitis and, 15
Tetracycline fibers, 72, 74
Tetracycline intake, one year post
  therapy associated with, *17*
Textured implant surface methods, 132
Theilade, E., 43
Thermal trauma, gingival recessions
  and, 14
Theses, 147
Thin knife edge interproximal area, 78
Three-unit partial denture, *59*
Tobacco use
  cessation, 33–34
    care pathway for dental practice,
      35
  history form, *36*
  journal, 34, *37*
  periodontal disease and, 27–28
Tongue piercing
  lingual gingival recessions due to
    chronic trauma from repeated
    contact with, *14*
  metallic barbell inserted after, *14*
Tooth brushing technique, mucogingival
  deformities/conditions and, 22
Tooth extraction dilemma, root canal
  therapy, fixed partial denture, or
  implant-supported crown,
  127–128
Tooth loss
  as tangible endpoint in periodontal
    therapy, 117
  tobacco use and, 27–28
Tooth malposition, 22
Toothpastes, allergic reactions to, 13
Torabinejad, 127
Toxic reactions, gingival reactions to, 13
TOXLINE, 150
TOXNET, 150
Trabecular bone
  composition of, 131
  healing of, after implant placement,
    132
Trace metals, periodontal health and, 32
Transitional partial dentures, 129
Traumatic lesions, 13–14
Trench mouth diseases, 19
Treponema denticola, 47, 70

Treponema-pallidum-associated lesions,
  10–11
Tsai, C. C., 88
Tufte, Edward, 160
Tumor necrosis factor-alpha, 25
Tunkel, J., 45
Tunnelization, 89, *95, 96*
Tunnelized lower left first molar, caries
  at, *96*
Type 1 diabetes mellitus, 9
Type 2 diabetes mellitus, 9

U
Ulcerative necrotizing gingivitis, in HIV
  patients, 12
Ultrasonic scalers, 43, 50, 51
  smaller tip size, *46*
Uniform Requirements for Manuscripts
  Submitted to Biomedical
  Journals, 151
Unilateral balance, 57
  group function or, *57*
Universal curettes, 43
  key differences in blade design
    between, *45*

V
Validity, scientific studies and, 155–156
Van der Weijden, G. A., 47
van Steenberghe, D., 62
van Winkelhoff, A. J., 70
Variability measures, 155
Variance, 155
Varicella-zoster infection, gingivitis and,
  11
Vascular diseases, 26
Veillonella parvula, 48
Vemino, A. R., 88
Verapamil, gingival diseases and, 9
Vincent's angina, 19
Viral infections, gingivitis caused by, 11
Vitamin C deficiency gingivitis, 10
Vitamins, periodontal health and, 32

W
Web of Science databases, 150
Widman flap surgery, 87
Wilderman, M., 86
World Workshop in Periodontics, 50
Writing, research and, 148
Writing Center, The (University of
  Wisconsin, Madison), 151
Wylam, J. M., 48, 49

X
Xenograft, 99, 100 (box 8.1)